Pathology at a Glance

CJF

To Rob, Ian and Emma

BATN

To Asma, my best friend

Pathology at a Glance

Caroline J. Finlayson

MBBS, FRCPath
Cellular Pathology Department
St George's Hospital Medical School
London, UK

Barry A. T. Newell

BSc, MBBS, MRCP, FRCPath
Cellular Pathology Department
St George's Hospital Medical School
London, UK

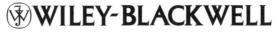
A John Wiley & Sons, Ltd., Publication

This edition first published 2009, © 2009 by Caroline J. Finlayson and Barry A.T. Newell

Blackwell Publishing was acquired by John Wiley & Sons in February 2007. Blackwell's publishing program has been merged with Wiley's global Scientific, Technical and Medical business to form Wiley-Blackwell.

Registered office: John Wiley & Sons Ltd, The Atrium, Southern Gate, Chichester, West Sussex, PO19 8SQ, UK

Editorial offices: 9600 Garsington Road, Oxford, OX4 2DQ, UK
The Atrium, Southern Gate, Chichester, West Sussex, PO19 8SQ, UK
111 River Street, Hoboken, NJ 07030-5774, USA

For details of our global editorial offices, for customer services and for information about how to apply for permission to reuse the copyright material in this book please see our website at www.wiley.com/wiley-blackwell

Library of Congress Cataloging-in-Publication Data
Finlayson, Caroline J.
    Pathology at a glance / Caroline J. Finlayson, Barry A.T. Newell.
      p. ; cm.
    Includes index.
    ISBN 978-1-4051-3650-1 (alk. paper)
    1. Pathology–Handbooks, manuals, etc.   I. Newell, Barry A. T.   II. Title.
    [DNLM: 1. Pathology–Handbooks. QZ 39 F512p 2008]
    RB118.F56 2008
    616.07–dc22
                                                                 2008009434

ISBN:978-1-4051-3650-1

A catalogue record for this book is available from the British Library.

Set in 9/11.5pt Times by Graphicraft Limited, Hong Kong
Printed in Singapore by Markono Print Media Pte Ltd

1   2009

Contents

Preface

Whenever medical students gather outside an examination hall in that strange, unpleasant hour or so before the challenge begins, it is interesting to observe the various manifestations which their anxiety may take.

Some students pace nervously, others stare fixedly into space, a few select an unobtrusive place in which to quiver and many thrash over those last few points and facts that always seem to refuse to stay in the memory, no matter how well the rest of the material has been grasped.

Some are laden with lever-arch files crammed with studiously crafted notes. There is always a cohort that ploughs fervently through textbooks in those tense last few moments before an exam. (The medical school librarians nod knowingly at each other as they gaze at their unusually sparsely occupied shelves.)

Members of the mixed group lacking textbooks may make forays to those who have laboured to the exam with weighty tomes, seeking to confirm that the fact they have already verified 10 times in the past week has not changed overnight.

Textbooks like *Pathology at a Glance* are popular at such tortured gatherings. They are light, require little space and come with the implication, however unsolicited by the authors, that they can somehow, in one-tenth of the number of pages of the larger textbooks, cover all that a student needs to know.

While it is true that one of the aims of *Pathology at a Glance* is to provide a summary of pathology that can be used to guide revision and to highlight the fundamental aspects of a particular topic, this book should also be considered as a guide and a low-scale map of the whole process of learning pathology, beginning with the student's first encounters with the subject.

One of the most common questions that students ask a tutor is, 'What do I need to know for the exam?' or its variant, 'If I learn what's in this book, will that be enough?' What we hope to achieve with *Pathology at a Glance* is a summary of the core information for the topics we have selected and to present a framework of understanding upon which the reader can add information that is gleaned from other sources.

Pathology is the study of disease and is fundamental to medicine. Time spent learning pathology can significantly reduce the effort required to learn about the presentation, clinical course and management of the vast array of diseases that exist. At first these may appear to be little more than a disparate collection of signs and symptoms and facts, to be added to the litany of lists that bedevil medical students. A sound knowledge of pathology provides an underlying basis that unifies many of these features and bestows a pattern on them.

Acknowledgements

Our thanks to the following, who provided advice on particular sections of the book:

- Dr Jennifer Else: renal disease.
- Professor Neil Shepherd: gastrointestinal pathology.
- Dr David Bevan: haemostasis.
- Professor Philip Butcher: tuberculosis.
- Professor Peter McCrorie: hypertension.
- Dr Jonathan Williams: breast disease.

Caroline J. Finlayson
Barry A.T. Newell

Abbreviations

AC	alternating current
ACE	angiotensin converting enzyme
ACTH	adrenocorticotrophic hormone
ADH	antidiuretic hormone
AIDS	acquired immune deficiency syndrome
AIH	autoimmune hepatitis
ALL	acute lymphoblastic leukaemia
ALP	alkaline phosphate
ALT	alanine aminotransferase
AML	acute myeloblastic leukaemia
ANCA	antineutrophil cytoplasmic antibody
APC	adenomatous polyposis coli
APTT	activated partial thromboplastin time
ARDS	adult respiratory distress syndrome
AST	aspartate aminotransferase
ATN	acute tubular necrosis
ATP	adenosine triphosphate
AV	atrioventricular
BCG	bacille Calmette–Guérin
BCR	B cell receptor
BMI	body mass index
cAMP	cyclic adenosine monophosphate
CBD	common bile duct
CCK	cholecystekinin
CF	cystic fibrosis
CFA	cryptogenic fibrosing alveolitis
CFTR	CF transmembrane receptor
CFU	colony forming unit
CIN	cervical intraepithelial neoplasia
CJD	Creutzfeld–Jakob disease
CLL	chronic lymphocytic leukaemia
CLO	columnar lined oesophagus
CML	chronic myeloid leukaemia
CMV	cytomegalovirus
CNS	central nervous system
CO	carbon monoxide
COPD	chronic obstructive pulmonary disease
CRC	colorectal carcinoma
CRP	C-reactive protein
CSF	cerebrospinal fluid
CT	computed tomography
CVA	cerebrovascular accident
DAD	diffuse alveolar damage
DAI	diffuse axonal injury
DC	direct current
DCC	deleted in colon cancer
DCIS	ductal carcinoma in situ
DIC	disseminated intravascular coagulation
DIP	desquamative interstitial pneumonia
DM	diabetes mellitus
DNA	deoxyribonucleic acid
DVT	deep venous thrombosis
EATCL	enteropathy-associated T cell lymphoma
EBV	Epstein–Barr virus
ENaC	epithelial sodium channel
ENT	ear, nose and throat
ER	endoplasmic reticulum
ERCP	endoscopic retrograde cholangiopancreatography
ET	endothelin
FDB	faecal occult blood
FDC	follicle dendritic cell
FEV_1	forced expiratory volume in first second
FFA	free fatty acid
FGF	fibroblast growth factor
FNA	fine needle aspiration
FSH	follicle-stimulating hormone
FVC	forced vital capacity
G6PD	glucose-6-phosphate dehydrogenase
GABA	gamma-aminobutyric acid
GBM	glomerular basement membrane
GDP	guanosine dephosphate
GFR	glomerular filtration rate
GGT	gamma glutamyl transferase
GH	growth hormone
GI	gastrointestinal
GN	glomerulonephritis
GORD	gastro-oesophageal reflux disease
GP	general practitioner
GTN	glyceryl trinitrate
GTP	guanosine triphosphate
HAART	highly active anti-retroviral therapy
HAV	hepatitis A virus
Hb	haemoglobin
HBcAg	hepatitis B core antigen
HBeAg	hepatitis B e antigen
HBsAg	hepatitis B surface antigen
HBV	hepatitis B virus
HCC	hepatocellular carcinoma
HCG	human chorionic gonadotrophin
HCV	hepatitis C virus
HDL	high density lipoprotein
HDV	hepatitis D virus
H&E	haematoxylin and eosin
HEV	hepatitis E virus
HIAA	hydroxyindoleacetic acid
HIV	human immunodeficiency virus
HLA	human leucocyte antigen
HNPCC	hereditary non-polyposis colorectal carcinoma
H_2O_2	hydrogen peroxide
HP	hydrostatic pressure
HPV	human papilloma virus
HRSC	Hodgkin–Reed–Sternberg cell
hsp	heat shock protein
5HT	serotonin/5-hydroxytryptamine
IBD	inflammatory bowel disease
ICAM	intercellular adhesion molecule
IDC	invasive ductal carcinoma
IFN	interferon
Ig	immunoglobulin
IL	interleukin

INR	international normalised ratio	POP	plasma oncotic pressure
IVC	inferior vena cava	PRV	polycythaemia rubra vera
JGA	juxtaglomerular complex	PSA	prostate-specific antigen
LAK	lymphokine-activated killer	PSC	primary sclerosing cholangitis
LDH	lactate dehydrogenase	PTH	parathyroid hormone
LDL	low density lipoprotein	PVC	polyvinyl chloride
LH	luteinising hormone	PVK	Plummer–Vinson–Kelly syndrome
LLETZ	long loop excision of the transformation zone	RF	rheumatoid factor
MALT	mucosa-associated lymphoid tissue	RNA	ribonucleic acid
MCHC	mean corpuscular haemoglobin concentration	ROS	reactive oxygen species
MCV	mean corpuscular volume	SA	sinoatrial
MEN	multiple endocrine neoplasia	SAME	syndrome of apparent mineralocorticoid excess
MGUS	monoclonal gammopathy of uncertain significance	SCC	squamous cell carcinoma
MHC	major histocompatibility complex	SIADH	syndrome of inappropriate antidiuretic hormone secretion
MI	myocardial infarction	SLE	systemic lupus erythematosus
MPTP	1-methyl-4-phenyl-1,2,3,6,tetrahydropyridine	SMA	superior mesenteric artery
MRCP	magnetic resonance cholangiopancreatography	SMC	smooth muscle cell
mRNA	messenger RNA	SRBCT	small round blue cell tumour
NADP	nicotinamide-adenine-dinucleotide phosphate	T4	thyroxine
NADPH	reduced NADP	TB	tuberculosis
NASH	non-alcoholic steatohepatitis	Tc	T cytotoxic (cell)
NHL	non-Hodgkin lymphoma	TCR	T cell receptor
NK	natural killer (cell)	TF	tissue factor
NLPHL	nodular lymphocyte predominant Hodgkin lymphoma	TDLU	terminal duct lobular unit
NO	nitric oxide	TGF	tumour growth factor
NOS	not otherwise specified	Th	T helper (cell)
NSAID	non-steroidal anti-inflammatory drug	TNF	tumour necrosis factor
NSGCT	non-seminomatous germ cell tumour	TSG	tumour suppressor gene
PAF	platelet activating factor	TSH	thyroid-stimulating hormone
PAH	polycyclic aromatic hydrocarbon	TT	thrombin time
PAN	polyarteritis nodosa	UIP	usual interstitial pneumonia
PBC	primary biliary cirrhosis	UTI	urinary tract infection
PE	pulmonary embolism	VEGF	vascular endothelial growth factor
PEG-IFN	pegylated interferon	VLDL	very low density lipoprotein
PGE	prostaglandin E	VSD	ventricular septal defect
PKD	polycystic kidney disease	vWF	von Willebrand factor
PMN	polymorphonuclear neutrophil	WCC	white cell count
PNET	primitive neuroectodermal tumour	5YSR	five-year survival rate

General pathology

1 The normal human cell

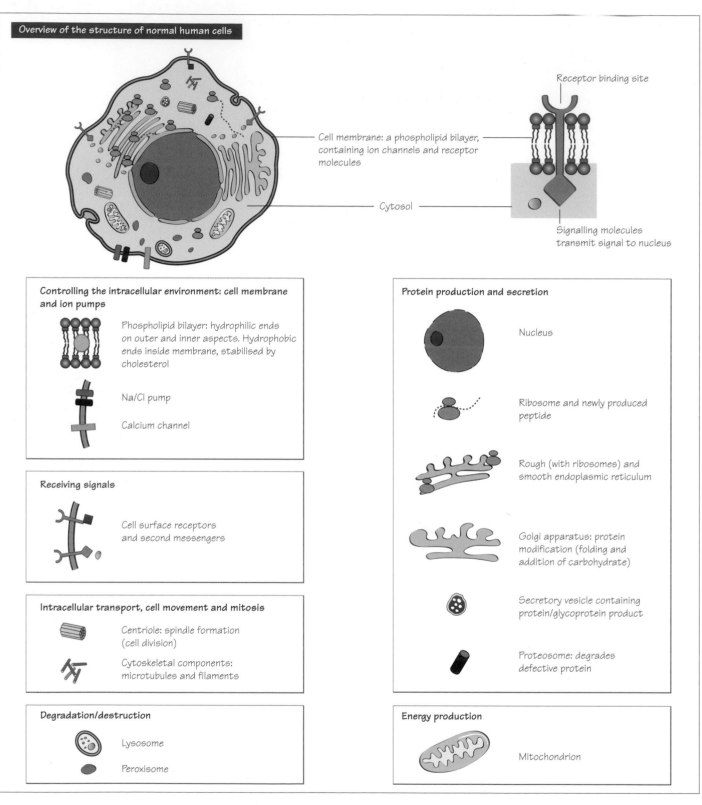

Overview of the structure of normal human cells

Receptor binding site

Cell membrane: a phospholipid bilayer, containing ion channels and receptor molecules

Cytosol

Signalling molecules transmit signal to nucleus

Controlling the intracellular environment: cell membrane and ion pumps

Phospholipid bilayer: hydrophilic ends on outer and inner aspects. Hydrophobic ends inside membrane, stabilised by cholesterol

Na/Cl pump

Calcium channel

Receiving signals

Cell surface receptors and second messengers

Intracellular transport, cell movement and mitosis

Centriole: spindle formation (cell division)

Cytoskeletal components: microtubules and filaments

Degradation/destruction

Lysosome

Peroxisome

Protein production and secretion

Nucleus

Ribosome and newly produced peptide

Rough (with ribosomes) and smooth endoplasmic reticulum

Golgi apparatus: protein modification (folding and addition of carbohydrate)

Secretory vesicle containing protein/glycoprotein product

Proteosome: degrades defective protein

Energy production

Mitochondrion

The important functions of the cell are: manufacture of proteins for local or distant use, energy generation, functions appropriate to tissue type and replication.

The main elements are the nucleus, the cytoplasm (cytosol), the cytoskeleton and the subcellular organelles, all bound by membranes.

Nucleus

The nuclear membrane contains pores to permit metabolites, RNA and ribosomal subunits in or out. It contains:
• DNA, the nuclear chromatin, which only forms about 20% of the nuclear mass.
• Nucleoli – ribosomal RNA synthesis and ribosome subunit assembly.
• Nucleoprotein, e.g. synthetic enzymes for DNA, RNA and regulatory proteins, all made in the cytoplasm and imported into the nucleus.
• Messenger, transfer and ribosomal RNA en route for the cytoplasm.

Cytosol

The nutritious fluid medium that bathes and supports the organelles, through which the cytoskeleton ramifies. Many reactions take place here.

Cytoskeleton

• Microtubules: organelles such as secretory vesicles or internalised receptors can be transported through the cell via the cytoskeleton.
• Microfilaments (actin, myosin): these stabilise cell shape and act as contractile proteins in muscle.
• Intermediate filaments, e.g. cytokeratin, desmin, neurofilament proteins and glial fibrillary acidic protein (the types differ between tissues and all are structural).

Organelles
Mitochondria

These are the main ATP/energy generating organelles and house the Krebs cycle and oxidative phosphorylation. They have their own ssDNA (maternally derived) which codes a minority of their proteins. A porous outer membrane and folded inner membrane are present.

Ribosomes

Nucleolus-produced ribosomal subunits aggregate in the cytosol and attach to the endoplasmic reticulum or lie loose in the cytosol, depending on the destination of the protein to be made (free ribosomes make proteins for inside the cell itself). Ribosomes translate RNA strands into a correctly assembled amino acid sequence (peptide molecule).

Endoplasmic reticulum (ER)

The ER is an irregular maze of membrane-bound tubules, saccules and cisterns which ramifies through the cell.
• **Rough ER** is studded with ribosomes. Proteins made by the rough ER pass into the rough ER cisternae and undergo secondary folding and early glycosylation before being incorporated into membranes for export from the cell, receptor molecules on the cell, or components such as lysosomes within the cell.
• **Smooth ER**: there is a further addition of carbohydrate moieties to protein, folding to achieve tertiary structure.

Golgi apparatus – see diagram.

Secretory vesicles

These membrane bound packets are moved via the cytoskeleton to fuse with the cell membrane to expel their contents outside.

Lysosomes

These are intracellular membrane-bound vesicles, containing destructive chemicals and enzymes, which fuse with phagosomes to release their contents into the phagolysosome and destroy pathogens. Lysosomes also degrade worn-out cell organelles (autophagy).

Peroxisomes

These small membrane-bound granules contain oxidative enzymes which make hydrogen peroxide plus its regulator catalase.

Proteasomes

These identify defective proteins and degrade them into their component peptides and amino acids for re-use by the cell. Portions of broken-down protein are bound by MHC class I molecules and displayed on the cell surface to Tc cells.

Centrosome

This contains the two linked centrioles, from which microtubules radiate into the cell. The centrioles duplicate and migrate to opposite ends of the cell during cell division, separating the duplicated chromosomes.

Membranes

Membranes are phospholipid barriers surrounding the cell itself and certain organelles. They isolate portions of the cell and permit several, often incompatible, metabolic processes to take place simultaneously.

The cell membrane

This phospholipid bilayer interacts with the extracellular world by assorted surface molecules. The centre is lipophilic and the surfaces hydrophilic, with cholesterol as a stabilising 'spacer' between them. The 'raft theory' suggests that intramembrane structures can float and be cross-linked around the perimeter of the cell.

Membrane proteins: proteins that project through the membrane outside the cell usually have attached carbohydrates. Glycolipids are carbohydrates attached to the lipid membrane and are important in cell recognition, cell–cell bonds and adsorbing molecules. Some tissues have a protective glycocalyx.

Transport through the cell membrane: The main mechanisms are:
• Passive diffusion (needs only a concentration gradient), e.g. lipids and lipid-soluble agents like ethanol.
• Facilitated diffusion: the binding of a molecule triggers a conformational change which moves the molecule across the membrane.
• Active transport: against a concentration gradient to maintain ion concentrations within the cell, e.g. the $Na^+/K^+/ATPase$ complex.
• Bulk transport: **endocytosis**, **transcytosis** and **exocytosis**. Endocytosis includes *receptor-mediated endocytosis* (ligands or viral particles) and *phagocytosis* (engulfing of particles). *Pinocytosis*, dendritic cell sampling of small quantities of tissue fluid is not receptor mediated.

Transmission of messages across the cell membrane:
• Lipid-soluble agents (e.g. steroids) diffuse directly across cell membranes.
• Receptor binding and activation of secondary messengers: applies to protein messenger molecules, which bind to a specific cell surface receptor (*ligand*), resulting in active transport of the molecule through the membrane or the triggering of intracellular cascade reactions.

Neurotransmitters: these are chemical messengers for neurones or myocytes that cause an electrical response in the target by receptor-mediated opening of an ion channel.

2 Fluid dynamics

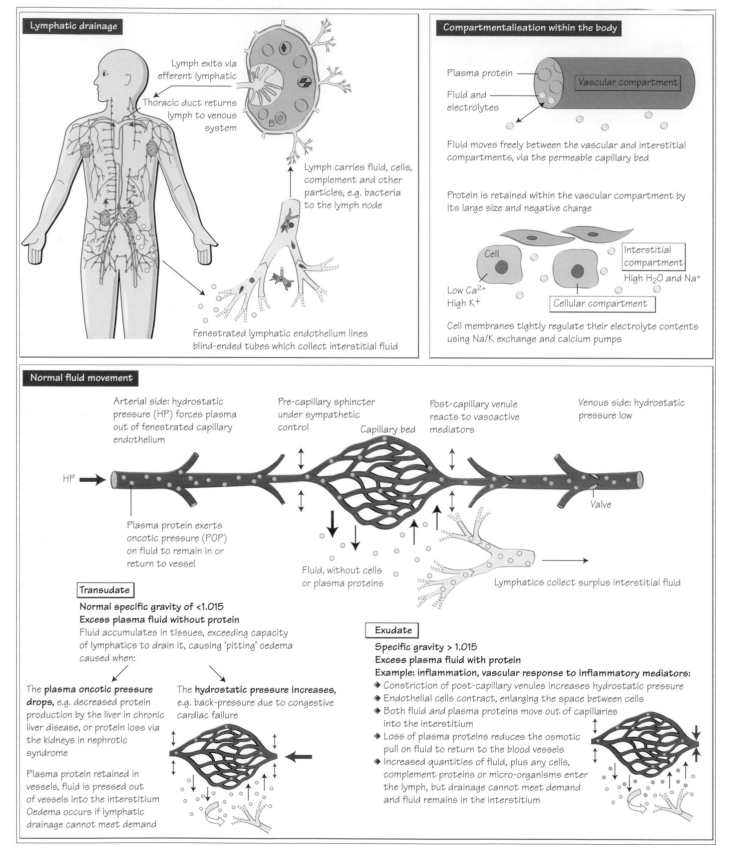

Lymphatic drainage

Lymph exits via efferent lymphatic

Thoracic duct returns lymph to venous system

Lymph carries fluid, cells, complement and other particles, e.g. bacteria to the lymph node

Fenestrated lymphatic endothelium lines blind-ended tubes which collect interstitial fluid

Compartmentalisation within the body

Plasma protein

Fluid and electrolytes

Vascular compartment

Fluid moves freely between the vascular and interstitial compartments, via the permeable capillary bed

Protein is retained within the vascular compartment by its large size and negative charge

Cell

Low Ca^{2+}
High K^+

Interstitial compartment
High H_2O and Na^+

Cellular compartment

Cell membranes tightly regulate their electrolyte contents using Na/K exchange and calcium pumps

Normal fluid movement

Arterial side: hydrostatic pressure (HP) forces plasma out of fenestrated capillary endothelium

Pre-capillary sphincter under sympathetic control

Capillary bed

Post-capillary venule reacts to vasoactive mediators

Venous side: hydrostatic pressure low

HP

Plasma protein exerts oncotic pressure (POP) on fluid to remain in or return to vessel

Fluid, without cells or plasma proteins

Valve

Lymphatics collect surplus interstitial fluid

Transudate

Normal specific gravity of <1.015
Excess plasma fluid without protein
Fluid accumulates in tissues, exceeding capacity of lymphatics to drain it, causing 'pitting' oedema caused when:

The **plasma oncotic pressure drops**, e.g. decreased protein production by the liver in chronic liver disease, or protein loss via the kidneys in nephrotic syndrome

The **hydrostatic pressure increases**, e.g. back-pressure due to congestive cardiac failure

Plasma protein retained in vessels, fluid is pressed out of vessels into the interstitium Oedema occurs if lymphatic drainage cannot meet demand

Exudate

Specific gravity > 1.015
Excess plasma fluid with protein
Example: inflammation, vascular response to inflammatory mediators:
◆ Constriction of post-capillary venules increases hydrostatic pressure
◆ Endothelial cells contract, enlarging the space between cells
◆ Both fluid and plasma proteins move out of capillaries into the interstitium
◆ Loss of plasma proteins reduces the osmotic pull on fluid to return to the blood vessels
◆ Increased quantities of fluid, plus any cells, complement proteins or micro-organisms enter the lymph, but drainage cannot meet demand and fluid remains in the interstitium

Approximately 70% of the body is composed of water. Water provides the essence of the fluid medium for the transport of cells, nutrients and waste products between organs, provides substance for cellular cytosol and is the solvent in which numerous chemical reactions occur. Disruptions of the quantity of water in the body and its distribution can have serious consequences.

Discussions of fluid balance tend to revolve around a compartmental model of fluid distribution. Three main compartments are described, the intracellular (66%), interstitial/intercellular (25%) and intravascular (7%). A fourth compartment of specialised fluids (2%) can also be considered and includes secretions of the GI tract, peritoneal and pleural fluids, cerebrospinal fluid, synovial fluid, intraocular fluid and the vestibulocochlear fluids. The fourth compartment is often amalgamated into the interstitial.

Fluid movement is dynamic between all of the compartments and tends to follow passive osmotic and hydrostatic gradients, provided that the membrane separating the compartments is water permeable. If water movement between body compartments is required, manipulation of these gradients is typically the method by which this is accomplished. For example, the secretion of sweat involves the pumping of sodium and chloride ions into the lumen of the sweat duct. Water then follows passively through membrane pores and intercellular junctions.

Electrolytes

Electrolytes are one of the main classes of solute within body water. The chief intracellular cation is potassium and the principal extracellular cation is sodium. This differential distribution of sodium and potassium is maintained by the $Na^+/K^+/ATPase$ that is present on effectively all cells. It is the basis for the electrical activity of neurones, skeletal muscle and cardiac muscle. Alterations in the extracellular concentration of either potassium or sodium can destabilise the electrically excitable membranes of these cells, generating aberrant electrical activity such as seizures, arrhythmias or muscle weakness.

Electrolyte concentrations are also vital in maintaing turgor within cells. If the osmolarity of extracellular fluid is disturbed, water will move in or out of cells accordingly, resulting in cell swelling (and ultimately rupture) or shrinkage. Such are the potentially catastrophic effects of this inappropriate movement of water that body osmolarity is extremely tightly regulated by the antidiuretic hormone (ADH) system. In extreme situations, homeostatic mechanisms will strive to preserve blood osmolarity (which is in equilibrium with that of the other compartments) even at the expense of electrolyte levels and other parameters.

Blood and blood filtration

The vascular compartment contains 70 ml of blood per kilogram body weight (hence 4900 ml for a 70 kg man). Cellular constituents (erythrocytes, leucocytes and platelets) comprise 40% of this volume, while the remaining 60% is plasma. Plasma is water in which electrolytes, numerous types of proteins and lipoproteins are dissolved. Blood serves as a transport medium to deliver nutrients to the tissues and to remove waste products from them. This movement of nutrients and metabolites occurs at the capillary level.

When blood reaches the capillaries, fluid and electrolytes can pass easily through the gaps between endothelial cells, but cells and larger molecules (proteins) cannot. This movement is bidirectional and the direction that dominates is regulated by the balance between the hydrostatic pressure (HP) exerted by the blood pressure generated by the heart and transmitted through the vascular tree and the plasma oncotic pressure (POP) generated by plasma proteins. The HP drives water from the blood into the tissues whereas the POP provides a gradient that draws fluid back into the blood from the extracellular space.

In the proximal capillary bed, HP exceeds POP and there is a net movement of fluid from the blood into the extracellular space. The interstitial fluid is in equilibrium with the intercellular fluid and there is ready movement of nutrients and metabolites between these two compartments. However, the HP falls across the capillary bed and on the distal side is overpowered by the oncotic pressure, causing a net movement of fluid and its accompanying solutes back into the blood. Nevertheless, the action of the POP is not complete and a small quantity of fluid remains in the extracellular space. This is lymph and is handled by the lymphatic drainage system.

Lymphatic system

Lymphatic vessels commence in the tissues as blind-ended tubes lined by fenestrated endothelium. The lymph is massaged through progressively larger and more valve-bearing, muscularised (non-leaky) vessels to the thoracic duct, which empties into the venous system via the superior vena cava, returning the fluid to the circulation. *En route*, lymph is sieved through lymph nodes and thus lymph has a vital role in presenting extracellular material to the immune system.

Transudates

A transudate is an abnormal accumulation of fluid that has a low concentration of protein (typically defined as less than blood albumin). Transudates may occur in numerous locations, including the pleural and peritoneal cavities, and arise for one of two reasons:
1 *Increased hydrostatic pressure*, typically back pressure within the venous system due to inadequate cardiac function. Fluid accumulates in the extracellular compartment and yields 'pitting' oedema of the skin. Pleural effusions may also be seen.
2 The *plasma oncotic pressure drops* due to either decreased hepatic protein synthesis (as in cirrhosis), or excessive protein loss via the kidneys (nephrotic syndrome). As well as pitting oedema, ascites and pleural effusions are common.

Exudate

An exudate is an abnormal collection of fluid that has a high protein concentration, typically greater than plasma albumin. Exudates are caused by inflammatory processes that markedly increase the leakiness of the capillary bed such that proteins that would not normally be able to leave the circulation are now able to. Constriction of post-capillary venules raises the hydrostatic pressure and also contributes to exudate formation.

3 Tissue types and the effects of tissue damage

Types of necrosis

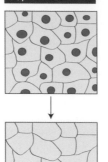
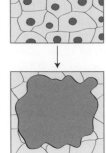
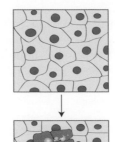
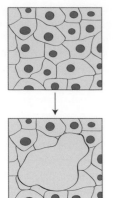
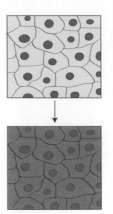
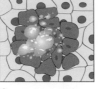

Coagulative necrosis
Example, renal infarct: cell outline preserved but cell contents degenerate

Liquefactive necrosis
Necrotic material liquefies, e.g. brain, abscess contents

Caseous necrosis
Tuberculosis – crumbly necrotic debris, combining coagulative and liquefactive features: granulomatous reaction

Fat necrosis
Follows trauma and forms hard nodule which can be mistaken for tumour (e.g. breast)

Gangrene
Blackened necrotic tissue liable to infection by anaerobic organisms (*Clostridium welchii* forms gas bubbles)

Watershed zone infarction

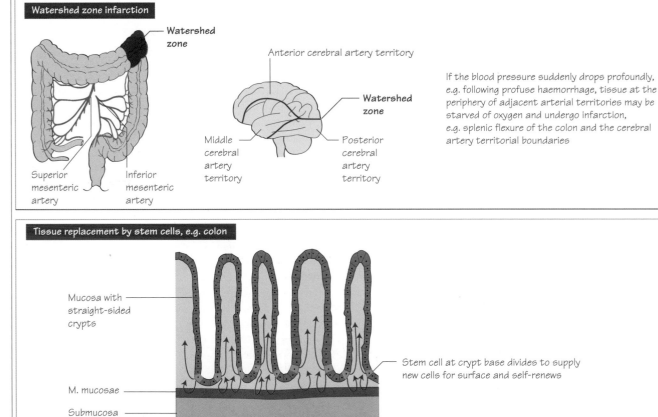

Watershed zone

Superior mesenteric artery

Inferior mesenteric artery

Anterior cerebral artery territory

Watershed zone

Middle cerebral artery territory

Posterior cerebral artery territory

If the blood pressure suddenly drops profoundly, e.g. following profuse haemorrhage, tissue at the periphery of adjacent arterial territories may be starved of oxygen and undergo infarction, e.g. splenic flexure of the colon and the cerebral artery territorial boundaries

Tissue replacement by stem cells, e.g. colon

Mucosa with straight-sided crypts

Stem cell at crypt base divides to supply new cells for surface and self-renews

M. mucosae

Submucosa

M. propria

Subserosal fat

• **Stem cells** are progenitor cells that can potentially form any tissue but respond to local hormones and cytokines to yield cells appropriate to the place in which they are generated. Stem cells divide to form a copy of themselves (and are thus immortal) plus a population of 'committed' progenitor cells. These divide into 'transit amplifying cells' and after several cell divisions yield terminally differentiated cells which die once their lifespan is over, to be replaced by further stem cell progeny.

Cell replacement in tissues with a high turnover is by stem cells. In tissues such as liver, with a low cell turnover, replacement of individually damaged cells is by division of adjacent cells, but larger amounts of hepatocyte loss requires stem cells for replacement. Each tissue has a compartment containing its own stem cell.

• **Labile tissues** readily regenerate and constantly proliferate in life, e.g. the epithelia of the skin, gastrointestinal tract, bronchus.

• **Stable tissues** include the liver and kidney, and can, if necessary, regenerate but usually show only very limited cell turnover. The liver has huge regenerative capacity – over half can be removed yet the remainder can undergo compensatory regeneration. Renal tubules are quick to regenerate following damage such as transient ischaemia.

• **Permanent tissues** show little to no regeneration so cell death can be catastrophic (e.g. cardiac myocytes, neurones).

Tissue necrosis

Necrosis is a form of cell death which has a variety of causes. The appearance of necrosis varies according to the stimulus and the tissue.

• **Coagulative necrosis** is commonest and usually appears as a firm, pale, wedge-shaped region of tissue reflecting the territory supplied by an occluded arteriole. Affected cells retain their shape but lose their nuclei and are known as 'ghost cells'.

• **Liquefactive necrosis** typically affects the central nervous system (CNS), often after a stroke. Once the damaged tissue has been cleared there is no healing and no scar – only a cystic space remains. Abscesses also show liquefactive necrosis, due to enzymic digestion of tissues.

• **Lytic necrosis** is the loss of single cells without any remaining evidence once the process is complete. It is often mediated by cytokines and typically occurs in the liver.

• **Caseation** is a white, crumbly, cottage-cheese-like appearance found in tuberculosis. It is a mixture of coagulative and liquefactive necrosis.

• **Gangrene**: 'dry gangrene' is black, dead, dry tissue caused by infarction, often seen in the toes of diabetic patients with severe atherosclerosis. 'Wet gangrene' occurs when the infarcted region becomes infected, particularly if there is oedema. 'Gas gangrene' follows infection of dead, anoxic tissue by gas-forming organisms, like *Clostridium welchii*.

• **Fat necrosis**: hard, bright yellow, nodules of fat necrosis occur, possibly secondary to trauma and may become calcified and resemble tumour clinically. Digestion of fat by pancreatic enzymes with fat necrosis and calcification is commonly seen in acute and chronic pancreatitis.

Infarction

Infarction is necrosis of a tissue or organ due to disruption of its blood supply. Infarction is either arterial, in which there is inadequate flow into the organ, or venous, in which venous outflow is obstructed which then prevents flow through the organ, causing congestion and stagnation. Arterial infarction is typically due to occlusion of the vessel by a thrombus or embolus; external compression is rare. Venous infarction often reflects compression of the veins, as occurs in strangulation of a hernia. The resulting congestion exacerbates the strangulation and therefore the degree of compression of the veins.

Normal tissue types
Epithelium

Epithelium, derived from embryonal ectoderm, lines the body's surfaces. It constantly regenerates and heals quickly.

1 Squamous: functions as a barrier and protects against friction.

• *Stratified squamous*: covers skin, pharynx and tongue, oesophagus, anus, vagina and external auditory canal; may be keratinised.

• *Simple squamous*: forms mesothelium lining the pleural and peritoneal cavities.

2 Transitional: this 'pseudostratified' epithelium lines the urinary tract. It contains umbrella cells that maintain the integrity of the surface on stretching to accommodate urine.

3 Glandular: lines all secretory organs. Its functions include:

• *Secretion*:
  • Non-specialised – e.g. mucin to facilitate food transport through the gut, or to trap bacteria in the nose.
  • Specialised – e.g. hormone secretion, acid secretion (gastric parietal) or absorption (gut, renal tubules).

• *Ion transfer*: renal tubules.

• *Clearance*: ciliated bronchial cells remove inhaled particles stuck in mucin (mucociliary escalator).

Neuroectodermal-derived tissue

This forms the central and peripheral nervous system. Scattered neuroendocrine cells populate various epithelia and secrete site-specific substances, e.g. skin melanocytes, gut hormone-secreting cells and in the bronchus (function is not known, but they are thought to give rise to pulmonary small cell carcinoma).

Connective tissue

Connective tissue forms structural tissues:

• **Fat** (adipo-) stores lipid, can regenerate and may secrete or respond to cytokines. Adipokines can drive inflammation.

• **Bone** (osteo-) consists mainly of matrix containing sparse osteocytes and is constantly remodelled by osteoblasts, which lay down matrix, and osteoclasts, which resorb it, in response to physical stresses and hormones (e.g. parathyroid hormone or calcitonin). It heals excellently.

• **Fibrous tissue** (fibro-), such as tendon, which consists mainly of acellular and avascular collagenous tissue and heals poorly.

• **Cartilage** (chondro-) consists mainly of avascular matrix, in which a few chondrocytes are embedded; it heals poorly.

• **Smooth muscle** (leio-) forms the walls of medium-sized and large blood vessels and lymphatics, the uterine myometrium, the vaginal wall and the muscular layers of the GI, respiratory and urological tracts. It can regenerate but often heals by scarring.

• **Striated muscle** ((rhabdo)myo-) forms voluntary muscle. Regeneration is limited.

• **Cardiac muscle** myocardium only; does not regenerate.

• **Endothelium** arises from 'blood islands' of the embryonal mesoderm. Different types line the blood vessels, lymphatics and the hepatic and splenic sinusoids. Endothelium readily regenerates.

Haemopoietic and lymphoreticular tissue

These tissues generate blood cells and form the immune system. They are discussed in Chapters 8–12.

Germ cells

These are the ovarian and testicular reproductive cells. They are constantly produced by the testis; the ovary contains a finite number from birth.

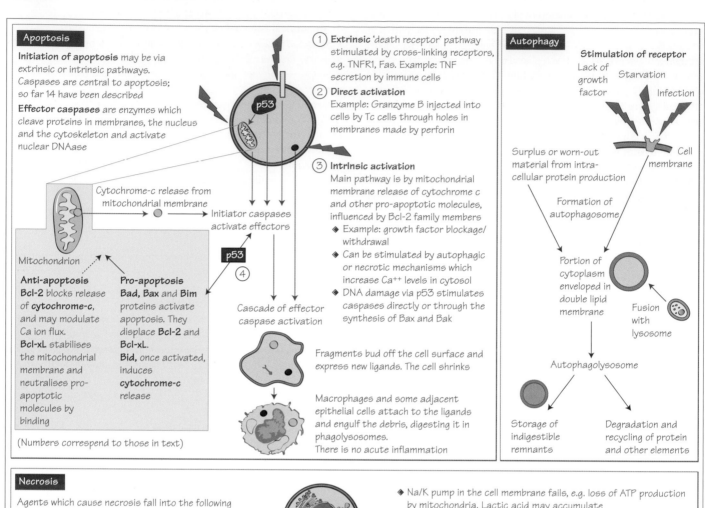

Apoptosis

Initiation of apoptosis may be via extrinsic or intrinsic pathways. Caspases are central to apoptosis; so far 14 have been described

Effector caspases are enzymes which cleave proteins in membranes, the nucleus and the cytoskeleton and activate nuclear DNAase

Cytochrome-c release from mitochondrial membrane → Initiator caspases activate effectors

Mitochondrion

Anti-apoptosis
Bcl-2 blocks release of **cytochrome-c**, and may modulate Ca ion flux.
Bcl-xL stabilises the mitochondrial membrane and neutralises pro-apoptotic molecules by binding

Pro-apoptosis
Bad, Bax and **Bim** proteins activate apoptosis. They displace **Bcl-2** and **Bcl-xL**.
Bid, once activated, induces **cytochrome-c** release

(Numbers correspend to those in text)

① **Extrinsic** 'death receptor' pathway stimulated by cross-linking receptors, e.g. TNFR1, Fas. Example: TNF secretion by immune cells

② **Direct activation**
Example: Granzyme B injected into cells by Tc cells through holes in membranes made by perforin

③ **Intrinsic activation**
Main pathway is by mitochondrial membrane release of cytochrome c and other pro-apoptotic molecules, influenced by Bcl-2 family members
◆ Example: growth factor blockage/ withdrawal
◆ Can be stimulated by autophagic or necrotic mechanisms which increase Ca⁺⁺ levels in cytosol
◆ DNA damage via p53 stimulates caspases directly or through the synthesis of Bax and Bak

Cascade of effector caspase activation

Fragments bud off the cell surface and express new ligands. The cell shrinks

Macrophages and some adjacent epithelial cells attach to the ligands and engulf the debris, digesting it in phagolysosomes.
There is no acute inflammation

Autophagy

Stimulation of receptor
Lack of growth factor
Starvation
Infection
Cell membrane

Surplus or worn-out material from intra-cellular protein production

Formation of autophagosome

Portion of cytoplasm enveloped in double lipid membrane

Fusion with lysosome

Autophagolysosome

Storage of indigestible remnants

Degradation and recycling of protein and other elements

Necrosis

Agents which cause necrosis fall into the following main categories:
◆ **Ischaemia, hypoxia or re-perfusion,** e.g. myocardial infarction
◆ **Infection,** e.g. bacterial, viral, fungal
◆ **Immune-mediated,** e.g. cross-reacting antibodies
◆ **Physical agents,** e.g. extreme heat or cold, electrocution, irradiation
◆ **Chemical agents,** e.g. strong acid or alkali, drugs which bind DNA
◆ **Nutritional,** e.g. folic acid/B12 deficiency

The generation of **free radicals** is a common effector pathway (oxidative stress occurs when there is more generation of reactive oxygen species (free radicals) than can be cleared by the available scavenging systems)

Reversible

Irreversible

◆ Na/K pump in the cell membrane fails, e.g. loss of ATP production by mitochondria. Lactic acid may accumulate
◆ Na⁺ enters the cell, passively accompanied by water. The cell swells
◆ Ca/Mg pump fails: excess cytosol Ca⁺⁺ activates enzymes which deplete ATP
◆ The membranes bleb and ribosomes dissociate from endoplasmic reticulum, cytoskeletal components clump
◆ The situation is still reversible
◆ Enzymes activated by Ca⁺⁺ digest the cell membrane, cytoskeleton and the nuclear chromatin
◆ The damage is irreversible
◆ Various nuclear changes may occur: it may shrink and get darker (pyknosis), fade away (karyolysis) or fragment (karyorrhexis). Similar nuclear changes are seen in apoptosis, particularly karyorrhexis. Some claim that this appearance is unique to apoptosis but it is disputed
◆ Release of cell contents stimulates acute inflammation. This adds to the damage by releasing further digestive enzymes and free radicals into the tissue
◆ If proteolytic digestion predominates there is less inflammation and the result is coagulative necrosis
If hydrolytic enzyme digestion predominates, the tissue undergoes liquefaction

In the living person, cell death occurs all the time and is often a necessary process. The two mechanisms that produce cell death are apoptosis and necrosis. It is becoming clear that these entities are not always distinct, but generalisations are made below.

Apoptosis

Apoptosis, often called 'programmed cell death', occurs during embryological development, as new tissues are formed and remodelled, or in physiological cycles such as the menstrual cycle. Apoptosis is characterised by the orderly breakdown of cellular constituents, which are packaged into membrane-bound vesicles and tagged for collection by phagocytes. This requires energy.

The initiation of apoptosis is as follows:

1 Binding of a 'death ligand' (e.g. TNFR1 or Fas) on the cell surface, e.g. direct binding by T cells or NK cells, or tumour necrosis factor (TNF) secretion by immune cells.

2 Membrane disruption by perforin, then intracellular injection of granzyme B by a cytotoxic T cell (Chapter 10).

3 Release of pro-apoptotic proteins, e.g. cytochrome *c*, from leaky mitochondrial membranes, a process largely regulated by pro- and anti-apoptotic proteins of the Bcl-2 family.

4 *p53*, a 'gatekeeper' gene in the cell cycle. p53 protein instigates apoptosis if there is a failure to repair DNA damage (Chapter 26).

Once started, apoptosis is generally irreversible, involving a final common pathway of an intracellular cascade of caspases. Proteolytic cleavage of cell contents and water loss causes cell shrinkage. Fragments bud off, enveloped by cell membrane, which expresses new ligands. Apoptosis does not stimulate an acute inflammatory response; instead, macrophages and adjacent cells bind the new ligands and phagocytose the fragments.

Necrosis

The death of a group of cells due to a noxious stimulus is referred to as necrosis. Necrosis is caused by many physical and chemical agents, amongst the most common of which are ischaemia, infection and drugs (e.g. chemotherapy). Necrotic cellular debris stimulates an acute inflammatory response which may increase the area of tissue damaged due to the leakage of lysosomal enzymes from polymorphs and macrophages.

It has been suggested that necrosis is what happens after cell death (i.e. irreversible damage) and that changes up to this point, which can be reversed, should be classed as cell damage. The point of no return is best recognised when there is a loss of membrane integrity and influx of calcium into the cytosol from the interstitial fluid or from the endoplasmic reticulum.

Factors that influence whether the damage is reversible include:

• **The duration of the stimulus**, e.g. ischaemia due to coronary artery thrombosis will cause myocardial infarction, but if the occlusion is rapidly cleared the area of cardiac muscle that dies will be reduced (Chapter 36). Reperfusion may cause problems due to the release of free radicals in the reperfused territory.

• **The dose of a chemical agent**: what can cause cell death in some people, does not in others due to genetic polymorphism (variation in inherited genes encoding the liver enzymes that metabolise the drugs).

• **The tissue type and its metabolic activity**: the neurones of the brain and cardiac muscle cells are highly metabolically active. Energy production from glycolysis via anaerobic pathways is available for liver or muscle (which store starch) but produces toxic lactic acid within the cell. Damage begins within minutes in the brain, but limb striated muscles can be deprived of oxygen for several hours. Cooling of tissues reduces their metabolism and increases survival time.

• **The state of health of the existing tissue**, e.g. iron overload in haemochromatosis renders the liver more susceptible to damage by other toxins, like alcohol.

Autophagy

The body attempts to preserve cells through times of adversity by undergoing autophagy, a particular type of cellular adaptation commonly seen in starvation and also in infection. It is also initiated by growth factor deprivation.

Portions of cytoplasm are bound by membranes to form a vesicle (autophagosome), which fuses with a lysosome and its contents, once degraded by hydrolase enzymes, are then recycled. The process is like hibernation and can be reversed once the lean times pass, but if taken to extreme because the stimulus persists, the cell dies, either by apoptosis or necrosis.

Pathological examples of diseases in which autophagy plays an important role include neurodegenerative diseases such as Alzheimer's, Parkinson's and Huntingdon's diseases. Much interest has recently developed in the role played by autophagy in cancer.

Free radicals

Free radicals are highly reactive anions with an unpaired outer orbital electron. They react with inorganic or organic chemicals to form further free radicals. Important examples are:

• Reactive oxygen species (ROS): hydrogen peroxide (H_2O_2), superoxide anion radical ($O^2 \cdot$) and hydroxyl ions ($OH\cdot$).

• Nitric oxide (NO) made by endothelium, macrophages, neurones and other cells.

Formation

• During normal cellular energy generation by oxygen reduction and electron transfer.

• Killing of pathogens by phagocytes: ROS are preformed in a membrane complex.

• Unwanted by-product of intracellular oxidase reactions.

• Radiation (generates hydroxyl and hydrogen free radicals by ionising water).

• Toxic by-product of drug/chemical metabolism by cellular enzymes, e.g. in the liver.

Harmful effects

• Lipid membrane damage by peroxidation (affects the cell membrane and the membranes of organelles).

• Protein damage by amino acid oxidation, cross-linkages or protein break down, e.g. microtubule aggregation.

• DNA damage can cause mutations and cancer.

Protection

• Natural decay to oxygen and H_2O_2.

• Antioxidants, e.g. glutathione and vitamins A, C and E.

• Binding of copper and iron to transport proteins.

• Scavenging enzymes that break down H_2O_2 and superoxide anion, e.g. catalase, superoxide dismutases or glutathione peroxidase.

5 Harmful agents in the environment

Cold-induced damage

- **Hypothermia** occurs when the core temperature is <35°C. **Frostbite** is localised freezing of exposed peripheries, e.g. nose, fingers

- The problems which affect resuscitation efforts are those of plasma volume depletion and alterations in ion concentration

- A cold-induced diuresis increases plasma viscosity and the blood becomes hyper-coagulable, increasing the risk of myocardial infarction and stroke on resuscitation

- Leakage of plasma also occurs across damaged capillary endothelium. Hypovolaemia may cause shock if a patient is warmed suddenly, without careful monitoring and fluid and electrolyte correction

- Plasma K^+ levels rise because of the loss of integrity of the cellular Na^+/K^+ pump - this normally functions to keep intracellular K^+ levels high and Na^+ low, while the reverse is true in the extracellular fluid. The high plasma K^+ levels may cause cardiac arrhythmias

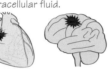

Heat-induced damage

Exogenous: high ambient temperatures and excessive exercise may cause **fluid and electrolyte loss and dehydration**. Treatment is by cooling and fluid and electrolyte replacement

Mixed exogenous/endogenous: high ambient temperatures and impaired heat-losing mechanisms cause **heat stroke**.
- Example: athletes exercising in extremely hot environments
- Infants, children and the elderly, especially those taking medication such as diuretics or tranquilisers
Treatment is with cooling, fluid and electrolyte replacement – antipyretics are ineffective

Many patients develop lactic acidosis, hypocalcaemia, muscle fibre damage and myoglobinuria, which may damage renal tubules

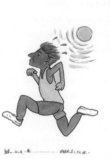

Endogenous:
Infections cause fever due to the release of cytokines, e.g. IL-1 and TNF, which affect the temperature control centre in the hypothalamus
- Example: the drenching sweats and high fevers seen in tuberculosis and some lymphoma patients (though why this is typically at night is not clear)
- Febrile convulsions are common in children with high temperatures
- An aberrant response to anaesthetic may cause 'malignant hyperthermia'

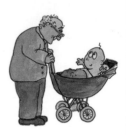

Radiation-associated disease

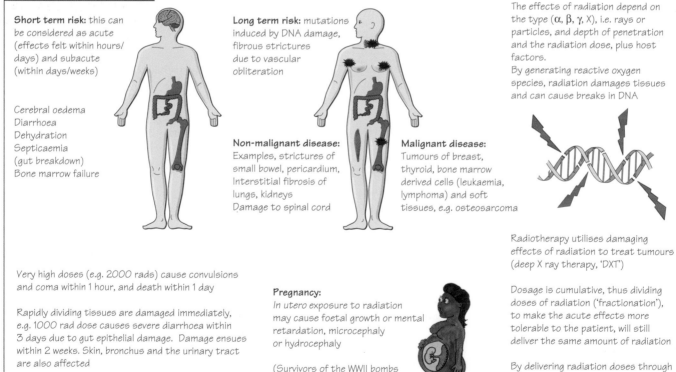

Short term risk: this can be considered as acute (effects felt within hours/days) and subacute (within days/weeks)

Cerebral oedema
Diarrhoea
Dehydration
Septicaemia
(gut breakdown)
Bone marrow failure

Long term risk: mutations induced by DNA damage, fibrous strictures due to vascular obliteration

Non-malignant disease:
Examples, strictures of small bowel, pericardium, Interstitial fibrosis of lungs, kidneys
Damage to spinal cord

Malignant disease:
Tumours of breast, thyroid, bone marrow derived cells (leukaemia, lymphoma) and soft tissues, e.g. osteosarcoma

The effects of radiation depend on the type (α, β, γ, X), i.e. rays or particles, and depth of penetration and the radiation dose, plus host factors.
By generating reactive oxygen species, radiation damages tissues and can cause breaks in DNA

Very high doses (e.g. 2000 rads) cause convulsions and coma within 1 hour, and death within 1 day

Rapidly dividing tissues are damaged immediately, e.g. 1000 rad dose causes severe diarrhoea within 3 days due to gut epithelial damage. Damage ensues within 2 weeks. Skin, bronchus and the urinary tract are also affected

The bone marrow cells are highly sensitive: a dose of 300 rads will cause marrow suppression and death within 3 weeks from anaemia, infection or widespread bleeding

Pregnancy:
In utero exposure to radiation may cause foetal growth or mental retardation, microcephaly or hydrocephaly

(Survivors of the WWII bombs in Japan were found to have no radiation-related problems with future pregnancies)

Radiotherapy utilises damaging effects of radiation to treat tumours (deep X ray therapy, 'DXT')

Dosage is cumulative, thus dividing doses of radiation ('fractionation'), to make the acute effects more tolerable to the patient, will still deliver the same amount of radiation

By delivering radiation doses through beams converging on the tumour site from different starting points, the tumour receives the highest possible dose whilst non-tumour tissues receive much lesser dosages

Physical agents

Electrocution

Electrocution may occur from lightning or contact with DC or AC currents from the domestic electricity supply. Electric currents are conducted through the body best by fluids with high ion content – blood and tissue fluids. They can also travel via the peripheral nerves. Electric currents within the body, well insulated by fatty tissue, generate a lot of heat very quickly and charring of the skin is often noticeable at the entry and exit points in the skin. Electric currents also interfere with the body's own electrical impulses – cardiac conduction is particularly vulnerable. Thus electrocution typically causes cardiac arrhythmia (often ventricular fibrillation) and severe burns, either of which may cause death.

This property is utilised in the treatment of ventricular fibrillation during cardiac arrest: a DC shock is applied to the praecordium and may shock the heart back into sinus rhythm.

Extremes of temperature

Extremes of temperature interfere with cellular homeostasis, which depends on temperature-sensitive enzyme reactions and the maintenance of ion concentrations within a fairly narrow range of normal values. The normal core temperature is maintained by the hypothalamus and is regulated by IL-1 release from macrophages and local prostaglandin production. Heat is generated by muscle and metabolic activity within the body and is lost through the skin, sweat and breath.

• **Excess heat**: A core temperature of 41–42°C causes severe confusion, problems with cardiac function and respiration; 42.5°C is virtually always fatal. The cause may be an increase in heat generation, an inability to lose heat or a disturbance of hypothalamic thermal regulatory mechanisms. The body responds by profound vasodilatation.

• **Burns**: Burns cause damage by coagulating the skin and variable amounts of subcutaneous tissue. Lipid membranes melt, enzymes denature and proteins precipitate. Burns are classified as 1st, 2nd or 3rd degree according to the depth of tissue damaged and the surface area of the body affected. Plasma and tissue fluid leak from the surfaces of the burned areas and may cause hypovolaemic shock if >70% of the body surface is involved with 3rd degree burns. The loss of vital protein molecules in the exudate impairs the acute inflammatory response and healing.

Inhalation of fire and smoke damages the respiratory tract mucosa and the alveolar walls, causing acute respiratory distress syndrome.

The damaging effect of heat is utilised in radiofrequency ablation.

• **Cold**: Hypothermia occurs when the core temperature drops to 35°C. If shivering and increased muscle activity fail to halt the fall in temperature, the respiration rate, pulse, blood oxygenation and tissue perfusion decreases. Blood sludges as plasma is lost by cold-induced diuresis and leaky endothelium. The patient becomes confused, then deeply unconscious. Death is usual by 28°C.

(Perfusion with cooled blood reduces metabolic demands and complications during cardiac transplant surgery. The transplanted heart will have been transported to the donor's hospital in a super-cooled state to reduce tissue deterioration.)

Sudden exposure to extreme cold, as seen in frostbite, causes hypothermic damage to exposed or less well-perfused parts, such as fingers, nose or toes. The fluid in the capillaries, cells and tissues freezes and thereby increases the volume of the cells. The plasma membranes rupture, as do those of the organelles. There is gangrenous ischaemic necrosis of the extremities. Treatment is by gradual warming. Often the extent of the damage is less than initially feared, so delay hasty amputation.

Radiation

Radiation damages tissues by causing ionisation of molecules in the tissue fluid, forming free oxygen radicals (reactive oxygen species). Risks are related to the type, extent and cumulative dose of radiation and the tissues exposed to it.

• **Short-term risk**: rapidly dividing tissues are damaged immediately, e.g. severe diarrhoea due to gut epithelial damage and bone marrow suppression.

• **Long-term risk**: development of malignant tumours due to mutations induced by DNA damage and fibrous strictures due to vascular obliteration (e.g. small bowel).

Radiation damages DNA by causing multiple breaks within it, or by cross-linkage (utilised therapeutically in the treatment of malignant tumours).

Chemical agents

Exposure to strong acid or alkali ruptures cell membranes, producing cell and tissue necrosis and capillary damage with leakage of blood into tissues. The effects can mimic burns. Healing of extensive wounds is often by scarring.

Many industries generate harmful substances as by-products. Some chemicals react with cellular constituents or are altered by normal metabolic pathways to create toxic metabolites, for example:

• Conjugation with glucuronide may render a molecule safe until it is excreted by the kidney, when the glucuronide is conserved and the urinary epithelium is exposed to the toxic metabolite.

• Volatile organic compounds, e.g. polycyclic aromatic hydrocarbons (PAHs), are generated by the petrochemical industry and by combustion of tars (e.g. soot), and are also found in cigarette smoke. When converted to epoxides by cytochrome p450 they can bind and mutate DNA. Smoking-related PAHs are strongly linked to the development of lung cancer. Soot was linked to scrotal cancer in chimney sweeps by Percival Pott in 1775.

• Vinyl chloride monomers, produced during PVC manufacture, may generate chloracetaldehyde when metabolised by hepatic cytochrome p450; this can bind and mutate DNA.

Cancer treatment employs drugs that interfere with DNA replication to attack dividing cells, working on the premise that more tumour than normal cells are usually proliferating at any one time, e.g. cyclosphosphamide alkylates DNA and causes nonsense mutations.

Water

Death by drowning is due to asphyxia. Diatoms from the water enter the blood and tissues. Death is four to five times faster in fresh water than salt water because the hypotonic fresh-water solution that enters the blood via the pulmonary capillary bed causes haemodilution, with low chloride and potassium levels, and later hyperkalaemia due to red cell lysis. Sea water may be almost isotonic, although usually it is hypertonic and the blood chloride level is increased, but haemolysis does not occur. For this reason, resuscitation efforts are more likely to be successful in people rescued from the sea. People who survive near-drowning may develop pneumonitis from organisms in dirty water.

Infectious agents

These will be covered elsewhere. In order to cause damage, these organisms must evade the body's primary defences and enter the tissues.

6 The effects of tobacco, alcohol and other drugs

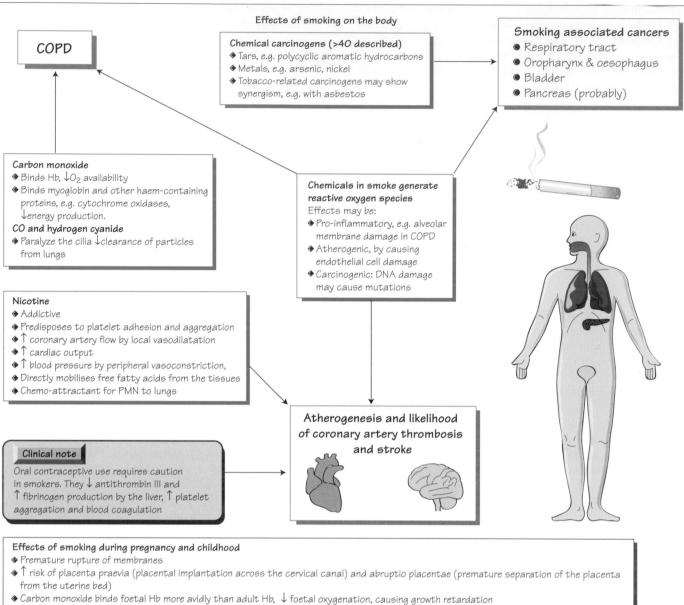

Effects of smoking on the body

COPD

Chemical carcinogens (>40 described)
- Tars, e.g. polycyclic aromatic hydrocarbons
- Metals, e.g. arsenic, nickel
- Tobacco-related carcinogens may show synergism, e.g. with asbestos

Smoking associated cancers
- Respiratory tract
- Oropharynx & oesophagus
- Bladder
- Pancreas (probably)

Carbon monoxide
- Binds Hb, $\downarrow O_2$ availability
- Binds myoglobin and other haem-containing proteins, e.g. cytochrome oxidases, $\downarrow$energy production.

CO and hydrogen cyanide
- Paralyze the cilia $\downarrow$clearance of particles from lungs

Chemicals in smoke generate reactive oxygen species
Effects may be:
- Pro-inflammatory, e.g. alveolar membrane damage in COPD
- Atherogenic, by causing endothelial cell damage
- Carcinogenic: DNA damage may cause mutations

Nicotine
- Addictive
- Predisposes to platelet adhesion and aggregation
- $\uparrow$ coronary artery flow by local vasodilatation
- $\uparrow$ cardiac output
- $\uparrow$ blood pressure by peripheral vasoconstriction,
- Directly mobilises free fatty acids from the tissues
- Chemo-attractant for PMN to lungs

Atherogenesis and likelihood of coronary artery thrombosis and stroke

Clinical note
Oral contraceptive use requires caution in smokers. They $\downarrow$ antithrombin III and $\uparrow$ fibrinogen production by the liver, $\uparrow$ platelet aggregation and blood coagulation

Effects of smoking during pregnancy and childhood
- Premature rupture of membranes
- $\uparrow$ risk of placenta praevia (placental implantation across the cervical canal) and abruptio placentae (premature separation of the placenta from the uterine bed)
- Carbon monoxide binds foetal Hb more avidly than adult Hb, $\downarrow$ foetal oxygenation, causing growth retardation
- Children exposed to passive smoking may develop asthma, recurrent respiratory tract and ear infections or sudden infant death syndrome

Tobacco

Tobacco is most damaging when smoked either directly or indirectly ('passive smoking'), but also has deleterious effects when chewed, or inhaled as snuff. It is addictive because of pleasurable effects such as increased feeling of well-being and alertness and decreased appetite. It has effects on children, the unborn foetus and on pregnancy itself. Long-term use causes cancer, cardiovascular disease and respiratory disease.

Tobacco smoke is absorbed into the blood via the alveolar capillaries or via the gastrointestinal tract in swallowed sputum. It has a direct effect on the mucous membranes lining the oropharynx, respiratory tract and oesophagus. The toxic effects of tobacco smoke are due to both gaseous and particulate agents.

Gaseous elements
• Carbon monoxide (CO) shows 200 times oxygen's affinity for haemoglobin and reduces oxygen availability to the tissues.
• CO or hydrogen cyanide may paralyse the cilia, impairing the removal of inhaled particles from the respiratory tract.

Particulate elements
1 Nicotine:
• Nictotine stimulates nicotine receptors in the brain to cause addiction.
• It increases blood pressure by direct catecholaminergic effects.
• It mobilises free fatty acids from the tissues, important in atherogenesis.
• Nicotine predisposes to platelet adhesion and aggregation, increasing the risk of coronary arterial thrombosis and myocardial infarction or cardiac arrhythmia.
• It is a chemoattractant, luring polymorphs and macrophages to the alveolar space.

2 Chemical carcinogens:
• Over 40 smoke-related carcinogens are known, chief of which are the polycyclic aromatic hydrocarbons, and also carcinogenic metals, such as arsenic and nickel.
• Smoking is linked to cancers of the respiratory tract, oropharynx, oesophagus, bladder and probably the pancreas.
• Tobacco-related carcinogens may act synergistically with each other, or with non-smoking-related carcinogens.
• Tobacco smoke contains reactive oxygen species (ROS), also known as free radicals.

3 Irritant substances:
• Cancer-promoting agents that stimulate cell turnover, increasing the risk of mutation induced by carcinogens, include acetaldehyde and phenol.
• These cause chronic obstructive pulmonary disease (COPD; Chapter 45) by inducing inflammation in the lung and respiratory tree, which can damage the delicate alveolar walls and cause emphysema or stimulate mucous cells to increase mucin secretion, which is difficult to clear if cilia function is impaired, resulting in chronic bronchitis.
• ROS stimulate the acute inflammatory response and cause further damage.

Combined effects
Tobacco smoke may syngergise with other agents to multiply the amount of damage either would cause independently.
• Occupational-related asthma or COPD: e.g. silicosis in coal miners, dust from grain in farm workers, or fumes from welding and asbestosis.
• Cancer related to occupational exposure: e.g. blue asbestos may cause primary lung cancer or mesothelioma (cancer of the pleura) but the risks are increased 20-fold in smokers.

Alcohol
Ethanol (ethyl alcohol)
Driving is illegal in the UK with blood alcohol levels >80 mg/dL. Unaccustomed drinkers are unconscious at 200 mg/dL; some chronic drinkers can tolerate 700 mg/dL, due to the induction of liver enzymes. Other drugs may compete with alcohol for these paths, rendering their effects unpredictable.

Ethanol directly damages cell membranes, e.g. skeletal muscle, cardiac muscle (ventricles dilate) and other sites. Hepatotoxic effects are probably from cytokine release by activated Kupffer cells, compounded in chronic alcoholics by amino acid deficiencies and cardiac failure. The metabolism of alcohol and its wider effects on tissue are further discussed in Chapter 58.

Other alcohols
Alcohol is often synonymous with ethanol, but there are other alcohols that may occasionally present as clinical problems.

1 Methanol (methyl alcohol): this is very slowly metabolised over many hours/days by the same pathway as alcohol, with the highly toxic end-product of formic acid. Although the initial sensation of inebriation is similar to ethanol, the meths drinker develops a severe metabolic acidosis, vomiting, dizziness, blurred vision and blindness and may die from respiratory depression.

2 Ethylene glycol: this is the main constituent of antifreeze, and reacts with metals in the body to form toxic aldehyde products. Patients who survive the initial insult often develop renal calcium oxalate stones and acute tubular necrosis.

Ironically, the treatment of methanol and ethylene glycol poisoning is ethanol, which competes for the metabolic pathways, giving the body more time to clear metabolites before toxic effects occur.

Commonly encountered therapeutic and addictive drugs
The mechanisms by which therapeutic and recreational drugs produce toxic effects are numerous. The pharmacological effects of the drug may be directly harmful (such as bone marrow suppression by chemotherapeutic agents), or the drug may have harmful side effects (e.g. diarrhoea induced by erythromycin or malignant neuroleptic syndrome caused by major tranquilisers). Recreational drugs can produce physical and/or psychological dependence, which can induce harmful patterns of behaviour that have deleterious psychological, physical and social consequences.

As well as the injuries produced by the drug itself, the metabolites may be harmful. Most drug metabolism occurs in the liver. The basic mechanisms are too detailed to be explored here, but the basic aims of the metabolism are to render the drug inactive and water soluble, the latter to facilitate excretion in the urine or bile. Both objectives are achieved by a set of enzymes that conjugate the drug by adding chemical groups to it. These include hydroxylation (cytochrome p450 system), glucuronidation and conjugation with glutathione. Paracetamol overdose is a very important example of a drug that is rendered toxic by metabolism but space again prevents elaboration of the detail; the reader should use other sources to ensure familiarity with the principles. Also important is that the xenobiotic enzymes show genetic polymorphism and can be induced or inhibited by other drugs.

7 # Nutritional disorders

General pathology

Under-nutrition

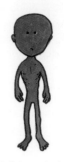

Marasmus
- Severe protein-calorie deficiency, body weight < 60% of normal for age and height
- Severe growth retardation
- Head appears huge because the rest of the body is emaciated, particularly the extremities, because of the extreme depletion of the subcutaneous fat and loss of skeletal muscle bulk
- Muscle is catabolised in order to maintain the serum albumin level, so oedema is not a feature (see fluid compartments; Chapter 2)

Kwashiorkor
- Weight 60–80% of normal (deficiency of protein, but carbohydrate sufficient)
- Skeletal muscle bulk appears normal; subcutaneous fat stores are maintained
- Black hair may appear red or alternating stripes of hyper- and hypo-pigmentation may be seen, and tufts of hair may fall out
- Flaky desquamation of skin may occur in patches
- Oedema in dependent parts due to low plasma albumin
- Chubby but apathetic, with no appetite
- Liver enlargement with severe fatty change
- Anaemia common, iron deficiency or mixed picture
- Thymic and lymphoid atrophy compromise immunity
- Small bowel undergoes villous atrophy. This adds malabsorption to the list of problems, and there may be secondary as well as primary deficiencies, often of vitamins

Over-nutrition

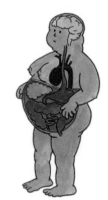

Obesity
- BMI>30

Health risks include:
- Cardiovascular disease: atherosclerosis, myocardial infarction and stroke
- Gastrointestinal disease: reflux oesophagitis, Barrett's oesophagus, adenocarcinoma of oesophagus, adenocarcinoma of colon, fatty liver disease and cirrhosis
- Endocrine disease: diabetes mellitus type II

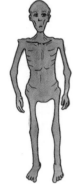

Cachexia
- Catabolism of skeletal muscle and visceral and subcutaneous fat stores leads to wasting, especially in deltoid muscles and upper limb girdle subcutaneous tissues
- Cytokines such as TNF, IL-1 and IL-6 implicated, released by some malignant tumours and in chronic inflammatory states such as tuberculosis and AIDS
- Dietary supplementation unsuccessful

24 *Pathology at a Glance.* By C.J. Finlayson and B.A.T. Newell. Published 2009 by Blackwell Publishing. ISBN: 978-1-4051-3650-1

Seven different classes of substance are essential in the diet:
- Water.
- Carbohydrates.
- Proteins (essential amino acids).
- Fat.
- Vitamins.
- Minerals.
- Fibre.

Carbohydrates, proteins and fats act as sources of both energy and structural materials, although proteins have predominantly structural roles and carbohydrates are mainly an energy source. Twenty amino acids are used in the body's proteins, of which nine cannot be synthesised and are therefore termed essential. The remaining 11 can be generated from the nine essential amino acids if they are not provided by the diet.

Vitamins and minerals do not provide energy but have specific roles in metabolic pathways (e.g. vitamin C and collagen synthesis), as prosthetic groups (e.g. iron in haemoglobin) and as substrates for vital molecules (e.g. vitamin A and rhodopsin).

The designation of fibre is sometimes debated. Fibre is not absorbed from the gut, but bulks out the contents of the GI tract lumen and facilitates peristalsis and the formation of stools. Nutritional fibre is a term used by some to mean substances absorbed from foodstuffs such as oats, which can increase high density lipoprotein (HDL) levels and thus reduce cholesterol.

Nutritional deficiency

Primary nutritional deficiency is due to a decrease in food intake where this reduction is not due to an underlying illness. The decrease may be generalised, as in marasmus and kwashiorkor, or selective, such as specific vitamin deficiencies or malabsorptive syndromes. The growth requirements of young children render them more susceptible to the more gross manifestations of nutritional deficiencies than adults. Pregnant women and adolescents are also more vulnerable.

Secondary causes of nutritional deficiency include reduced food intake secondary to another condition (e.g. chronic alcoholism or cancer cachexia) or defective absorption of food. Malabsorption disorders can cause either selective or global nutritional deficiencies. The psychiatric disorders of appetite and eating behaviour, anorexia and bulimia, tend only to be seen in the developed world.

Protein energy malnutrition

This term can refer to a variety of conditions in which there is a generalised nutritional deficiency, although it is employed most commonly in relation to marasmus and kwashiorkor.

Marasmus: There is marked calorie deficiency, with a body weight less than 60% of normal for age and height. Children are severely growth retarded.
- The head appears huge because the rest of the body is emaciated, particularly the extremities, because of extreme depletion of the subcutaneous fat and loss of skeletal muscle bulk.
- Muscle is catabolised in order to maintain the serum albumin level, so oedema is not a feature.
- There is usually anaemia, which may be iron deficiency type or a mixed picture. Vitamin deficiencies may manifest.

Kwashiorkor: The patient's weight is between 60% and 80% of normal, because the problem is a relative deficiency of protein, whilst carbohydrate intake may be adequate. The problem is seen particularly in African and Southeast Asian children who are weaned from the breast when a new baby arrives and for whom the only available diet is composed almost exclusively of carbohydrate. The absence of essential amino acids prevents new protein synthesis by the liver and its protein stores become depleted.

Patients with severe malnutrition often have deficient immunity due to lack of dietary protein substrates for immune molecules and may have one or more infections at presentation. The cytokine release and energy demands resulting from the inflammatory response may compromise the patient's status further.

Cachexia

This is a catabolic process resulting from chronic disease such as malignancy, AIDS or tuberculosis. The clinical picture is similar to marasmus, but the cause is not primarily an inadequate diet. Instead, the process is driven by cytokines such as tumour necrosis factor (TNF) and interferons (IL-1 and IL-6 are particularly implicated) secreted by or in response to the underlying condition. There are some cancers that appear more likely than others to generate this distressing phenomenon, which undoubtedly reduces a patient's chances of treatment response – e.g. carcinoma of stomach, pancreas and bronchus. Current interest centres on the catabolic pathways activated by these cytokines and their manipulation.

The patient is emaciated due to loss of body fat around the arms, shoulders, chest wall and even in the hand, plus a marked reduction in skeletal muscle bulk seen particularly in the deltoid and quadriceps. Dependent oedema can occur.

Obesity

While malnutrition tends to affect the Third World, various circumstances can lead to it afflicting people in developed countries. However, obesity is a far greater nutritional disorder in the First World. The causes are complex, but revolve around a more sedentary lifestyle and readily available carbohydrate and fat-rich processed foods.

Obesity, as defined by a body mass index (BMI) of over 30 kg/m^2 (overweight is $25.0\text{--}29.9 \text{ kg/m}^2$), can cause many health problems. High blood cholesterol is a major risk factor for atherosclerosis. Lifestyles that lead to obesity also predispose to colorectal adenocarcinoma. Gastro-oesophageal reflux disease is exacerbated by obesity. Marked obesity may produce degenerative joint disease.

Metabolic syndrome

This is a pro-atherogenic, low-grade inflammatory syndrome characterised by visceral obesity and hyperlipidaemia which gives rise to type II diabetes mellitus that features insulin resistance, hyperinsulinism and hyperglycaemia. It tends to occur in inactive, middle-aged or older people (>45 years). It is thought that physical inactivity leads to a chronic catabolic state in which insulin resistance develops as an adaptation to decreased tissue energy requirements. Adipose tissue itself is metabolically active and can release adipokines, which modulate inflammation and insulin resistance. Insulin has an anti-inflammatory action, thus insulin resistance may be one reason that these patients develop a chronic low-grade, acute inflammatory state. Endothelial action is also impaired.

The metabolic syndrome has been implicated in the causation of atheroma, cardiovascular disease and stroke, hypertension and non-alcoholic fatty liver disease.

8 The body's natural defences

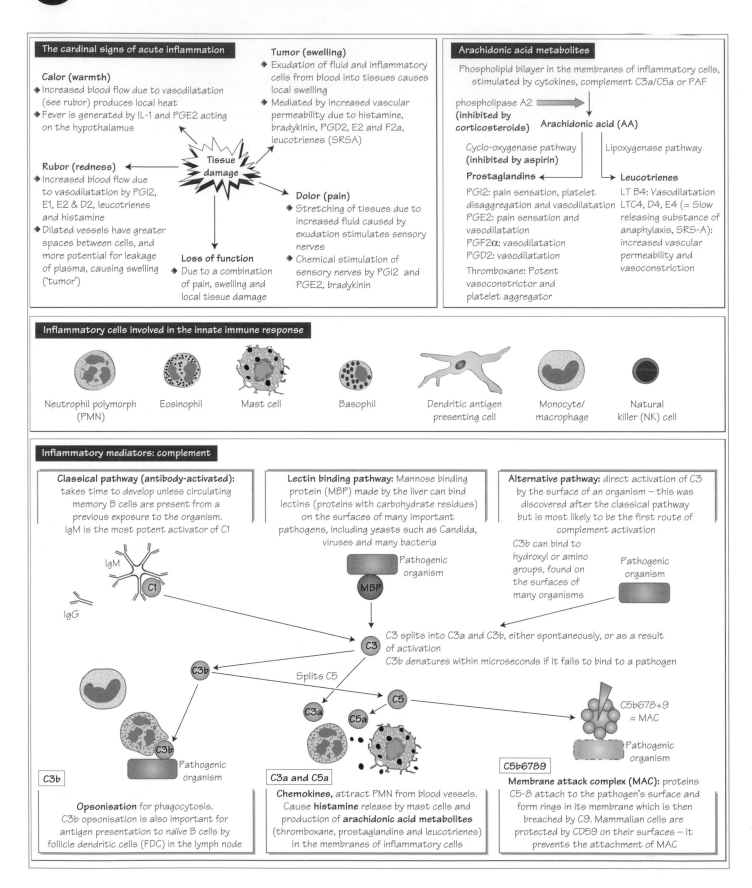

The cardinal signs of acute inflammation

Calor (warmth)
- Increased blood flow due to vasodilatation (see rubor) produces local heat
- Fever is generated by IL-1 and PGE2 acting on the hypothalamus

Rubor (redness)
- Increased blood flow due to vasodilatation by PGI2, E1, E2 & D2, leucotrienes and histamine
- Dilated vessels have greater spaces between cells, and more potential for leakage of plasma, causing swelling ('tumor')

Tissue damage

Tumor (swelling)
- Exudation of fluid and inflammatory cells from blood into tissues causes local swelling
- Mediated by increased vascular permeability due to histamine, bradykinin, PGD2, E2 and F2a, leucotrienes (SRSA)

Dolor (pain)
- Stretching of tissues due to increased fluid caused by exudation stimulates sensory nerves
- Chemical stimulation of sensory nerves by PGI2 and PGE2, bradykinin

Loss of function
- Due to a combination of pain, swelling and local tissue damage

Arachidonic acid metabolites

Phospholipid bilayer in the membranes of inflammatory cells, stimulated by cytokines, complement C3a/C5a or PAF

phospholipase A2 (inhibited by corticosteroids) → Arachidonic acid (AA)

Cyclo-oxygenase pathway (inhibited by aspirin)

Prostaglandins
PGI2: pain sensation, platelet disaggregation and vasodilatation
PGE2: pain sensation and vasodilatation
PGF2α: vasodilatation
PGD2: vasodilatation

Thromboxane: Potent vasoconstrictor and platelet aggregator

Lipoxygenase pathway

Leucotrienes
LT B4: Vasodilatation
LTC4, D4, E4 (= Slow releasing substance of anaphylaxis, SRS-A): increased vascular permeability and vasoconstriction

Inflammatory cells involved in the innate immune response

Neutrophil polymorph (PMN) — Eosinophil — Mast cell — Basophil — Dendritic antigen presenting cell — Monocyte/ macrophage — Natural killer (NK) cell

Inflammatory mediators: complement

Classical pathway (antibody-activated): takes time to develop unless circulating memory B cells are present from a previous exposure to the organism. IgM is the most potent activator of C1

IgM
IgG
C1

Lectin binding pathway: Mannose binding protein (MBP) made by the liver can bind lectins (proteins with carbohydrate residues) on the surfaces of many important pathogens, including yeasts such as Candida, viruses and many bacteria

Pathogenic organism
MBP

Alternative pathway: direct activation of C3 by the surface of an organism – this was discovered after the classical pathway but is most likely to be the first route of complement activation

C3b can bind to hydroxyl or amino groups, found on the surfaces of many organisms

Pathogenic organism

C3 splits into C3a and C3b, either spontaneously, or as a result of activation
C3b denatures within microseconds if it fails to bind to a pathogen

C3
C3b
Splits C5
C3a
C5a
C5
C5b678+9 = MAC
Pathogenic organism

C3b
Pathogenic organism

C3a and C5a

C5b6789

C3b
Opsonisation for phagocytosis. C3b opsonisation is also important for antigen presentation to naïve B cells by follicle dendritic cells (FDC) in the lymph node

Chemokines, attract PMN from blood vessels. Cause **histamine** release by mast cells and production of **arachidonic acid metabolites** (thromboxane, prostaglandins and leucotrienes) in the membranes of inflammatory cells

Membrane attack complex (MAC): proteins C5-8 attach to the pathogen's surface and form rings in its membrane which is then breached by C9. Mammalian cells are protected by CD59 on their surfaces – it prevents the attachment of MAC

Innate immunity

The innate immune system provides the initial resistance to infection. It responds more quickly than the acquired immune system but lacks the advantages of the memory and specificity of the acquired system.

Barriers

The body's first line of defence is its protective epithelial surfaces, which are the skin, cornea and conjunctiva, respiratory tract, gastro-intestinal tract, urinary tract and reproductive systems. In each case, the epithelium provides a physical barrier to the entry of organisms, but this barrier is reinforced by additional mechanisms.

With the exception of the skin, all the other barriers are bolstered by the movement of fluid over the epithelial surface, such as tears in the eye, the mucociliary escalator in the lung and menstruation in the uterus. This flushes the surface and prevents organisms from penetrating and establishing a foothold.

The barriers are further enhanced by secretions. Tears are again an example as they contain lysozyme. Gastric acid has a powerful antibacterial action. Mucus in the GI tract and lungs also serves to oppose micro-organisms, as well as entrapping them to cause them to be cleared by the flow processes mentioned above.

Although primarily a component of the innate system, barriers are supported by the acquired system, in the form of mucosal-associated lymphoid tissue and the secretion of immunoglobulin A.

Cells

The cells of the innate immune system operate in the front line of the body's defences and are the first to engage the infection.

Neutrophil polymorphs: These constitute 70% of peripheral blood leucocytes, are produced from myeloid precursors in the bone marrow, and attempt to kill invaders by phagocytosis and release of their granules. They contain lysozyme, reactive oxygen species (ROS), myeloperoxidase and other harmful agents. They are programmed to live 5 days, but once in the blood live for only about 10 hours. If involved in an acute inflammatory response, they die within minutes to a few hours, depending on their activity (e.g. they die after phagocytosing about 12 organisms).

Eosinophils: Eosinophils are also derived from the myeloid lineage. Like neutrophils, they possess granules, although their granules contain histamine, heparin, major basic protein and bactericidal eosinophil cationic protein, amongst others. They do not phagocytose organisms but instead release their granules and are therefore important against large pathogens. They are recruited by IL-5.

Mast cells and basophils: These are also myeloid leucocytes. They are closely related granulated cells and basophils may be thought of as a circulating form of mast cells. Mast cells live in the tissues for years and secrete serotonin by degranulation. Degranulation is stimulated by the binding of multiple molecules of IgE. As with eosinophils, they are deployed against larger pathogens. Basophils are recruited into the tissue to become mast cells by IL-4. While in the blood, their granules do not contain serotonin but instead release peroxidase, heparin, histamine and kallikrein if provoked. Their lifespan is only a few days.

Monocytes and macrophages: Monocytes complete the myeloid leucocytes. They initially enter the blood but within 20–40 hours move to tissues, where they are known as macrophages or histiocytes and survive for weeks/months. They are versatile cells that normally function as scavengers, phagocytosing and breaking up tissue debris, necrotic material, particulate matter and apoptotic debris. However, if activated, macrophages enlarge, develop enhanced phagocytic and killing properties (using toxic granules similar to those in neutrophils) or differentiate to present antigen to other inflammatory cells, as well as secreting TNF and other cytokines and activating other cells (including endothelial cells). Activated macrophages also function as antigen presenting cells and are vital in assisting the cells of the acquired system. Microbial products in the tissue fluid, IL-1 and bound C3b, can all activate macrophages.

Humoral mediators

Complement system: The complement system is a protein cascade that functions to lyse pathogens. It may be activated directly by the organism or after being stimulated by antibodies. In addition to its lytic effects, complement can also assist cells of the innate system. Complement component C3b renders the pathogen more readily phagocytosed (opsonisation) while C5a and C3a are chemokines that attract acute inflammatory cells.

Arachidonic acid: This can be metabolised to yield a variety of vasoactive metabolites that in addition to their role in blood flow and coagulation may be utilised by the immune response.

Cytokines (interleukins and tumour necrosis factors): These encompass numerous different molecules that are elaborated by assorted cells of the immune response and have varied actions. Different cells release different molecules, which in turn have differing cellular targets.

Acquired immunity

The acquired immune system is slower to enter the fray than the innate system but compensates for this by possessing specificity for different pathogens and an ability to remember previous encounters. Therefore, while the innate immune system will mount the same magnitude of response to a given pathogen on the tenth exposure as the first, the acquired system will have learnt from the previous encounter and be ready to respond much more powerfully after the initial exposure. The acquired immune system comprises B lymphocytes and T lymphocytes. The latter, in particular, employ a wide variety of cytokines to co-ordinate the immune response of both the innate and acquired systems. The acquired immune system will be discussed in more detail in the next few chapters.

Cerebral cortex

Behaviour such as hand washing, bathing and other elements of personal hygiene, plus proper preparation of food, has preventative impacts against infection and, therefore, the brain could be considered to be part of the immune system. This role extends beyond that of the brain in the individual and into that of society. Vaccinations, sewerage systems and public sanitation all act to oppose infection and are products of the cerebral cortex, both in terms of their inception and in organising society to provide them.

General pathology

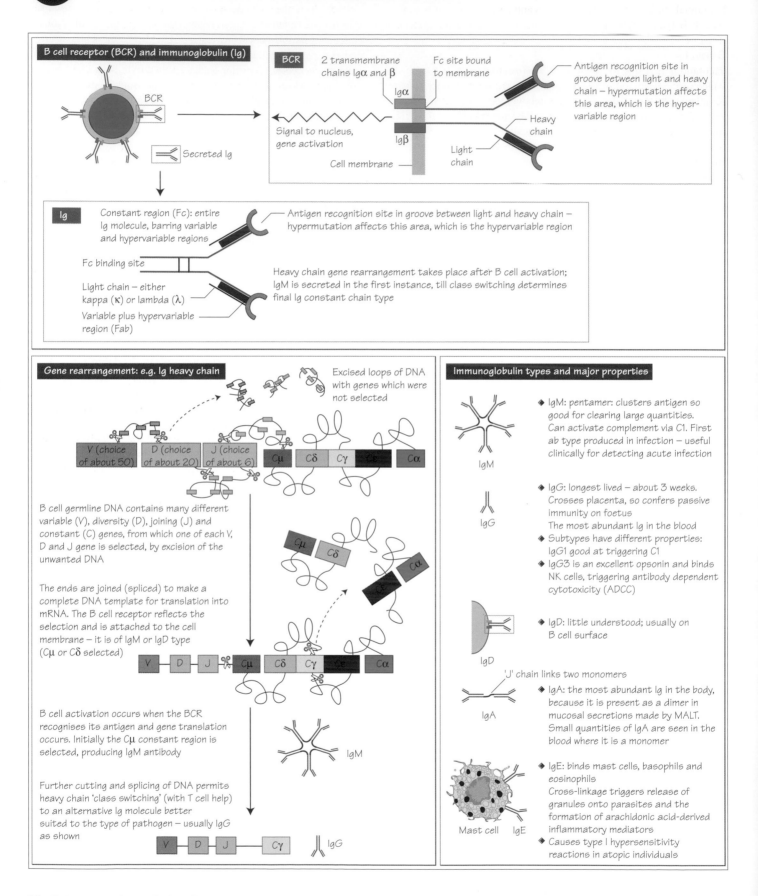

B cell receptor (BCR) and immunoglobulin (Ig)

BCR

Secreted Ig

BCR

2 transmembrane chains Igα and β

Igα

Igβ

Fc site bound to membrane

Signal to nucleus, gene activation

Cell membrane

Antigen recognition site in groove between light and heavy chain – hypermutation affects this area, which is the hyper-variable region

Heavy chain

Light chain

Ig

Constant region (Fc): entire Ig molecule, barring variable and hypervariable regions

Fc binding site

Light chain – either kappa (κ) or lambda (λ)

Variable plus hypervariable region (Fab)

Antigen recognition site in groove between light and heavy chain – hypermutation affects this area, which is the hypervariable region

Heavy chain gene rearrangement takes place after B cell activation; IgM is secreted in the first instance, till class switching determines final Ig constant chain type

Gene rearrangement: e.g. Ig heavy chain

Excised loops of DNA with genes which were not selected

V (choice of about 50) D (choice of about 20) J (choice of about 6) Cμ Cδ Cγ Cε Cα

B cell germline DNA contains many different variable (V), diversity (D), joining (J) and constant (C) genes, from which one of each V, D and J gene is selected, by excision of the unwanted DNA

The ends are joined (spliced) to make a complete DNA template for translation into mRNA. The B cell receptor reflects the selection and is attached to the cell membrane – it is of IgM or IgD type (Cμ or Cδ selected)

Cμ Cδ

Cε

Cα

V D J Cμ Cδ Cγ Cε Cα

B cell activation occurs when the BCR recognises its antigen and gene translation occurs. Initially the Cμ constant region is selected, producing IgM antibody

IgM

Further cutting and splicing of DNA permits heavy chain 'class switching' (with T cell help) to an alternative Ig molecule better suited to the type of pathogen – usually IgG as shown

V D J Cγ   IgG

Immunoglobulin types and major properties

IgM

IgG

IgD

'J' chain links two monomers

IgA

Mast cell   IgE

- IgM: pentamer: clusters antigen so good for clearing large quantities. Can activate complement via C1. First ab type produced in infection – useful clinically for detecting acute infection

- IgG: longest lived – about 3 weeks. Crosses placenta, so confers passive immunity on foetus
  The most abundant Ig in the blood
- Subtypes have different properties: IgG1 good at triggering C1
- IgG3 is an excellent opsonin and binds NK cells, triggering antibody dependent cytotoxicity (ADCC)

- IgD: little understood; usually on B cell surface

- IgA: the most abundant Ig in the body, because it is present as a dimer in mucosal secretions made by MALT. Small quantities of IgA are seen in the blood where it is a monomer

- IgE: binds mast cells, basophils and eosinophils
  Cross-linkage triggers release of granules onto parasites and the formation of arachidonic acid-derived inflammatory mediators
- Causes type I hypersensitivity reactions in atopic individuals

28 *Pathology at a Glance*. By C.J. Finlayson and B.A.T. Newell. Published 2009 by Blackwell Publishing. ISBN: 978-1-4051-3650-1

B lymphocytes are part of the acquired immune system and are responsible for generating the immunoglobulin response to pathogens. Immunoglobulins are also referred to as antibodies.

• Each B lymphocyte produces only one immunoglobulin molecule structure. This immunoglobulin is specific for a particular antigen. Generation of this structure is a complex process that occurs during maturation of the B cell.

• Once optimisation of its immunoglobulin molecule has been completed, the B cell can either become a memory cell, which acts as a form of reserve force, ready to be deployed if a response to that specific antigen is required, or the B cell can mature into a plasma cell. Plasma cells secrete large quantities of immunoglobulins.

By binding to antigens, immunoglobulins provide various defence mechanisms:

• Bound immunoglobulin opsonises the pathogen for phagocytosis and also acts as a target for the activation of complement.

• NK cells employ immunoglobulin in cytotoxic killing.

• Immunoglobulin molecules bound to different organisms can cross-link, thereby agglutinating the pathogens and neutralising them.

• Binding of immunoglobulins to toxins can also curtail the ability of the toxin to interact with cells.

Immunoglobulin structure and subtypes

Five different immunoglobulin molecules exist: IgG, IgM, IgA, IgE and IgD. IgG is the commonest and is typically used to illustrate the basic structure. All immunoglobulins share a Y-shaped basic design. IgG, IgE and IgG consist of only one Y unit, whereas IgA has two units cross-linked and IgM has five linked units. The arms of the Y bear the antigen recognition sites (Fab) so that each Y unit has two antibody binding sites. The structure of the Fab region undergoes considerable variation during development of the B cell in order to allow a huge variety of different antibodies to be generated. The stem is the constant region (Fc). Its sequence is more fixed, allowing it to provide interaction with other elements of the immune response. In parallel to the Fab and Fc structure are the heavy and light chains, of which there are two per immunoglobulin. The light chains contribute only to the Fab region, whereas the heavy chains form the Fc region and complete the Fab region. Two light chain subtypes, kappa and lambda, exist. Any one B cell utilises only one light chain subtype. Furthermore, there are four IgG subclasses and two IgA subclasses.

Immunoglobulins are an integral part of the B cell receptor (BCR). The BCR enables the lymphocyte to recognise when it is exposed to its target antigen and to initiate activation. The BCR features either IgD or IgM.

Beyond its role in the BCR, the function of IgD is unclear. By contrast, IgM is important in the antibody response within the blood.

Its pentameric structure allows IgM to be particularly effective at agglutinating antigens. IgG is found in blood and tissues. Whereas IgM levels tend to subside after the acute infection is resolved (but can reappear on re-exposure), there is some preservation of a reserve of IgG. Assaying for specific IgG and IgM molecules (e.g. against Epstein–Barr virus) can be useful in determining if a person has been previously exposed to an antigen and if the infection is acute or past. IgA is mainly secreted by mucosa-associated lymphoid tissue and assists in defending mucosal surfaces such as the GI tract and airways. IgE is integral to the activation of the mast cell response.

Immunoglobulin variability

In order for the immunoglobulin response to be effective, a myriad of different immunoglobulins, each with a Fab sequence that will bind avidly to a particular antigen, must be available. At least 100 000 000 different antibody permutations are possible. It is clearly beyond the scope of the genome to provide genes specific for each of these 100 000 000 structures. Instead, the genome provides a toolkit of genes that can be assembled in various combinations to begin the generation of diversity. The heavy chain is selected from four categories of gene: variable (V), diversity (D), joining (J) and constant (C). There are up to 50 different V genes, 20 D genes, six J genes and five C genes arranged in a long line along the chromosome. The C gene determines the immunoglobulin subtype. By default, B cells select the IgM C gene, but T helper cells can initiate a switch to IgG, IgA or IgE as necessary.

The VDJ variability alone is inadequate to give sufficient antibody diversity. B cells are unique in being encouraged to mutate in a controlled manner. The VDJ genes mutate so as to try to optimise the antibody Fab configuration. This process occurs during B cell maturation and is akin to the training of troops in a barracks. B cells that fail to make the grade are killed by apoptosis. Those that show promise undergo repeated mutation (hypermutation) to hone their antibody.

An antigen is a complex structure, with several possible antibody binding sites (epitopes). Because multiple different immunoglobulin configurations are directed against it, the immunoglobulin response to a given antigen is polyclonal.

Limitation of the B cell response

Once an infection has been repelled, the immune response must be stood down. Antibody-bound antigen is either phagocytosed in the tissues, or enters the lymph and is trapped by follicle dendritic cells (FDCs) and presented to further naive B cells. B cells continue to be activated in this way until no further opsonised antigen reaches the FDCs. Antibody survives for about 3 weeks. Hence, removal of the antigen limits the B cell response, providing self-regulation.

General pathology

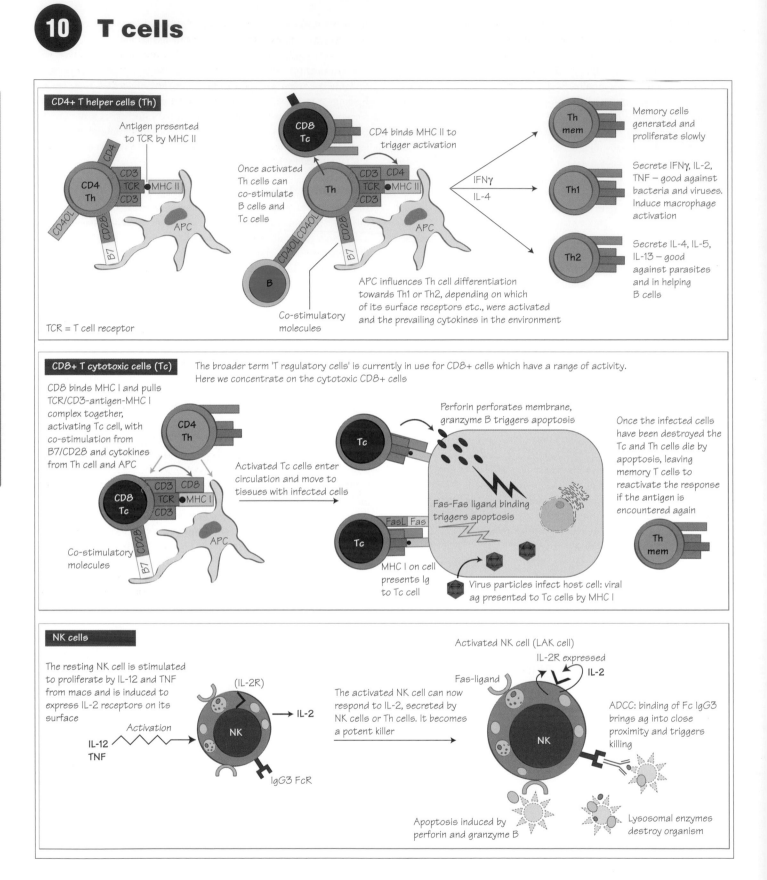

T lymphocytes are also part of the acquired immune response. They are central to the co-ordination of the immune system's response to an infection, and if their function is inadequate the immune response as a whole may be defective, even if the other components are otherwise fully operational.

Three main classes of T cells exist: CD4+ T helper (Th) cells, CD8+ T cytotoxic (Tc) cells and natural killer (NK) cells. CD8+ cells are also referred to as 'T regulatory cells' as not all are cytotoxic.

Natural killer cells ('large granular lymphocytes')

These are larger than other lymphocytes and share characteristics with neutrophils and macrophages. Although they lack T cell receptors (TCRs), NK cells are considered to be T cells.

Like neutrophils and macrophages, NK cells kill pathogens by release of the contents of their toxic lysosome granules. However, they can also induce apoptosis in the target cell using the Fas ligand, as well as employing perforin and granzyme B injected into the target cell. Recognition of IgG3 bound to an antigen can trigger NK activity.

Relative to B cells and other T cells, NK cells are in a state of increased alertness and do not require co-stimulation by other molecules or co-operation with other cells. Nevertheless, they can be induced to proliferate by TNF and IL-12 and are activated by Il-2. Bacterial lipopolysaccharides activate NK cells.

As well as their killing properties, NK cells release interferon γ (IFNγ) to activate macrophages. Activated NK cells enlarge and increase their killing activity and are known as LAK (lymphokine-activated killer) cells.

T cell receptor (TCR)

Central to the function of Th and Tc cells is the TCR. It consists of two chains (α and β in 95%, γ and δ in 5%) that are complexed with the CD3 molecule. CD3 spans the membrane to provide the mechanism by which receptor binding of antigen is signalled to the nucleus. The TCR is also associated with either CD4 in Th cells or CD8 in Tc cells.

The 5% of γδ-chain T cells do not interact with the major histocompatibility complex (MHC), but can kill pathogens directly. They line mucosal surfaces.

Helper T cells (Th cells)

Th cells do not kill organisms, but are crucial to the activation of Tc cells, the hypermutation and class-switching of B cell antibody production, and the general co-ordination of the immune response.

Th cells do not recognise raw antigen, only processed antigen that is presented to them by antigen presenting cells (APCs). These cells include dendritic APC, activated macrophages and activated B cells, all of which bear surface MHC II molecules.

A Th cell is activated when its TCR is presented with and binds its cognate antigen (the antigen specific for the TCR). Successful binding requires the CD4 molecule and co-stimulatory molecules. It takes far more co-stimulation to activate a naive Th cell than a memory Th cell that has previously experienced its cognate antigen.

Once activated, Th cells proliferate but require a week to develop into effector Th cells. Hence the innate system is important as it begins to fight pathogens immediately, allowing the T cells time to organise.

Effector Th cells secrete cytokines such as IL2, which co-stimulate Tc activation and co-stimulate B cells via CD40. Th cell–B cell interaction is essential in the production of hypermutated antibody with optimal antigen binding ability. Antibody class-switching cannot occur without Th cell co-operation and neither can the production of memory B cells.

Effector Th cells differentiate into cells that produce specific types of cytokines (Th1 or Th2 'profiles'). Th2 processes will lean towards antibody production, useful against bacteria; Th1 favours cell-mediated immunity, useful against viruses and parasites.

Self-renewing memory cells are generated and maintain their Th1 or Th2 profile. They can be quickly activated, with less need for co-stimulation, when they next encounter their cognate antigen.

Cytotoxic T cells (Tc cells)

The Tc cell is a powerful killing machine, which often eliminates infected host cells, so it must not be launched without many safeguards. Naive Tc cells must be activated before they gain their ability to kill. The Tc TCR/CD3 complex recognises and binds to its matching antigen presented in the groove of the MHC I molecule on the APC (mainly dendritic APC). CD8 attaches to and stabilises MHC I; co-stimulatory molecules such as B7/CD28 bind; IL-2 secreted by Th cells interacts with receptors on the Tc surface and activation is triggered. However, the APC interact first with Th cells, which secrete cytokines to upregulate the number of MHC I molecules expressed by the APC. Activated Th cells also secrete cytokines, such as IL-2, which promote the proliferation of activated Tc cells.

The Tc cell only needs this extensive co-stimulation and cytokine stimulation on its first exposure to antigen. Memory Tc cells require only the presence of Th cells and their cognate antigen presented to be reactivated.

Once activated, Tc cells proliferate in the lymph node, and then enter the blood and migrate to antigen-containing sites. The TCR recognises antigen displayed by MHC I molecules on tissue cells; CD8 binds the complex close and triggers killing. Tc cells kill by inducing apoptosis via the Fas pathway and by secreting perforin, which creates holes in the membrane of the target cell, allowing the T cell to inject granzyme B which also induces apoptosis. One Tc cell can kill many infected cells.

Limiting the T cell response

Co-stimulatory molecules, essential for lymphocyte activation, are also important in limiting the duration of infection. Activated T cells in the circulation begin to express new CTLA-4 receptors, which deactivate the T cell.

11 The major histocompatibility complex

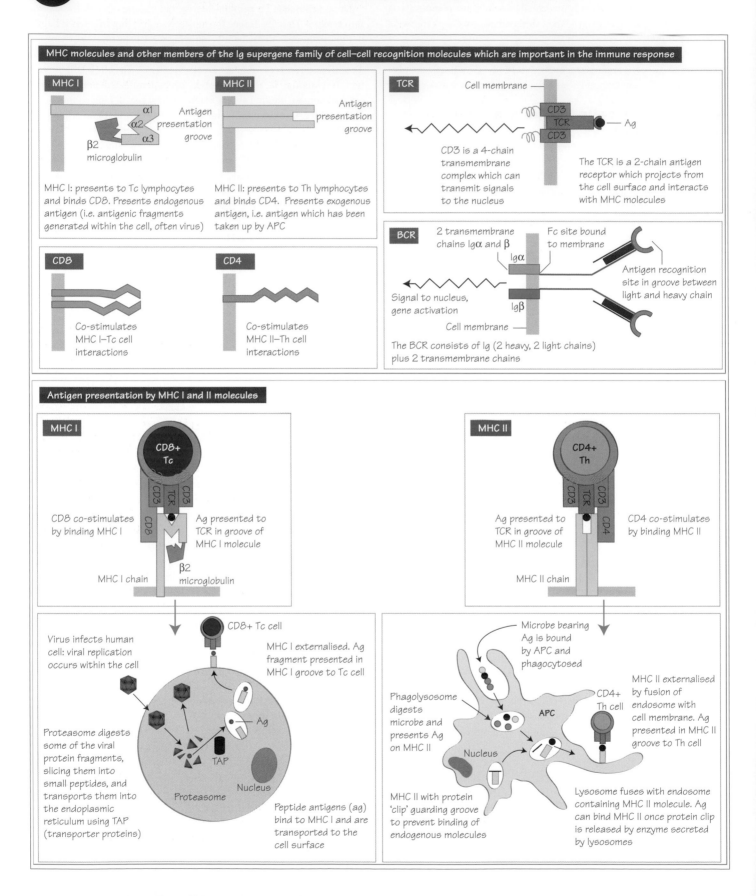

MHC molecules and other members of the Ig supergene family of cell–cell recognition molecules which are important in the immune response

MHC I

α1
α2
α3
β2 microglobulin

Antigen presentation groove

MHC I: presents to Tc lymphocytes and binds CD8. Presents endogenous antigen (i.e. antigenic fragments generated within the cell, often virus)

MHC II

Antigen presentation groove

MHC II: presents to Th lymphocytes and binds CD4. Presents exogenous antigen, i.e. antigen which has been taken up by APC

CD8

Co-stimulates MHC I–Tc cell interactions

CD4

Co-stimulates MHC II–Th cell interactions

TCR

Cell membrane

CD3
TCR
CD3

Ag

CD3 is a 4-chain transmembrane complex which can transmit signals to the nucleus

The TCR is a 2-chain antigen receptor which projects from the cell surface and interacts with MHC molecules

BCR

2 transmembrane chains Igα and β

Igα

Fc site bound to membrane

Antigen recognition site in groove between light and heavy chain

Signal to nucleus, gene activation

Igβ

Cell membrane

The BCR consists of Ig (2 heavy, 2 light chains) plus 2 transmembrane chains

Antigen presentation by MHC I and II molecules

MHC I

CD8+ Tc

CD3 TCR CD3
CD8

CD8 co-stimulates by binding MHC I

Ag presented to TCR in groove of MHC I molecule

MHC I chain

β2 microglobulin

MHC II

CD4+ Th

CD3 TCR CD3
CD4

Ag presented to TCR in groove of MHC II molecule

CD4 co-stimulates by binding MHC II

MHC II chain

Virus infects human cell: viral replication occurs within the cell

CD8+ Tc cell

MHC I externalised. Ag fragment presented in MHC I groove to Tc cell

Proteasome digests some of the viral protein fragments, slicing them into small peptides, and transports them into the endoplasmic reticulum using TAP (transporter proteins)

Ag

TAP

Nucleus

Proteasome

Peptide antigens (ag) bind to MHC I and are transported to the cell surface

Microbe bearing Ag is bound by APC and phagocytosed

Phagolysosome digests microbe and presents Ag on MHC II

APC

CD4+ Th cell

MHC II externalised by fusion of endosome with cell membrane. Ag presented in MHC II groove to Th cell

Nucleus

MHC II with protein 'clip' guarding groove to prevent binding of endogenous molecules

Lysosome fuses with endosome containing MHC II molecule. Ag can bind MHC II once protein clip is released by enzyme secreted by lysosomes

Interactions between the cell adhesion molecules of the immunoglobulin supergene family are vital in acquired immunity. The immunoglobulin molecule itself and the T and B cell receptors have been mentioned in previous chapters, where allusion has also been made to the major histocompatibility complex (MHC).

The MHC molecules are integral in the presentation of antigen to T cells, a process which is essential for the T cell to respond to the antigen. MHC molecules are encoded by the HLA (human leucocyte antigen) genes of which there are four main classes: HLA-A, -B and -C encode MHC I molecules, and HLA-D (subclasses -DR, -DP, -DQ and -DW) encodes MHC II molecules.

MHC class I molecules

MHC class I molecules are expressed on all nucleated cells in the body. They present endogenous antigen, such as peptides from within the cell, to T cytotoxic (Tc) cells. Proteasomes within a host cell break down redundant protein and, using transporter proteins, select short fragments to be transported into the endoplasmic reticulum where they are bound by type I MHC molecules and transported to the surface, on which the MHC I/antigen complex is displayed. This permits lymphocytes patrolling the body to monitor what is happening within the cell at a particular time.

As there is a constant turnover of MHC molecules, if a cell is infected by a virus it is able to display antigenic fragments of that virus to Tc cells, which then kill the host cell by inducing apoptosis.

MHC class II molecules

MHC II molecules present exogenous antigen, peptides derived from the environment, to T helper (Th) cells. This reaction is vital to the entire system of acquired immunity, hence the devastating effect of the HIV virus, which causes AIDS when it infects and destroys CD4+ Th cells.

Under normal circumstances MHC II molecules are only expressed on antigen presenting cells (macrophages and dendritic APCs) and B cells. However, in some disease states, type II MHC molecule expression can be induced in other cells, e.g. epidermal keratinocytes in patients with graft versus host disease.

Because MHC II exists to present pathogenic material to Th cells, it must not be permitted to bind self-generated peptides, and an elaborate 'clip' system has evolved to block the MHC molecule until it can be certain of presenting pathogenic material. Macrophages and APCs engulf antigenic material or whole organisms from the external tissue environment by endocytosis or phagocytosis. A phagolysosome is formed and lysosomal enzymes degrade the material. At this stage, the APC's MHC II cytoplasmic molecules are sealed by a clip that prevents antigen from binding to it. An endosome containing the clip-sealed MHC II molecule fuses with the phagolysosome, where an enzyme releases the clip, exposing the binding site. MHC II can bind slightly larger peptide fragments than MHC I.

The MHC II/antigen complex is then transported to the surface, where it interacts with the TCR/CD3 complex of CD4+ Th cells, again requiring the binding of co-stimulatory molecules for T cell activation.

Note that APCs, mainly dendritic APCs, also express MHC I molecules, allowing them to present exogenous antigens to Tc cells.

Tissue transplantation

The HLA genes were first discovered after it was realised that tissue transplants between people with compatible blood groups were being rejected by an unknown mechanism. It was soon realised that closely related donor–recipient combinations worked best, with identical twins being the optimal match.

MHC I molecules identify 'self' and MHC II molecules present 'non-self' to immune cells. Thus a tissue transplant which is as close as possible to the recipient's own MHC I make-up has the best chance of being accepted by the MHC II expressing cells.

There are several types of rejection, best exemplified in renal transplants:
• **Hyperacute rejection**: this antibody-mediated reaction occurs almost immediately in patients presensitised to an antigen present in the graft. The recipient may have anti-blood type or anti-HLA antibodies circulating in the blood due to a previous graft or blood transfusion that contained the mismatched antigens.
• **Acute rejection**: this evolves within days and is driven by both humoral (antibody) and cell-mediated (T cell) reactions. T cells reject the cells they encounter first, usually vascular endothelium, and antibodies react with the endothelium, causing severe local inflammatory damage to the elastic and muscle of the vessel walls. This type of rejection reflects HLA mismatch and occurs if the patient is not sufficiently immunosuppressed relative to the degree of HLA mismatch.
• **Chronic rejection**: this occurs over several months, usually as a result of insufficient immunosuppression and is a cell-mediated reaction that results in progressive narrowing of the blood vessels in the graft, due to intimal fibrosis. This causes hypoxic damage to the grafted organ.

Bone marrow transplantation

In bone marrow transplantation, HLA mismatch can also have harmful consequences, but in this situation the lymphocytes of the donor mount an immune response against the recipient, causing graft versus host disease. The recipient's own immune system will already have been ablated by chemotherapy and radiotherapy.

12 The reticuloendothelial system

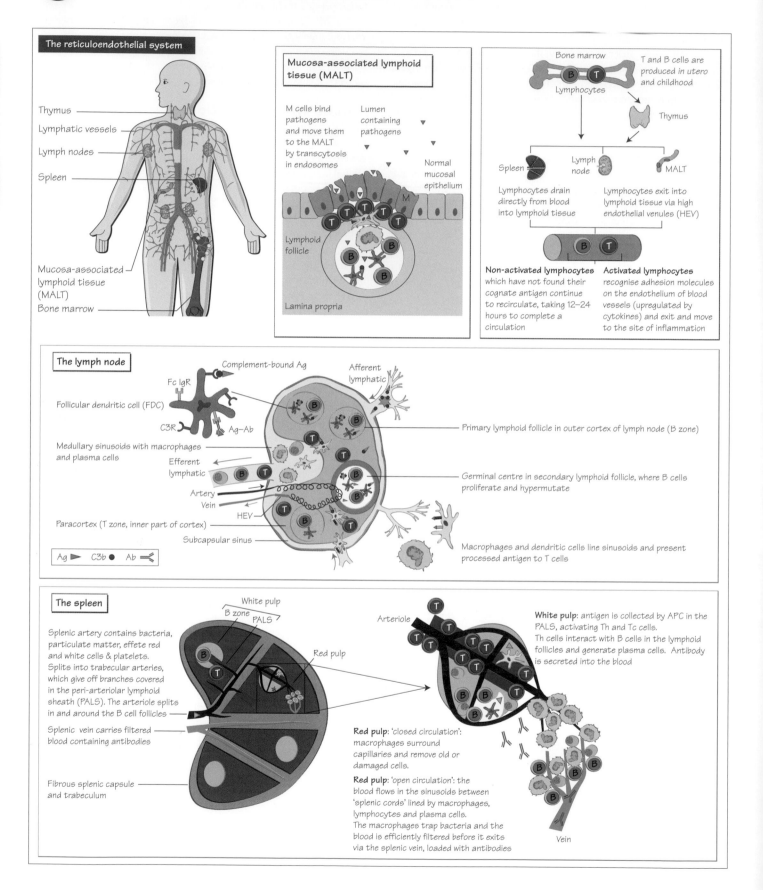

The reticuloendothelial system

Thymus
Lymphatic vessels
Lymph nodes
Spleen
Mucosa-associated lymphoid tissue (MALT)
Bone marrow

Mucosa-associated lymphoid tissue (MALT)

M cells bind pathogens and move them to the MALT by transcytosis in endosomes

Lumen containing pathogens

Normal mucosal epithelium

Lymphoid follicle

Lamina propria

Bone marrow

Lymphocytes

T and B cells are produced in utero and childhood

Thymus

Spleen
Lymph node
MALT

Lymphocytes drain directly from blood into lymphoid tissue

Lymphocytes exit into lymphoid tissue via high endothelial venules (HEV)

Non-activated lymphocytes which have not found their cognate antigen continue to recirculate, taking 12–24 hours to complete a circulation

Activated lymphocytes recognise adhesion molecules on the endothelium of blood vessels (upregulated by cytokines) and exit and move to the site of inflammation

The lymph node

Complement-bound Ag
Afferent lymphatic
Fc IgR
Follicular dendritic cell (FDC)
C3R
Ag–Ab
Medullary sinusoids with macrophages and plasma cells
Efferent lymphatic
Artery
Vein
HEV
Paracortex (T zone, inner part of cortex)
Subcapsular sinus

Primary lymphoid follicle in outer cortex of lymph node (B zone)

Germinal centre in secondary lymphoid follicle, where B cells proliferate and hypermutate

Macrophages and dendritic cells line sinusoids and present processed antigen to T cells

Ag ▶   C3b ●   Ab ≺

The spleen

White pulp
B zone   PALS
Red pulp
Arteriole

Splenic artery contains bacteria, particulate matter, effete red and white cells & platelets. Splits into trabecular arteries, which give off branches covered in the peri-arteriolar lymphoid sheath (PALS). The arteriole splits in and around the B cell follicles

Splenic vein carries filtered blood containing antibodies

Fibrous splenic capsule and trabeculum

White pulp: antigen is collected by APC in the PALS, activating Th and Tc cells.
Th cells interact with B cells in the lymphoid follicles and generate plasma cells. Antibody is secreted into the blood

Red pulp: 'closed circulation': macrophages surround capillaries and remove old or damaged cells.

Red pulp: 'open circulation': the blood flows in the sinusoids between 'splenic cords' lined by macrophages, lymphocytes and plasma cells. The macrophages trap bacteria and the blood is efficiently filtered before it exits via the splenic vein, loaded with antibodies

Vein

This is a body-wide system of haemopoietic tissue (bone marrow) and lymphoid organs (lymph nodes, spleen, thymus and mucosa-associated lymphoid tissue (MALT) with lymphoid tissue organised into T and B cell areas), connected by lymphatics and blood vessels. It is responsible for generating acquired immunity.

Dendritic antigen presenting cells

These highly effective antigen presenting cells (APCs) are found at potential pathogen entry points in the spleen and liver (Kupffer cells), skin (Langerhans cells), kidney (mesangial cells), brain (microglial cells) and mucosal and joint surfaces. They also populate bone marrow, lymph nodes and thymus. They live for weeks/months and sample tissue fluid by endocytosis. They are activated when pathogens are detected via one of several receptors, which include:

• **Toll-like receptors**, e.g. for lipopolysaccharide from Gram-negative bacteria, proteins from Gram-positive bacteria, viral coat proteins, viral double-stranded RNA and the bacterial DNA protein CpG.
• **Heat shock protein (hsp) receptors**: hsp is released by damaged or dying cells.
• **Cytokine receptors**.

The activated APCs migrate via the lymphatics to the lymph nodes to present antigen to Th cells.

Bone marrow

In adults, haematopoiesis occurs in the spongy trabeculae of the bone marrow, mainly of the long bones, vertebra and skull. The proportion of haematopoietic marrow tissue declines with age. Foetal haematopoiesis occurs in the yolk sac, then in islands dotted through the liver and later the spleen.

Haematopoietic stem cells are pluripotent and can differentiate to become either myeloid or lymphoid self-renewing stem cells. Stem cell division generates a new stem cell and committed progenitor cells, which produce colony forming units (CFUs). Five myeloid CFUs exist: for erythrocytes, megakaryocytes, granulocyte-macrophages, basophils and eosinophils.

As the progenitors mature they have increasingly limited mitotic capacity; the most mature cells are purely functional. Haematopoietic growth factors and locally and distantly produced cytokines, including colony stimulating factors, erythropoietin (renal origin), thrombopoietin (hepatic origin) and interleukins, govern their production.

The bone marrow stroma contains fat, fibroblasts and abundant blood vessels and macrophages. Fat and fibroblasts secrete substances which nurture haematopoietic cells.

Lymphoid organs
Lymph nodes

Unstimulated T and B cells arrive via the blood and enter the node through high endothelial venules, attaching to endothelial cells by specific cell adhesion molecules. Here the endothelial cells are loosely attached to each other, facilitating lymphocyte entry.

Tissue lymph, containing opsonised antigen, arrives via afferent lymphatic vessels and trickles through the subcapsular sinus, the cortical B zone, the paracortical T zone and the medullary sinusoids. Lymph exits via a single efferent lymphatic. The efferent lymphatic joins others. Eventually lymph reaches the thoracic duct, which empties back into the bloodstream via the superior vena cava.

Follicular dendritic cells reside in the B zone and do not travel beyond it. They form during the second trimester and are not of bone marrow origin. Follicular dendritic cells possess receptors for complement (C3R) and the immunoglobulin Fc component, allowing any opsonised antigen that arrives to be gathered for presentation to B cells.

APCs are resident in the sinusoids, but also arrive in the lymph, bearing processed antigen, on their surface MHC II molecules to activate T helper cells and on their surface MHC I molecules to interact with T cytotoxic cells. If their cognate antigens are displayed the lymphocytes bind and are activated, proliferate, and then exit the node to migrate to their target site.

After B cell activation, pale germinal centres form (secondary follicles). Those cells with B cell receptors showing good affinity for antigen proliferate, while the others undergo apoptosis; macrophages clear the debris. People who lack C3 cannot form germinal centres and have a deficient B cell response.

If unstimulated, lymphocytes leave the node through the efferent lymphatic and continue to circulate, each tour lasting 12–24 hours.

Spleen

The spleen, like lymph nodes, is a specialised filter, but for blood arriving via the splenic artery, as opposed to lymph. Blood passes through the white pulp lymphoid tissue, then the red pulp. The cleaned blood rejoins the circulation via the splenic vein.

The white pulp is zoned: the T cell zone surrounds the arterioles as the periarteriolar lymphoid sheath; the follicular B zone is nearby. The interaction between APCs and lymphocytes is similar to that in the lymph nodes. White pulp is a major plasma cell generation site; once produced they remain in the spleen and secrete antibody into the blood. Activated lymphocytes enter the blood to reach sites where they are needed.

The red pulp is lined by macrophages that scavenge damaged or old cells, particularly erythrocytes, and break them down. The haem iron is returned to the body's stores. Bacteria in the bloodstream are removed. Splenic macrophages are particularly effective at dealing with encapsulated bacteria like *Streptococcus pneumoniae*. Splenectomised patients are at increased risk from such bacteria if they do not already have antibodies. The red pulp's capacious sinuses can store surplus neutrophils and erythrocytes for times of need.

Mucosa-associated lymphoid tissue

MALT defends against organisms entering via the respiratory and gastrointestinal tracts and is also present beneath other epithelial surfaces. The gut MALT is present as large, organised Peyer's patches in the terminal ileum and in small, less well defined aggregates throughout the small and large intestines.

MALT comprises lymphoid nodules – B cell follicles containing follicular dendritic cells, adjacent T zones containing APCs and high endothelial venules to carry lymphocytes to them – covered by specialised epithelial 'M' cells that have receptors for commonly encountered organisms. When these are bound, they are engulfed in endosomes and transported from the luminal surface to the APCs for presentation to lymphocytes. B cells are activated to become plasma cells that synthesise antibody, almost always IgA, which is secreted into the lumen for mucosal protection.

13 Acute inflammation

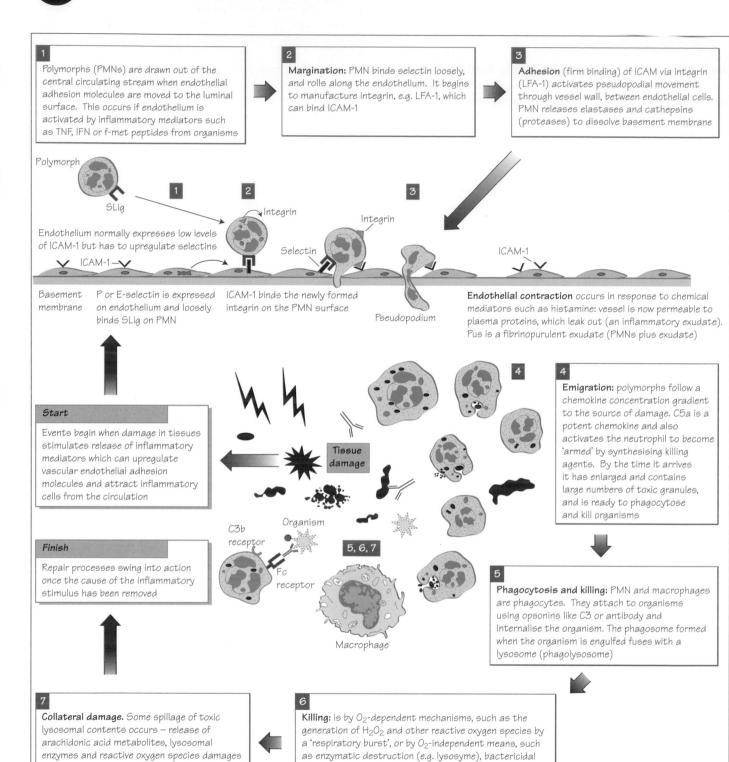

1 Polymorphs (PMNs) are drawn out of the central circulating stream when endothelial adhesion molecules are moved to the luminal surface. This occurs if endothelium is activated by inflammatory mediators such as TNF, IFN or f-met peptides from organisms

2 **Margination:** PMN binds selectin loosely, and rolls along the endothelium. It begins to manufacture integrin, e.g. LFA-1, which can bind ICAM-1

3 **Adhesion** (firm binding) of ICAM via integrin (LFA-1) activates pseudopodial movement through vessel wall, between endothelial cells. PMN releases elastases and cathepsins (proteases) to dissolve basement membrane

Polymorph

SLig

1

2 Integrin

Integrin

3

Endothelium normally expresses low levels of ICAM-1 but has to upregulate selectins

ICAM-1

Selectin

ICAM-1

Basement membrane

P or E-selectin is expressed on endothelium and loosely binds SLig on PMN

ICAM-1 binds the newly formed integrin on the PMN surface

Pseudopodium

Endothelial contraction occurs in response to chemical mediators such as histamine: vessel is now permeable to plasma proteins, which leak out (an inflammatory exudate). Pus is a fibrinopurulent exudate (PMNs plus exudate)

4

4 **Emigration:** polymorphs follow a chemokine concentration gradient to the source of damage. C5a is a potent chemokine and also activates the neutrophil to become 'armed' by synthesising killing agents. By the time it arrives it has enlarged and contains large numbers of toxic granules, and is ready to phagocytose and kill organisms

Start

Events begin when damage in tissues stimulates release of inflammatory mediators which can upregulate vascular endothelial adhesion molecules and attract inflammatory cells from the circulation

Tissue damage

C3b receptor

Organism

Fc receptor

5, 6, 7

Macrophage

Finish

Repair processes swing into action once the cause of the inflammatory stimulus has been removed

5 **Phagocytosis and killing:** PMN and macrophages are phagocytes. They attach to organisms using opsonins like C3 or antibody and internalise the organism. The phagosome formed when the organism is engulfed fuses with a lysosome (phagolysosome)

7 **Collateral damage.** Some spillage of toxic lysosomal contents occurs – release of arachidonic acid metabolites, lysosomal enzymes and reactive oxygen species damages host tissue and perpetuates the acute inflammatory response

6 **Killing:** is by O_2-dependent mechanisms, such as the generation of H_2O_2 and other reactive oxygen species by a 'respiratory burst', or by O_2-independent means, such as enzymatic destruction (e.g. lysozyme), bactericidal permeability-inducing protein, elastases, proteases and many others

Acute inflammation is a complex response to infection, or tissue damage from another source, that involves various components of the immune and vascular systems. It provides a rapid response to the infection/injury.

Acute inflammation features increased blood flow to the affected area. The capillaries become leakier, allowing fluid and inflammatory humoral mediators to enter the tissue, as well as facilitating the migration of blood-borne leucocytes into the tissue. The hyperaemia yields redness (rubor) and calor (heat). The oedema causes swelling (tumor). Pain (dolor) arises from tissue damage and cytokine release. These cardinal signs of acute inflammation were first described by Celsus in 1 AD. Virchow added loss of function (laesio functae) in the late 1800s.

Various factors can trigger acute inflammation and include complement, foreign antigens, endothelial cell damage and tissue damage. Any acute inflammatory event is likely to be initiated by more than one stimulus.

Among the causes of the vasodilatation is histamine released from damaged mast cells. Histamine relaxes the vascular smooth muscle of post capillary venules. Another mast cell product, serotonin, causes endothelial cell contraction. This increases the space between them and increases vascular permeability. Activation of phospholipase enzymes in platelets and mast cell membranes creates arachidonic acid metabolites, some of which contribute to the vascular changes. Activated endothelial cells also participate. Bacterial molecules can initiate the complement cascade and thereby bring another set of mediators into play.

Under the influence of tumour necrosis factor α (TNFα), endothelial cells upregulate cell surface adhesion molecules called selectins. These loosely bind neutrophils in the bloodstream and pull them gently to the wall. Neutrophils are stimulated to manufacture and express integrins, which bind firmly to endothelial intercellular adhesion molecules (e.g. ICAM-1). The binding process activates neutrophil intermediate filaments and neutrophils emigrate through the wall of the vessel. Once within the extravascular space, neutrophils follow a concentration gradient of chemokines (chemotaxis), such as C5a and f-met peptide, to the war zone. The bone marrow generates more neutrophils in response to the IL-1 and IL-6 secreted by macrophages and NK cells.

As the neutrophils migrate, they become activated, enlarging and increasing their content of toxic granules. The activated neutrophils and macrophages, as well as mast cells, phagocytose C3b-tagged ('opsonised') microbes and destroy them. If the organism has been encountered before, there may be circulating antibodies. These can also opsonise microbes, facilitating the function of neutrophils, macrophages and complement.

Killing by neutrophils and macrophages is by fusing the phagosome with lysosomes containing preformed toxic chemicals and enzymes, or by a 'respiratory burst' mechanism that generates highly toxic superoxide radicals, which damage the microbial membranes. Phagocytes often leak enzymes, toxins and peptides from microbial walls into the tissues, causing damage.

The same endothelial signalling system used for neutrophils allows NK cells to migrate into inflamed tissues. NK cells can be activated by IL-12 secreted by activated macrophages and in turn secrete large quantities of IL-1, which further activates the macrophages. NK cells kill microbes or viral-infected cells, being particularly useful in viral infections. NK cells have a complex and not wholly understood means of selecting targets and are also valuable in killing tumour cells.

Acute inflammation produces numerous dead bacteria and damaged and dying neutrophils, macrophages and tissue cells situated in a fibrin-rich fluid. Together, these ingredients form the yellow fibrinopurulent exudate known as pus, the hallmark of acute inflammation.

Systemic effects
Acute phase response
Circulating IL-1 and IL-6 stimulate the liver to form acute phase proteins (the 'acute phase response'). C-reactive protein (CRP), probably another opsonin, is used clinically to monitor inflammation and is an indicator of intercurrent infection, since blood levels rise early, particularly in bacterial-induced inflammation, but fall almost as quickly due to a short half-life. Hepatic output of clotting factors, complement, mannose binding protein and transport proteins, such as haptoglobins, which may regulate the levels of amines and oxygen free radicals, is elevated. Anti-proteases are also increased. Transferrin elevation is typical, as neutrophils use ferrous iron in generating antimicrobial OH^- ions. Many other acute phase proteins are produced but their role is unclear.

Viral infection is a poor inducer of acute phase proteins, whereas bacterial infections are potent, probably because bacterial endotoxins raise TNFα levels.

Fever
Fever is often present, particularly in bacterial infections but also in most viral infections. The body temperature of 37°C is controlled by the hypothalamus, but can be 'reset' by pyrogens – either endogenous (e.g. TNF, IL-1, noradrenaline, IFNα, PGE1, PGE2) or exogenous (e.g. bacterial and viral molecules). Exogenous pyrogens probably work by stimulating IL-1 release. Aspirin inhibits cyclo-oxygenase and this interferes with prostaglandin production, so is an effective antipyretic. Fever causes vasodilatation and sweating. The rigors of septicaemia are likely to be a direct response to bacterial products. Fever is said to be potentially beneficial in that the immune system operates more effectively at the higher temperature while the enzymes of pathogens are subjected to suboptimal conditions.

Hormone production
There is also elevated production of hormones such as growth hormone, prolactin, antidiuretic hormone, adrenocorticotrophic hormone and adrenaline, causing increased break down of glycogen and alterations in fatty acid metabolism and sodium/potassium transport. This results in the malaise, weakness, appetite loss and other systemic manifestations often seen in viral and bacterial infection or after injury. Interleukins are also instrumental in producing these systemic symptoms.

Acute inflammatory response
The acute inflammatory response is short-lived and self-limiting. Neutrophils live an average of 12–36 hours after formation in the bone marrow and die within seconds to hours after activation and killing organisms. Once the reason for generating the agents responsible for summoning neutrophils has subsided, the influx will cease. Surviving macrophages return to their preactivated state. All the molecular cascades have inbuilt negative feedback loops, and some even generate agents that lead to their own break down. Healing and repair can now be instigated.

14 Chronic inflammation

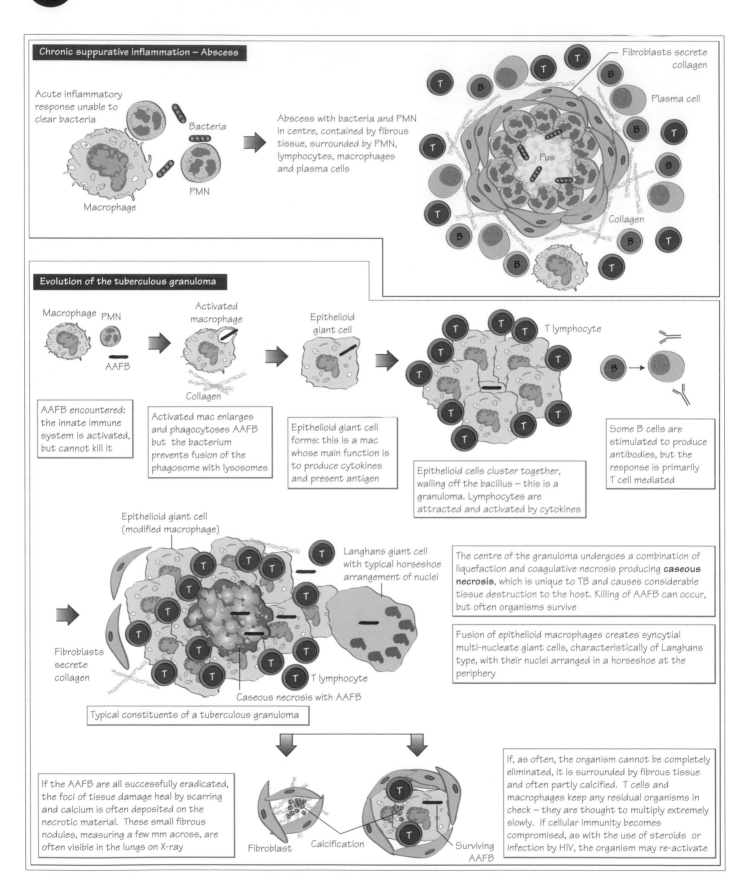

Chronic suppurative inflammation – Abscess

Acute inflammatory response unable to clear bacteria

Bacteria

Macrophage

PMN

Abscess with bacteria and PMN in centre, contained by fibrous tissue, surrounded by PMN, lymphocytes, macrophages and plasma cells

Fibroblasts secrete collagen

Plasma cell

Pus

Collagen

Evolution of the tuberculous granuloma

Macrophage PMN

AAFB

Activated macrophage

Collagen

Epithelioid giant cell

T lymphocyte

AAFB encountered: the innate immune system is activated, but cannot kill it

Activated mac enlarges and phagocytoses AAFB but the bacterium prevents fusion of the phagosome with lysosomes

Epithelioid giant cell forms: this is a mac whose main function is to produce cytokines and present antigen

Epithelioid cells cluster together, walling off the bacillus – this is a granuloma. Lymphocytes are attracted and activated by cytokines

Some B cells are stimulated to produce antibodies, but the response is primarily T cell mediated

Epithelioid giant cell (modified macrophage)

Langhans giant cell with typical horseshoe arrangement of nuclei

Fibroblasts secrete collagen

T lymphocyte

Caseous necrosis with AAFB

Typical constituents of a tuberculous granuloma

The centre of the granuloma undergoes a combination of liquefaction and coagulative necrosis producing **caseous necrosis**, which is unique to TB and causes considerable tissue destruction to the host. Killing of AAFB can occur, but often organisms survive

Fusion of epithelioid macrophages creates syncytial multi-nucleate giant cells, characteristically of Langhans type, with their nuclei arranged in a horseshoe at the periphery

If the AAFB are all successfully eradicated, the foci of tissue damage heal by scarring and calcium is often deposited on the necrotic material. These small fibrous nodules, measuring a few mm across, are often visible in the lungs on X-ray

Fibroblast

Calcification

Surviving AAFB

If, as often, the organism cannot be completely eliminated, it is surrounded by fibrous tissue and often partly calcified. T cells and macrophages keep any residual organisms in check – they are thought to multiply extremely slowly. If cellular immunity becomes compromised, as with the use of steroids or infection by HIV, the organism may re-activate

The cells involved in chronic inflammation are B and T lymphocytes (B and T cells), plasma cells and antigen presenting cells (APCs), including macrophages, and an infiltrate of these cells within the affected organ is the essence of the histopathological features. Specific histopathological nuances may be found in particular diseases.

There are two main situations in which chronic inflammation is the usual picture.

Viral infection: Viruses infect cells and reproduce within them, screened from the surveillance of the sentries of the innate immune system. They are not accessible to acute inflammation, nor are they detectable by complement, macrophages or mannose binding protein.

Viral proteins from within the infected host cell are displayed on its surface using MHC type I antigen presenting molecules. T cytotoxic cells (Tc cells) whose receptors match the antigen presented by MHC I then bind and cause the death of the infected cell.

The process is not quite that simple, since Tc cells have to be activated first by APC and T helper cells (Th cells), and the response takes about 10 days or so to be effective the first time the virus is detected. In order for this response to occur, viral fragments need to be taken up by APCs or follicle dendritic cells (FDCs) in lymphoid tissue in order to be presented to Th cells. Th cells then 'help' the Tc cells to become activated and to proliferate.

B cells are also stimulated to form antibody against viral proteins: their activation is achieved in the lymphoid tissues, where FDCs trap and present antigen to B cells. Antibody production occurs when activated B cells differentiate into plasma cells. Circulating memory B and T cells are quick to respond on second exposure to the antigen.

Autoimmune disease: Sometimes the immune system 'tolerance' of the 'self' antigens on the body's own cells breaks down. Such immune-mediated diseases begin with a chronic inflammatory stimulus and they are usually characterised by a plasma cell and lymphocyte-rich cellular infiltrate within the affected tissues. Later, the presence of antibody/antigen complexes, as occurs in systemic lupus erythematosus, may stimulate acute inflammation.

Special types of chronic inflammation
Chronic suppurative inflammation
This follows the failure of the acute inflammatory response to clear an inflammatory stimulus. In this circumstance there is persistent acute inflammation, which lasts more than a few days and it is termed 'chronic' due to its duration. Examples include:
• **Persistent bacterial infection** that cannot be contained, as in necrotising fasciitis. This is due to bacterial secretion of enzymes that facilitate the spread of the infection through the connective tissues, e.g. hyaluronidase secretion by *Streptococcus pyogenes*.
• **Abscess formation**: a wall of fibrous tissue surrounds an acute inflammatory focus, which develops a liquefied centre full of pus due to the presence of numerous dead and dying polymorphonuclear neutrophils (PMNs) and bacteria. As mentioned earlier, PMNs have a very short half-life and their presence in such foci indicate a continuing stimulus (i.e. continual secretion of acute inflammatory cellular and chemical mediators), which ensures continuing recruitment of PMNs from the blood and their production by the bone marrow.
• **Sequestration of acute inflammation**: this is similar to abscess formation, but occurs in bone, a difficult site from which to clear infection (osteomyelitis). A wall of new bone forms around the site, but there are usually 'leaks' and acute inflammation can spread either to adjacent bone, to the skin surface as a fistula, or into the blood.

Granulomatous inflammation
A granuloma is a collection of five or more epithelioid macrophages, with or without attendant lymphocytes and fibroblasts. Epithelioid giant cells are altered macrophages, which have turned themselves over to becoming giant phagocytosing and killing machines. They often fuse to become multinucleate giant cells – it is thought that this may occur when two or more cells attempt to phagocytose the same particle and their membranes merge.

Granulomatous inflammation is typically seen when an infective agent with a digestion-resistant capsule (e.g. *Mycobacterium tuberculosis* or the ova of *Schistosoma mansoni*) or a piece of inert foreign material (such as suture material or glass) is introduced into the tissue. A transient acute inflammatory response occurs and when this is ineffective in eradicating the stimulus, chronic inflammation supervenes. These agents primarily stimulate a macrophage response and larger and larger clusters of enlarging macrophages accumulate.

Granulomas are a feature of the type IV hypersensitivity response. Exactly why granulomas form in some diseases but not others is not clear, but cytokines appear to play a role: IL-1 is said to be important in initiating granuloma formation, IL-2 can cause them to enlarge and TNF maintains them. In parasitic disease, IL-5 attracts eosinophils, whereas IL-6 is important in tuberculous granulomas.

Some typical causes of granulomatous chronic inflammation
1 Infective:
• Tuberculosis.
• Parasitic infection, e.g. schistosomiasis.
• Leprosy.
• Syphilis (occasionally).
• Cryptococcus.
2 Foreign material:
• Silica (glass).
• Talc.
• Suture material.
3 Unknown:
• Sarcoidosis.
• Crohn's disease.
4 Drug related:
• Many drugs can cause small granulomas to develop in the liver.
5 Autoimmune disease:
• Primary biliary cirrhosis.
• Rheumatoid arthritis ('rheumatoid nodules').
6 Tumour related (cause unascertained):
• Hodgkin lymphoma.
• Lymph nodes draining tumour sites.

15 Wound healing and repair

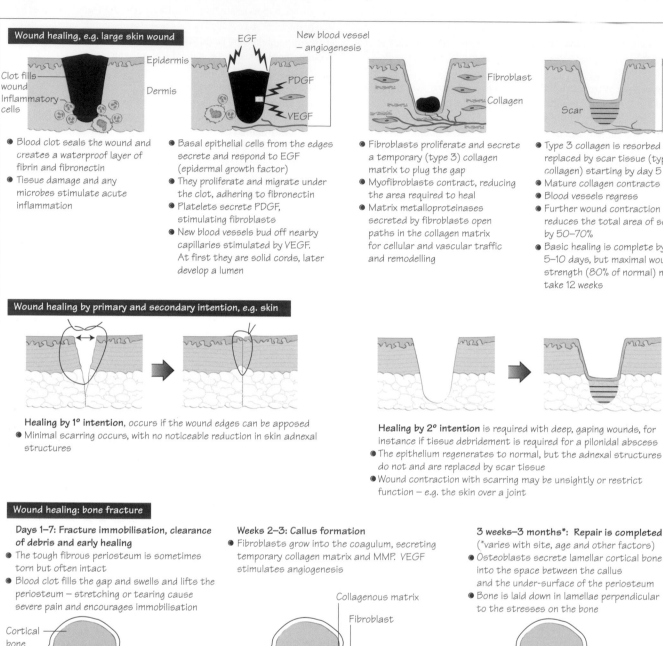

Wound healing, e.g. large skin wound

Epidermis
Clot fills wound
Inflammatory cells
Dermis

EGF
New blood vessel – angiogenesis
PDGF
VEGF

Fibroblast
Collagen

Scar

- Blood clot seals the wound and creates a waterproof layer of fibrin and fibronectin
- Tissue damage and any microbes stimulate acute inflammation

- Basal epithelial cells from the edges secrete and respond to EGF (epidermal growth factor)
- They proliferate and migrate under the clot, adhering to fibronectin
- Platelets secrete PDGF, stimulating fibroblasts
- New blood vessels bud off nearby capillaries stimulated by VEGF. At first they are solid cords, later develop a lumen

- Fibroblasts proliferate and secrete a temporary (type 3) collagen matrix to plug the gap
- Myofibroblasts contract, reducing the area required to heal
- Matrix metalloproteinases secreted by fibroblasts open paths in the collagen matrix for cellular and vascular traffic and remodelling

- Type 3 collagen is resorbed and replaced by scar tissue (type 1 collagen) starting by day 5
- Mature collagen contracts
- Blood vessels regress
- Further wound contraction reduces the total area of scarring by 50–70%
- Basic healing is complete by 5–10 days, but maximal wound strength (80% of normal) may take 12 weeks

Wound healing by primary and secondary intention, e.g. skin

Healing by 1° intention, occurs if the wound edges can be apposed
- Minimal scarring occurs, with no noticeable reduction in skin adnexal structures

Healing by 2° intention is required with deep, gaping wounds, for instance if tissue debridement is required for a pilonidal abscess
- The epithelium regenerates to normal, but the adnexal structures do not and are replaced by scar tissue
- Wound contraction with scarring may be unsightly or restrict function – e.g. the skin over a joint

Wound healing: bone fracture

Days 1–7: Fracture immobilisation, clearance of debris and early healing
- The tough fibrous periosteum is sometimes torn but often intact
- Blood clot fills the gap and swells and lifts the periosteum – stretching or tearing cause severe pain and encourages immobilisation

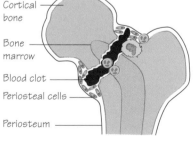

Cortical bone
Bone marrow
Blood clot
Periosteal cells
Periosteum

- Periosteal cells are activated by PDGF, FGF and other factors in the blood clot
- They grow across the surface of the coagulum, attaching via fibronectin derived from the plasma
- Phagocytes remove the debris

Weeks 2–3: Callus formation
- Fibroblasts grow into the coagulum, secreting temporary collagen matrix and MMP. VEGF stimulates angiogenesis

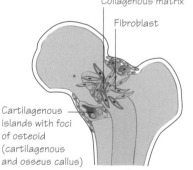

Collagenous matrix
Fibroblast
Cartilagenous islands with foci of osteoid (cartilagenous and osseus callus)

- Some fibroblasts differentiate into chondrocytes and lay down islands of cartilage (cartilaginous callus)
- Osseous metaplasia within the cartilage yields osseus callus, formed of rigid, but weak, woven bone
- Callus replaces the marrow space

3 weeks–3 months*: Repair is completed
(*varies with site, age and other factors)
- Osteoblasts secrete lamellar cortical bone into the space between the callus and the under-surface of the periosteum
- Bone is laid down in lamellae perpendicular to the stresses on the bone

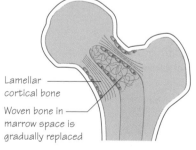

Lamellar cortical bone
Woven bone in marrow space is gradually replaced

- Bony trabeculae develop in the marrow space
- The woven bone of the osseous callus is resorbed by osteoclasts; osteoblasts secrete new lamellar bone
- The marrow space is repopulated to normal by fat and haemopoietic cells

Limitation of acute inflammation is necessary before effective healing processes can occur. Acute inflammation is limited by various factors:
• The inflammatory response is signal-driven: once the initial stimulus has been removed, the secretion of cytokines and chemokines from the damaged cells ceases.
• Once micro-organisms have been eliminated, phagocytosed and degraded fragments shed from their coats are no longer present to attract inflammatory cells.
• The molecular mediators of inflammation, and polymorphs, have a short half-life (from minutes to hours to days).
• Longer lived inflammatory cells return to their normal quiescent state once activation signals cease.

Resolution by regeneration produces a complete return to normality, but in most tissues the result of injury is repair by granulation tissue, followed by scar formation. Perfect resolution is rare, but is seen in bone healing, lobar pneumonia and acute liver damage. Repair is required if the organ's connective tissue framework is damaged.

Wound healing

The process of healing starts almost immediately after injury but may take weeks to complete. The following are essential for good healing:
• An adequate blood supply to deliver inflammatory cells to remove debris and provide nutrition and oxygen to the regenerating tissue.
• Nutrients to supply building materials.
• Vitamins, especially vitamin C, used in the manufacture of tropocollagen.
• Immobilisation of the healing tissues.
• The absence of infection or other destructive processes.
• Viable cells that can undertake the process of clearing debris and replacing the damaged tissue.

Healing by primary intention: A neat, incisional wound, such as a surgical incision, damages little underlying dermal and subcutaneous tissue and heals relatively quickly (healing by primary intention). Suturing of a surgical wound apposes and immobilises the edges.

Healing by secondary intention: A ragged, deep, gaping wound needs longer to heal and produces more scarring (healing by secondary intention). An example of such healing is the surgical debridement of a pilonidal abscess, a deep inflammatory response to ingrowing hair shafts in the perianal region, for which apposition of the edges is neither possible nor desirable since closure of the wound may permit the abscess to reaccumulate. The actual process of healing is similar in each case, but healing by secondary intent leaves a scar, whereas scarring is sometimes almost undetectable in that by primary intent.

Haematoma: A haematoma is a swelling composed of extravasated blood, which can develop in a closed wound. Traumatic damage to blood vessels releases blood into subcutaneous or deep tissue. A large, solid, blood clot may form – for instance within skeletal muscle (a clot is coagulated extravascular blood; thrombus is intravascular coagulation). Although the healing processes of fibroblastic invasion, angiogenesis and organisation are attempted at the periphery, sometimes the centre remains a mass of erythrocytes, which can undergo dystrophic calcification or become a nidus for infection. It may be necessary to drain or excise a haematoma.

Fracture repair

The principles are similar to healing elsewhere, but the aim is resolution rather than repair – i.e. replacement bone *must* develop, not scar tissue. Bone repair is so effective that usually there is complete restitution of normality within a few months. Healing depends on factors such as the patient's age, the type and site of the fracture and whether it is a long bone, composed largely of lamellar bone, or a flat bone, such as scapula (mainly woven bone), that is affected.

It is essential that bone is properly aligned and immobilised during healing. Malunion results from misalignment, with consequent shortening of the bone and effects on the rest of the skeleton, possibly causing arthritis in the long term.

The pain engendered by periosteal stretching ensures that most patients stay still initially, but splinting is required to prevent movement over the following weeks while cartilaginous and osseous callus form. In extreme cases the moving bony ends, instead of fusing, may become lined by cartilaginous caps to form a false joint (pseudoarthrosis). Alternatively, the ends may fail to ossify and continuity is provided by fibrous scar tissue – a 'fibrous union' – a far weaker option than bone, and prone to pliability or refracture.

Wound healing at other sites

Brain: The brain undergoes liquefactive degeneration after major injury, such as a stroke. Survivors have cystic spaces within their brains. No significant regeneration of neurones occurs, but 're-wiring' of neuronal pathways is possible to a limited extent. Minor injuries related to infective organisms may heal by 'gliosis', the nervous system equivalent of scarring, but collagen formation is not seen.

Peripheral nerves: Axonal damage must be repaired by regeneration from the nerve cell body, a slow process which proceeds at about 1 mm per day. Schwann cells can regenerate myelin to form the nerve's insulation. The muscle may have atrophied beyond repair by the time regeneration is complete and so must be kept stimulated. A problem occurs when axonal fibres are completely severed – it is usually impossible for them to follow their original route back to their target muscle. Proliferation at the site of injury may cause a painful tumour-like nodule of nerve fibres and myelin – a traumatic neuroma (common at amputation sites).

Muscle: Smooth muscle and striated muscle can regenerate and repair when necessary, though re-innervation may be a problem after major trauma. Cardiac muscle cannot regenerate and scarring is normal after damage such as a myocardial infarction.

Complications of healing

• **Scar contractures**, e.g. burns or wounds over joints.
• **Keloid formation**: a potentially disfiguring hypertrophic scar, seen particularly in Afro-Caribbeans.
• **Failure to heal**: abscess or empyema formation.
• **Failure to unite** (skin, muscle, fascia): wound break down.
• **Bone fracture**: malunion, fibrous union or pseudoarthrosis (see above).
• **Traumatic neuroma**.

16 Infection and immunodeficiency

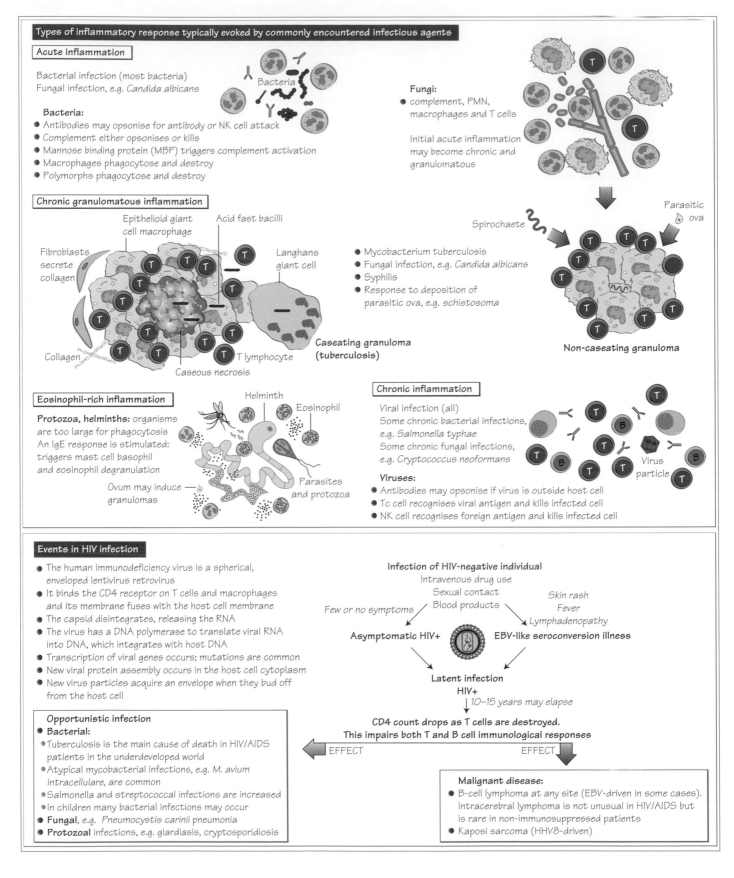

Types of inflammatory response typically evoked by commonly encountered infectious agents

Acute inflammation

Bacterial infection (most bacteria)
Fungal infection, e.g. *Candida albicans*

Bacteria:
- Antibodies may opsonise for antibody or NK cell attack
- Complement either opsonises or kills
- Mannose binding protein (MBP) triggers complement activation
- Macrophages phagocytose and destroy
- Polymorphs phagocytose and destroy

Bacteria

Fungi:
- complement, PMN, macrophages and T cells

Initial acute inflammation may become chronic and granulomatous

Chronic granulomatous inflammation

Epithelioid giant cell macrophage
Acid fast bacilli
Fibroblasts secrete collagen
Langhans giant cell
Collagen
Caseous necrosis
T lymphocyte

Spirochaete
Parasitic ova

- Mycobacterium tuberculosis
- Fungal infection, e.g. *Candida albicans*
- Syphilis
- Response to deposition of parasitic ova, e.g. schistosoma

Caseating granuloma (tuberculosis)

Non-caseating granuloma

Eosinophil-rich inflammation

Protozoa, helminths: organisms are too large for phagocytosis
An IgE response is stimulated: triggers mast cell basophil and eosinophil degranulation

Helminth
Eosinophil
Ovum may induce granulomas
Parasites and protozoa

Chronic inflammation

Viral infection (all)
Some chronic bacterial infections, e.g. *Salmonella typhae*
Some chronic fungal infections, e.g. *Cryptococcus neoformans*

Viruses:
- Antibodies may opsonise if virus is outside host cell
- Tc cell recognises viral antigen and kills infected cell
- NK cell recognises foreign antigen and kills infected cell

Virus particle

Events in HIV infection

- The human immunodeficiency virus is a spherical, enveloped lentivirus retrovirus
- It binds the CD4 receptor on T cells and macrophages and its membrane fuses with the host cell membrane
- The capsid disintegrates, releasing the RNA
- The virus has a DNA polymerase to translate viral RNA into DNA, which integrates with host DNA
- Transcription of viral genes occurs; mutations are common
- New viral protein assembly occurs in the host cell cytoplasm
- New virus particles acquire an envelope when they bud off from the host cell

Infection of HIV-negative individual
Intravenous drug use
Sexual contact
Blood products

Skin rash
Fever
Lymphadenopathy

Few or no symptoms

Asymptomatic HIV+

EBV-like seroconversion illness

Latent infection
HIV+
10–15 years may elapse

CD4 count drops as T cells are destroyed.
This impairs both T and B cell immunological responses

EFFECT   EFFECT

Opportunistic infection
- Bacterial:
  - Tuberculosis is the main cause of death in HIV/AIDS patients in the underdeveloped world
  - Atypical mycobacterial infections, e.g. M. avium intracellulare, are common
  - Salmonella and streptococcal infections are increased
  - In children many bacterial infections may occur
- Fungal, e.g. Pneumocystis carinii pneumonia
- Protozoal infections, e.g. giardiasis, cryptosporidiosis

Malignant disease:
- B-cell lymphoma at any site (EBV-driven in some cases). Intracerebral lymphoma is not unusual in HIV/AIDS but is rare in non-immunosuppressed patients
- Kaposi sarcoma (HHV8-driven)

 Pathology at a Glance. By C.J. Finlayson and B.A.T. Newell. Published 2009 by Blackwell Publishing. ISBN: 978-1-4051-3650-1

Infective agents
Bacteria
The ubiquitous distribution of bacteria in the environment and their tendency not to need a specific vector for infection makes them a common problem for the immune system. The cutaneous and mucosal barriers of the innate system offer a good first line of defence. Colonisation of these surfaces by commensal organisms, such as in the gastrointestinal tract, provides an extra level of defence as these bacteria occupy the territory and limit colonisation by harmful strains.

On occasion, the mucosal defences are breached and infection develops. The hallmark of the response to bacterial infection is acute inflammation. As small extracellular organisms, bacteria are ideal targets for phagocytosis by neutrophils and macrophages. Complement assists the cellular response.

The antibodies of the acquired system are also highly effective against bacteria and enhance the innate response. Antibodies opsonise bacteria for phagocytosis, recruit complement into the fray, bind toxins and even agglutinate the bacteria.

Mycobacteria
Mycobacteria, as exemplified by *Mycobacterium tuberculosis*, have evolved an advantageous resistance to neutrophil-based killing mechanisms and are even able to withstand the contents of macrophage lysosomes to survive inside lysosomes. Faced with such a challenge, macrophages unite to form giant cells. T cells are essential to co-ordinate this response and for their cytotoxic ability to kill infected cells.

Often, the body's response is to contain the infection in a 'prison zone' formed by a granulomatous macrophage response, lymphocytic infiltrate and fibrosis. Thus, mycobacterial infections are characterised by chronic granulomatous inflammation and fibrosis.

Viruses
Viruses are primarily intracellular organisms and therefore have to be eliminated by a system that can target cells. This is provided by T cells. The innate immune system and B cells can assist in dealing with extracellular virus particles, as well as helping to target infected cells, with antibodies and complement that bind to virally derived particles expressed on the cell surface. However, an effective T cell response is essential to clear the infection by removing the infected cells, which act as virus factories. Hence, chronic inflammation is the main response to viral infection. Therefore, an acute viral infection, like hepatitis A, shows chronic, not acute, inflammation.

Fungi
Most fungal infections tend to affect only mucosal surfaces. Fungi can be extracellular (e.g. *Candida*) or intracellular (e.g. histoplasma) and require a co-ordinated response from all aspects of the immune system. Of particular note is the characteristic presence of neutrophils within the epithelium of squamous mucosal surfaces infected by *Candida*. Granulomas may occur with invasive fungal infection.

Protozoa
Although uncommon in the UK, the global burden of protozoal disease is considerable. Approximately one-third of the planet's population reside in malaria-endemic areas. The life cycles of protozoa are more complex than those of bacteria and they exhibit both intracellular and extracellular forms. In addition, protozoa, including malaria, can incorporate host antigens into their surfaces as a form of disguise. Hence, all components of the innate and acquired immune system are necessary to combat the infection. Simple elements such as mucosal barriers should not be underestimated, as many protozoa require an insect vector to infect the host. The features of the antihelminth response mentioned below are also sometimes important.

Helminths
Helminths range in size from millimetres to metres. The organisms are too large to be phagocytosed, even by the giant cell forms of macrophages. Instead, eosinophils are recruited to set up an artillery bombardment with their granules. The acquired system augments the response with IgE-mediated mast cell degranulation.

Helminthic infection is complicated by the presence of their eggs. These are smaller than the parent helminths and typically elicit a granulomatous and fibrous response. Extensive granulomatous inflammation and fibrosis can compromise organ function.

Immunodeficiency
Innate immune system deficiencies
If the neutrophil or complement systems are impaired, bacteria tend to be the principal organisms that take advantage. Patients suffer repeated pyogenic infections, often including abscesses. Severe deficiencies render patients susceptible to systemic fungal infections, notably aspergillosis. This is a serious complication of profound neutropenia and pyrexia in neutropenic patients should be taken very seriously.

Examples include chronic granulomatous disease, myeloperoxidase deficiency, leukocyte adhesion protein deficiency and acquired neutropenia.

T cell disorders
While HIV/AIDS is the most common T cell disorder, assorted inherited forms also exist and include Wiskott–Aldrich syndrome and diGeorge syndrome.

Although T cells are vital in combating viral and mycobacterial infection, such that these pose particular problems in people with defective T cell function, the integral role of T cells in co-ordinating the whole immune response means that there is a susceptibility to all types of infection. Furthermore, those organisms that would not normally cause pathogenic infections can produce problems, such as *Pneumocystis carinii* pneumonia in AIDS. This is known as opportunistic infection.

Impaired T cell immunity also curtails the detection of malignant cells and their removal before they can establish a tumour. Thus, patients with defective T cell immunity have an increased risk of developing certain tumours (like lymphoma).

B cell deficiencies
Isolated B cell deficiencies tend to relate to defective synthesis of immunoglobulins and include the inherited disorders X-linked agammaglobulinaemia and selective IgA deficiency. The paraprotein load in myeloma can suppress the synthesis of other immunoglobulins.

Defective B cell-mediated immunity is characterised by repeated bacterial infections.

Combined B and T cell deficiencies
In these inherited disorders, known as severe combined immunodeficiency, the body is extremely susceptible to all classes of infection. Examples include adenosine deaminase deficiency and deficiencies of MHC molecules.

General pathology

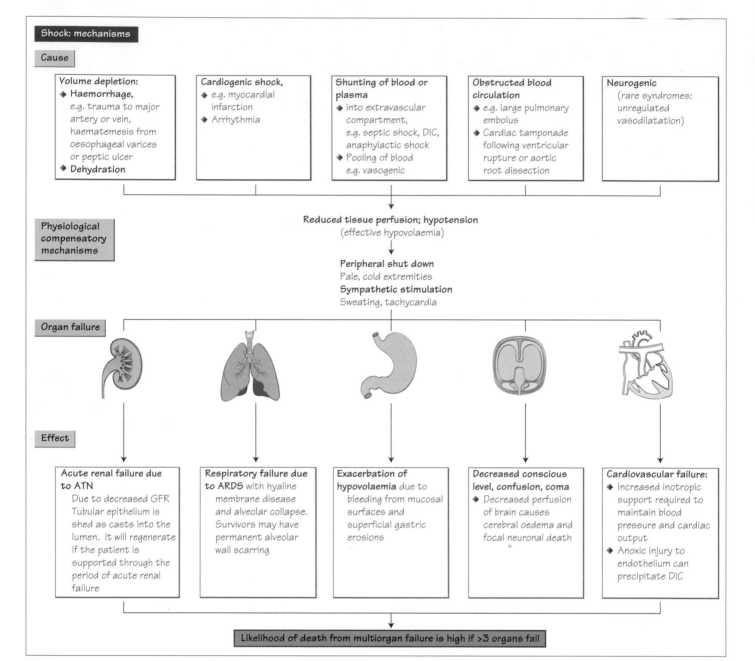

Shock: mechanisms

Cause

Volume depletion:
- Haemorrhage,
  e.g. trauma to major
  artery or vein,
  haematemesis from
  oesophageal varices
  or peptic ulcer
- Dehydration

Cardiogenic shock,
- e.g. myocardial
  infarction
- Arrhythmia

**Shunting of blood or
plasma**
- into extravascular
  compartment,
  e.g. septic shock, DIC,
  anaphylactic shock
- Pooling of blood
  e.g. vasogenic

**Obstructed blood
circulation**
- e.g. large pulmonary
  embolus
- Cardiac tamponade
  following ventricular
  rupture or aortic
  root dissection

Neurogenic
(rare syndromes:
unregulated
vasodilatation)

Reduced tissue perfusion; hypotension
(effective hypovolaemia)

**Physiological
compensatory
mechanisms**

Peripheral shut down
Pale, cold extremities
Sympathetic stimulation
Sweating, tachycardia

Organ failure

Effect

**Acute renal failure due
to ATN**
Due to decreased GFR
Tubular epithelium is
shed as casts into the
lumen. It will regenerate
if the patient is
supported through the
period of acute renal
failure

**Respiratory failure due
to ARDS** with hyaline
membrane disease
and alveolar collapse.
Survivors may have
permanent alveolar
wall scarring

**Exacerbation of
hypovolaemia** due to
bleeding from mucosal
surfaces and
superficial gastric
erosions

**Decreased conscious
level, confusion, coma**
- Decreased perfusion
  of brain causes
  cerebral oedema and
  focal neuronal death

Cardiovascular failure:
- Increased inotropic
  support required to
  maintain blood
  pressure and cardiac
  output
- Anoxic injury to
  endothelium can
  precipitate DIC

Likelihood of death from multiorgan failure is high if >3 organs fail

Definition

Shock is the clinical and pathological syndrome that results when there is generalised inadequate perfusion of the body's organs. Patients are pale, cold and clammy and are often slightly confused. There is hypotension and tachycardia.

Causes

The basic mechanism of shock is either inadequate circulating volume (hypovolaemia) or inadequate vascular tone. In some situations, both mechanisms apply. The following are specific causes.

Volume depletion:
• **Haemorrhage**: this depletes blood volume rapidly and faster than the body can compensate by redistributing water from the other compartments. In an individual without cardiovascular disease, a typical sequence of responses occurs at specific volumes of blood loss:

  15%: tachycardia
  20%: postural hypotension (often the first sign to be manifested in fit young adults)
  30%: supine hypotension
  40%: renal failure
  50%: death

In addition to the pressure effects of volume loss, the problem of hypoperfusion is exacerbated by the loss of erythrocytes. Fluid redistribution can occur, but recruitment of additional erythrocytes requires more time and, in that interval, their relative concentration and thus the oxygen carrying capacity of the blood is reduced.

• **Dehydration**: there is basal water loss from the body through the processes of urination (0.5 ml/kg/h, average 800–900 ml/day), respiration (500 ml/day), GI secretions (200 ml) and sweating (200 ml). More generally, at least 2000 ml of water intake per day are required to maintain normal hydration. If water intake is inadequate, or there is excessive fluid loss (e.g. copious sweating in hot weather), dehydration can result. Given the relative volume of the extravascular compartment to the intravascular, if a person has hypovolaemia due to dehydration, their actual fluid deficit is many litres.

Cardiogenic shock: This is pump failure. The typical cause is a myocardial infarction, but acute myocarditis and other myocardial diseases can be responsible. The heart cannot maintain a blood pressure that is adequate to perfuse vital organs.

Shunting of blood or plasma:
• **Septic**: overwhelming infection can yield hypotension by massive vasodilatation that is mediated by a combination of bacterial toxins and the body's cytokines. Some organisms, such as strains of *Staphylococcus aureus*, release specific toxins that can induce shock at lower infectious loads.
• **Anaphylaxis**: this extreme form of a type I hypersensitivity response plummets blood pressure such that organ perfusion is insufficient.
• **Disseminated intravascular coagulation**: see Chapter 38.
• **Vasogenic**: inappropriate vasodilatation may be mediated by mechanisms other than anaphylaxis or sepsis.

Obstructed blood circulation:
• **Large pulmonary embolus**: see Chapter 41.
• **Cardiac tamponade**: see Chapter 40.

Neurogenic: Rarely, autonomic function and homeostasis are defective and vascular tone is inadequately maintained.

Clinical consequences

• Inadequate organ perfusion impairs organ function. Prolonged hypoperfusion leads to damage that is ultimately irreversible. Different organs have different thresholds for moving through these stages.
• The initial response to shock is to preserve blood pressure and cardiac output by vasoconstriction and increasing the heart rate. Vasoconstriction in the splenic and hepatic reservoirs can restore small volume losses. If these actions are unsuccessful, the vasonstriction becomes more pronounced, with shunting of blood from the skin and the splanchnic circulation. The sympathetic activation underlying this also causes clamminess via sweating.
• If the response is still inadequate, organ function deteriorates. This is seen particularly in the kidney where glomerular filtration, which is perfusion dependent, falls and urine output drops. Inadequate delivery of oxygen to the tissues causes anaerobic metabolism, yielding a lactic acidosis.
• Persistence of the hypoperfusion leads to organ failure. Once three organ systems have failed, the prognosis is very poor.

Acute tubular necrosis (ATN)

The renal tubular epithelium has a very high metabolic activity. Hypoperfusion sufficient to decrease the glomerular filtration rate (GFR) significantly also causes ischaemic death of the tubular epithelial cells. The dead cells are shed into the lumen, forming casts that are detectable in the small residual volume of urine formed until renal failure is total (anuria). Sometimes these cellular casts obstruct the tubules and impede urine flow.

If the patient survives the acute episode, the tubular epithelium will regenerate and, in a few weeks, renal function will be restored. The recovery phase is marked by diuresis, where GFR is normal but the regenerating epithelium has yet to regain full reabsorptive capacity.

Although acute tubular necrosis is usually caused by hyopvolaemic/hypotensive shock, it can also be due to direct damage by toxins such as paraquat, or by large quantities of the haem prosthetic group from myoglobin (massive rhabdomylosis) or haemoglobin (massive haemolysis) entering the renal filtrate.

Adult respiratory distress syndrome (ARDS, 'shock lung')

This devastating complication of many types of shock, particularly septic shock and massive trauma (bone marrow fat emboli may shower the lungs after long bone fracture), results from a combination of exudation of fibrin-rich fluid from the capillaries into the alveolar spaces and injury to the alveolar lining epithelial cells.

The fibrin-rich pulmonary oedema and debris from damaged cells form 'hyaline membranes'. These line the alveolar wall, impede gas exchange and cause collapse of the air spaces by loss of surfactant (due to damage to the surfactant-secreting epithelium and to its lack of access to the alveolar surface). Inflammatory cells may be attracted to the site. The microscopical features are termed diffuse alveolar damage (DAD).

Efforts by the lungs to repair the damaged epithelium produces hyperplasia of type II pneumocytes (these can secrete surfactant but are wider than type I pneumocytes and so impair gas exchange). Type II respiratory failure develops (the arterial $p\mathrm{O}_2$ is decreased and $p\mathrm{CO}_2$ is increased).

Patients are severely dyspnoeic (breathless) and require ventilatory support. Half the patients will die; survivors often have residual respiratory impairment due to alveolar septal scarring.

18 Tolerance and autoimmune disease

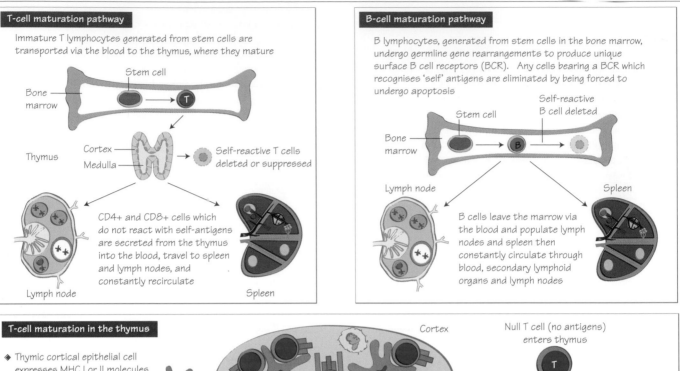

T-cell maturation pathway

Immature T lymphocytes generated from stem cells are transported via the blood to the thymus, where they mature

Stem cell

Bone marrow

Thymus — Cortex — Medulla → Self-reactive T cells deleted or suppressed

CD4+ and CD8+ cells which do not react with self-antigens are secreted from the thymus into the blood, travel to spleen and lymph nodes, and constantly recirculate

Lymph node

Spleen

B-cell maturation pathway

B lymphocytes, generated from stem cells in the bone marrow, undergo germline gene rearrangements to produce unique surface B cell receptors (BCR). Any cells bearing a BCR which recognises 'self' antigens are eliminated by being forced to undergo apoptosis

Stem cell

Self-reactive B cell deleted

Bone marrow

Lymph node

Spleen

B cells leave the marrow via the blood and populate lymph nodes and spleen then constantly circulate through blood, secondary lymphoid organs and lymph nodes

T-cell maturation in the thymus

◆ Thymic cortical epithelial cell expresses MHC I or II molecules. It presents peptide antigens to naïve T cells and selects out those that are non-reactive by inducing apoptosis

◆ Death of T cells which fail to develop CD4 & CD8 and cannot interact with MHC I or II molecules occurs

◆ Macrophages phagocytose antigenic particles from the blood to prevent tolerance to pathogens developing. They also clear apoptotic debris from deleted T cells

◆ Dendritic cells from the bone marrow test the lymphocytes against self-MHC molecules in the medulla

◆ T cells which bind strongly to self-antigens presented by bone-marrow-derived dendritic cells are deleted

◆ Hassall's corpuscles are the remnants of degenerate epithelial cells. They are often partly calcified

◆ T lymphocytes enter blood and travel to lymph nodes, spleen and other lymphoid tissue sites

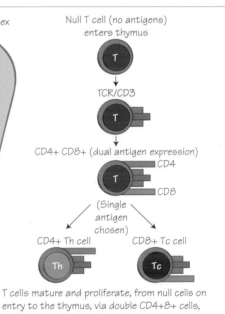

Cortex

Medulla

Null T cell (no antigens) enters thymus

TCR/CD3

CD4+ CD8+ (dual antigen expression)

CD4

CD8

(Single antigen chosen)

CD4+ Th cell

CD8+ Tc cell

T cells mature and proliferate, from null cells on entry to the thymus, via double CD4+8+ cells, to individual CD4 OR CD8+ cells within the cortex. **Positive selection** for cells which can recognise peptide bound to MHC molecules occurs in the cortex **Negative selection** against cells which bind self MHC molecules without peptide (in the medulla)

Non-autoreactive cells which can interact with antigen displayed on an appropriate MHC molecule move to the medulla and are secreted into the blood

The T and B lymphocytes, which exist to recognise and eliminate pathogens, must not attack host antigens. The deletion or suppression of anti-self-reacting cells is known as tolerance and develops in two phases – 'central' and 'peripheral' tolerance.

B cell tolerance

B cells develop from stem cells in the bone marrow. B lymphocytes whose B cell receptor (BCR) reacts against host antigens that are expressed by cells in the bone marrow are deleted by apoptosis. The B cells that have survived this selection process are then secreted into the blood, from where they home to lymph nodes, spleen and other secondary lymphoid tissues.

Until B cells are stimulated by contact with their specific cognate antigen within the lymphoid tissues they do not leave this circulation pathway, otherwise they would run the risk of encountering self-antigens in the tissues to which they have not been tolerised. Activated lymphocytes express cell surface adhesion molecules that will bind appropriate endothelial receptors and allow them to cross into the tissues. Any B cells that accidentally enter the tissues before they have been officially activated by exposure to exogenous antigen are 'anergised' or caused to undergo apoptosis, or die after chronic overstimulation.

T cell tolerance

Immature T cells made from stem cells in the bone marrow ('null cells') are taken by the blood to the thymus. They do not express the T cell receptor (TCR), let alone CD4 or CD8. They proliferate in the thymic cortex and acquire the TCR/CD3 complex as their TCR gene rearrangements occur. Soon afterwards they acquire both CD4 and CD8 complexes.

The role of the cortex is to supply the correct environment to permit the maturing T cells to develop their appropriate phenotypes and to select only lymphocytes that are capable of responding to an antigenic stimulus presented on MHC molecules. The cortical thymocytes expose the maturing T cells to 'self' (i.e. HLA) antigens. Until they have been educated to ignore self, naive T cells must not encounter pathogens, so macrophages line the capillaries that carry the naive T cells to the thymus from the bone marrow and phagocytose antigenic particles.

The first round of deletion occurs when CD4/8+ cells are tested for binding with cortical thymocytes – these are thymic epithelial cells, which express both MHC I and II molecules. They present antigenic peptides on their MHC molecules to the immature T cells. If any T cells *do not* bind to the thymocytes, they are deleted, since it is necessary to produce an end population of cells that can respond to antigen presented by MHC molecules.

The successful cells select one complex, either CD4 or CD8, and express the mature phenotype before they leave the cortex to enter the medulla. Here they are tested against bone marrow-derived dendritic cells. Those cells that bind strongly to the MHC antigens expressed by these cells are deleted. This step leaves cells that react to peptide presented on MHC complexes, but not just to the MHC molecules themselves or to self-antigens.

Mature T cells enter the circulation and home to lymphoid organs. They are programmed to respond to antigen presented on MHC molecules by cells with co-stimulatory molecules, such as B7, to authenticate the signal. If the newly arrived unstimulated T cells accid-

Table 18.1 Common autoimmune diseases.

Organ specific (or limited)
- Graves' disease
- Hashimoto's thyroiditis
- Diabetes mellitus
- Goodpasture's syndrome
- Pernicious anaemia
- Bullous pemphigoid
- Pemphigus

Non-organ specific
- Systemic lupus erythematosus
- Primary biliary cirrhosis
- Rheumatoid arthritis
- Autoimmune hepatitis
- Scleroderma

entally enter the tissues they may become overstimulated by antigens, and die. Alternatively, they display 'anergy' to self-antigens because the co-stimulatory molecules required for full T cell activation, such as B7, are not expressed since other inflammatory cells are not stimulated.

The thymus, of huge importance in the education of newly formed T lymphocytes in the neonate and child, atrophies to a barely detectable streak of lymphoid tissue in the anterior mediastinum of the adult. This is because the majority of T cells have been made by then and very few new cells are produced.

Autoimmune diseases

Autoantibodies or anti-self, cytotoxic lymphocytes develop if the tolerance mechanisms break down, particularly those that involve 'anergy'. There is a variety of autoimmune disease, which affects approximately 7% of the population. The typical patient is a middle-aged female, for reasons not yet elucidated.

Autoimmune diseases are conventionally considered in terms of those that are organ specific, such as Graves' disease, and those in which many organs are affected, such as systemic lupus erythematosus.

The mechanisms by which autoimmune diseases occur vary, and include:
- Cross reactivity between host antigens and those found on microbial organisms – e.g. rheumatic fever, which involves anti-streptococcal antibodies that cross-react with soft tissues, particularly the subendocardial tissues of the heart.
- Exposure, e.g. by trauma, of 'hidden' antigenic self-proteins, such as spermatozoa or lens protein, to which the cells have not been previously exposed in the bone marrow or thymus.
- Induction of antigenic presenting capability in cells that do not normally have this function, e.g. the epidermis in graft versus host disease.
- Abnormal immune cell regulation, e.g. due to mutation in key genes.
- Generalised (polyclonal) B cell activation is a function of some viral infections, such as Epstein–Barr virus; the stimulation of a wide range of B cells to form antibody in the absence of a specific antigenic stimulus may lead to self-reacting antibody being produced.

The effector mechanisms vary, depending on the type of cell involved and the stimulus.

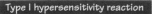

19 Hypersensitivity reactions

General pathology

Type I hypersensitivity reaction

IgE antibodies produced – they stick to eosinophils, mast cells and basophils

Antigen presented by APC to Th cells

Antigen, with repeated epitopes

First exposure to allergen: IgE antibodies are generated instead of IgG, an aberrant reaction in atopic people

Eosinophil

Basophil

IL-4

Mast cell

Antigen recognised by IgE

IL-4 attracts basophils and eosinophils from blood and stimulates their production by bone marrow

IgE is quickly formed by the action of memory B and Th2 cells, interacting with APC

Second exposure to allergen: IgE is formed by activation of memory B-cells; some primed mast cells are present in tissues from previous exposure

Effects of type I hypersensitivity reaction
- Skin rashes
- Nausea, vomiting, diarrhoea
- Tissue oedema
- Bronchospasm, wheezing
- Hypotension
- Death: hypotensive shock, laryngeal obstruction, status asthmaticus

Cross-linked IgE triggers degranulation and production of arachidonic acid metabolites
Anaphylactic reactions are more likely if antigen enters the systemic circulation, e.g. bee sting

Type II hypersensitivity reaction

Goodpasture's syndrome occurs when antibodies develop against glomerular and pulmonary basement membrane – the antibodies bind to basement membrane, which is effectively opsonised, generating an acute inflammatory reaction at the site

Antibody

Capillary endothelium

Polymorphs and complement

Antigen fixed in basement membrane, with bound antibody

Necrosis and tissue destruction

Type III hypersensitivity reaction

Antigen enters blood, e.g. via alveolar capillaries or directly

Initial exposure leads to the formation of antibody and memory B cells

Re-exposure causes a rapid antibody response

Immune complexes form and circulate

When antibodies greatly outnumber antigen the complexes precipitate out of solution at their site of entry to the bloodstream

Soluble complexes, with roughly equal numbers of antibody and antigen (e.g. SLE) frequently lodge in the kidneys, where they are trapped in the basement membrane. Glomerulonephritis occurs

The immune complexes lodge in capillary walls and elicit a destructive acute inflammatory reaction

First exposure

Antigen

Second exposure

Polymorphs and complement

Capillary endothelium

Delayed-type hypersensitivity (Type IV)

Tuberculin is a non-infective, purified protein derivative of Mycobacterium tuberculosis. In the Mantoux and Heaf tests, it is injected into the skin

Tuberculin protein

In a previously exposed patient, memory T cells are activated by tuberculin antigens. Cytokine release causes local redness and swelling

A red inflammatory reaction occurs at the injection site 2–3 days later in a patient who has previously experienced TB. The more rapid and vigorous the response, the more likely it is that a patient has active TB

Tuberculin protein

Re-testing with tuberculin will now be positive

In a patient who has never been infected with tuberculosis, there is no skin reaction. Vaccination can therefore be offered

APC

BCG vaccination: this cocktail of attenuated tuberculosis antigens activates Langerhans cells which process the antigen and display it to Th cells – immunity is generated within 3 weeks

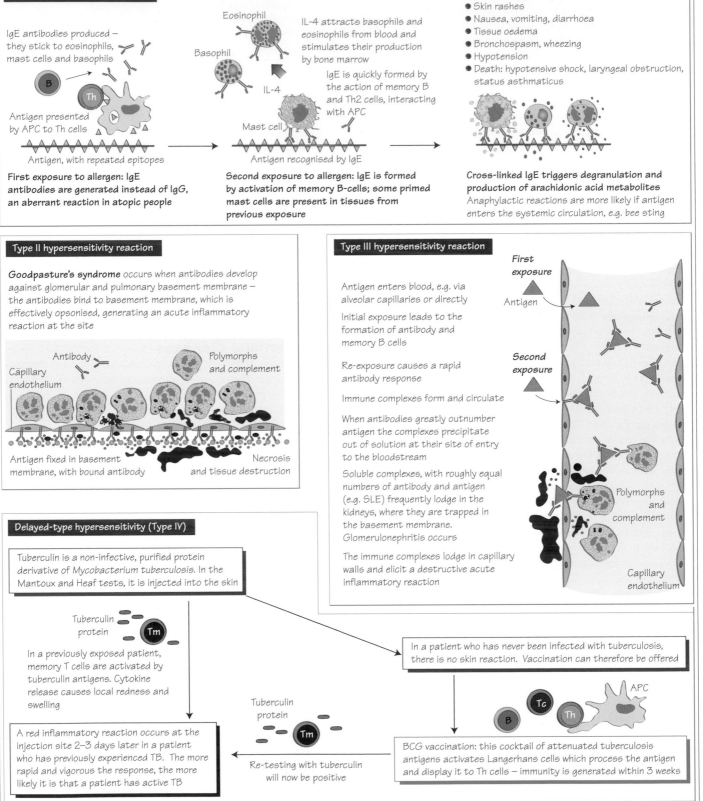

Hypersensitivity reactions are exaggerated or inappropriate versions of the normal immune response. Four types are recognised: types I–III involve antibody-mediated damage, whilst type IV is due to T cells.

Type I hypersensitivity (allergic and anaphylactic responses)

This is due to the inappropriate production of IgE antibodies. It is thought that 'atopic' people have a tendency to generate Th2 rather than Th1 helper T cells. Current thinking is that exposure to pathogens in early childhood is important in preventing this from occurring – too hygienic a household may lead to less childhood infections, but a lifelong allergy problem.

IgE is usually synthesised by B cells when interleukins 4, 5 and 10, secreted by Th2 cells, signal the presence of parasites at the stage of B cell immunoglobulin class switching.

Mast cells, basophils, eosinophils and monocytes specifically bind the Fc region of IgE. All these cells, except the monocytes, contain granules of substances that are toxic to parasites. Binding and cross-linking of two or more of these IgE molecules by antigens on the surface of a parasite triggers the release of toxic granules onto the parasite, injuring or killing it. The production of arachidonic acid metabolites in the mast cell membrane is also initiated.

In atopic individuals, IgE is aberrantly made instead of IgG in response to a variety of antigens. The common feature of these antigens is the presence of large numbers of repeat epitopes, to which multiple antibodies can bind, allowing antibody cross-linking and cell degranulation. Such antigens include bee stings, nuts, pollen grains or house dust mites.

Immediate effects: These are seen within 5–30 minutes and last for around 1 hour, and are due to the release of preformed mediators in granules:
• Histamine (vasodilatation and pain).
• Proteases, which cause tissue damage.
• Chemokines, which attract other inflammatory cells.
• 5HT (vascular permeability).

Delayed effects: These occur after 8–12 hours and reflect the time taken to manufacture arachidonic acid derivatives. These effects may be sustained over 2–3 days and are caused by:
• Platelet activating factor (vascular permeability, vasodilatation, neutrophil adhesion and platelet aggregation).
• Leukotrienes (bronchospasm).
• Prostaglandins (widespread effects, often opposing each other).

The delayed effects of allergy, as encountered in asthma, reflect recruitment of eosinophils from the bone marrow, via blood. Thus the finding of increased eosinophils in a patient's peripheral blood suggests either parasitic infection or an allergic response.

The effects of an allergy can be mildly irritating – for instance hay fever – or life-threatening, as in status asthmaticus or anaphylactic shock.

Asthma is often used to illustrate the concept of a type I hypersensitivity disease and its pathology may be encapsulated as 'a condition in which there is bronchial hyper-reactivity due to a type 1 hypersensitivity reaction that leads to reversible bronchoconstriction and increased mucus production'.

Anaphylactic shock

An allergen such as bee sting that can enter the bloodstream can trigger a body-wide allergic response, anaphylactic shock, in which there is bronchospasm and increased permeability of blood vessels coupled with vasodilatation. The clinical features are wheezing, laryngeal oedema, profound hypotension and clinical shock.

Death may ensue if a vasopressor response cannot be achieved (with adrenaline) or the inflammatory mediators are not damped by antihistamines (in the initial minutes – histamine's effects last approximately 15 minutes) or steroids. Laryngeal obstruction due to oedema may require an emergency tracheotomy.

Type II hypersensitivity

This is caused by antibody directed against a tissue element, i.e. a 'fixed' antigen.

In Goodpasture's disease, anti-type IV collagen antibodies bind to the basement membrane of the lung and renal glomerulus, causing haemoptysis and glomerulonephritis. This is because complement binds to the Fc component of IgG and either acute inflammation, phagocytosis or antibody-dependent NK cell cytotoxicity occurs. The original stimulus to antibody formation is not known.

Transfusion reactions and Rhesus disease of the newborn are other examples. In Rhesus disease, there is destruction of fetal erythrocytes by maternally derived antibodies against the Rhesus blood group antigen. This occurs if a Rhesus-negative mother becomes pregnant with a Rhesus-positive baby and has previously developed antibodies to the Rhesus antigen. The development of these antibodies has usually occurred in a previous Rhesus-positive pregnancy due to fetomaternal haemorrage in labour. To reduce the risk of this complication, which can be fatal to the fetus, Rhesus-negative mothers are given large doses of anti-Rhesus immunoglobulins at delivery to suppress their own endogenous production.

Type III hypersensitivity

This is due to antibody directed against an 'unfixed' antigen, with the formation of immune complexes that lodge in capillaries and elicit an acute inflammatory reaction.

The condition can occur in people with chronic antigen exposure. The initial exposure leads to the formation of antibody and memory B cells. These quickly proliferate and secrete large quantities of antibody if the antigen is encountered again. Acute inflammatory damage is caused to the organs in which the antibody/antigen complexes lodge.

Examples include systemic lupus erythematosus (SLE), post-streptococcal glomerulonephritis and extrinsic allergic alveolitis.

Type IV hypersensitivity (delayed hypersensitivity)

This develops in people who have developed an aberrant, predominantly T cell immune response to a particular antigen. This reaction takes time to develop: 3 weeks if the patient has not previously been sensitised and 3–5 days if sensitised already.

The reaction is utilised clinically in the tuberculin test to identify patients with active tuberculosis (TB). A tuberculin skin test after BCG vaccination should be positive. An exception to bear in mind clinically is that a patient with overwhelming tuberculosis may be anergic (show no response).

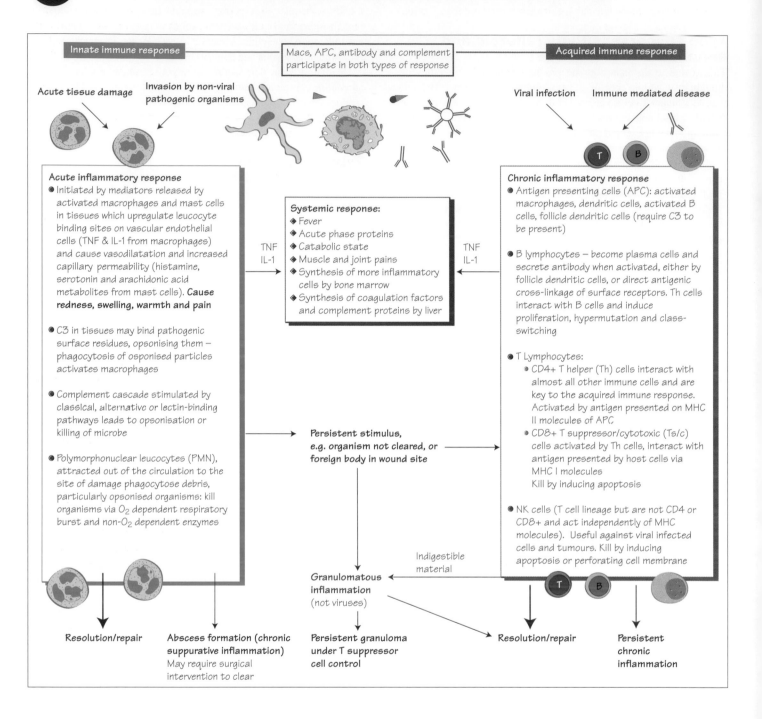

Innate immune response

Macs, APC, antibody and complement participate in both types of response

Acquired immune response

Acute tissue damage

Invasion by non-viral pathogenic organisms

Viral infection   Immune mediated disease

T   B

Acute inflammatory response
- Initiated by mediators released by activated macrophages and mast cells in tissues which upregulate leucocyte binding sites on vascular endothelial cells (TNF & IL-1 from macrophages) and cause vasodilatation and increased capillary permeability (histamine, serotonin and arachidonic acid metabolites from mast cells). **Cause redness, swelling, warmth and pain**

- C3 in tissues may bind pathogenic surface residues, opsonising them – phagocytosis of opsonised particles activates macrophages

- Complement cascade stimulated by classical, alternative or lectin-binding pathways leads to opsonisation or killing of microbe

- Polymorphonuclear leucocytes (PMN), attracted out of the circulation to the site of damage phagocytose debris, particularly opsonised organisms: kill organisms via O_2 dependent respiratory burst and non-O_2 dependent enzymes

Systemic response:
- Fever
- Acute phase proteins
- Catabolic state
- Muscle and joint pains
- Synthesis of more inflammatory cells by bone marrow
- Synthesis of coagulation factors and complement proteins by liver

TNF IL-1   TNF IL-1

Chronic inflammatory response
- Antigen presenting cells (APC): activated macrophages, dendritic cells, activated B cells, follicle dendritic cells (require C3 to be present)

- B lymphocytes – become plasma cells and secrete antibody when activated, either by follicle dendritic cells, or direct antigenic cross-linkage of surface receptors. Th cells interact with B cells and induce proliferation, hypermutation and class-switching

- T Lymphocytes:
  - CD4+ T helper (Th) cells interact with almost all other immune cells and are key to the acquired immune response. Activated by antigen presented on MHC II molecules of APC
  - CD8+ T suppressor/cytotoxic (Ts/c) cells activated by Th cells, interact with antigen presented by host cells via MHC I molecules Kill by inducing apoptosis

- NK cells (T cell lineage but are not CD4 or CD8+ and act independently of MHC molecules). Useful against viral infected cells and tumours. Kill by inducing apoptosis or perforating cell membrane

Persistent stimulus, e.g. organism not cleared, or foreign body in wound site

Indigestible material

Granulomatous inflammation (not viruses)

T   B

Resolution/repair

Abscess formation (chronic suppurative inflammation) May require surgical intervention to clear

Persistent granuloma under T suppressor cell control

Resolution/repair

Persistent chronic inflammation

Inflammation and immunity are intimately related processes. Acute and chronic inflammation are typically the consequences of a response by the immune system to infection, but are also encountered in other forms of tissue damage, such as infarction.

Immune system: The immune system is a highly complex army of diverse elements, each of which provides different skills and functions for dealing with a threat.

Co-ordinating and leading the behaviour of the army are the CD4+ T helper (Th) cells, which act as the senior officers. They do not engage directly in killing, but their recognition of the enemy and issuing of orders through various humoral mediators allows the immune system to function efficiently. Without Th cells, the individual units of the army can still execute their specific functions, but these will be at a suboptimal and possibly ineffective level.

The CD8+ T cytotoxic (Tc) cells, natural killer (NK) cells and B cells are the junior officers. The Tc and NK cells engage in direct hand-to-hand (cell-to-cell) combat, while the B cells exert their effects by releasing intelligent homing missiles in the form of antibodies. Any individual antibody locks onto one specific target only and is therefore briefed to execute a very specific mission. Once it has bound to its target, the antibody serves as a beacon and focus of attack for other elements in the army.

Antigen presenting cells (APCs) like follicular dendritic cells and macrophages constitute the intelligence division. They gather and process data about the enemy in the form of antigens. They then present these antigens, suitably digested, to the other officers, particularly the T cells, in order to alert the cells to the threat and permit the officers to develop a strategy against it.

Acquired immune system: The T and B cell officers constitute the acquired immune system. This is a powerful and sophisticated element of the army that has memory and creates specific strategies, in the form of molecular-specific antibodies and T cell receptors, against individual classes of enemy. Once a strategy has been developed, it is stored and latent, ready for use should the incursion recur, when it can be mobilised rapidly. However, during the initial encounter, the gathering of intelligence and division of the strategy requires time – up to 3 weeks. During this interval, a rapid response unit is essential and this rapid response force remains available to be brought into the campaign plan that the officers later develop.

Innate immune system: The innate immune system is the rapid response force. While it lacks the specificity of the acquired response and the ability of the acquired system to adapt, it provides an immediate counter to any invader and provides the frontline troops. The basic infantry are the neutrophils, armed with phagocytic capacity and toxic granule weaponry. They converge on the enemy and unleash a burst of killing. Eager to enter the carnage, their life expectancy is proportionately short. Weighing in alongside the neutrophils is the limpet mine ordnance that is complement, an archaic system of proteins that nevertheless remains effective against many organisms.

Supporting the neutrophils are the macrophages. They are also frontline troops, but are more seasoned campaigners that are more resilient in the chaos of battle and have a more versatile function. When faced with a particularly implacable foe, macrophages can band together to form giant cells, uniting forces to create a more powerful phagocytic unit. They can either destroy the contents of the phagosome or present portions to the officers of the acquired immune system.

Special forces exist in the shape of eosinophils and mast cells. These only come into their own when faced with certain opponents, usually parasites, but offer an artillery option in the form of toxic granules that are packed with assorted proteins and other agents, which can assail invaders that would otherwise resist the efforts of the other troops.

Summary

The non-leucocytic cells of the body may constitute the civilian population, but are not idle bystanders in the war. Their MHC molecules serve as a form of identity badge, letting the immune army recognise them as friend. Chemical signals that they secrete or liberate can alert the immune system to points of invasion and footholds established by the invaders. Endothelial cells are especially active in this context and provide vital guidance for neutrophils towards the infectious organisms as well as regulating blood flow to allow an influx of leucocytes into the battle zone, thus serving as landing strips, bridges and roads.

Numerous signals must pass between the cellular components of the immune system and these are provided by a myriad of cytokines, each of which encodes specific instructions that can only be read by cells expressing the appropriate cell surface receptors.

Standing fortifications in the shape of cutaneous and mucosal barriers and the rivers of the mucociliary escalator, peristalsis and tears, all act as physical obstacles employed by the immune system to oppose the invasion at the first opportunity, before troops are deployed.

Once the chaos is concluded, the battlefield must be cleared and attempts made to restore it to its previous normal function. In this regard, macrophages, having already served as intelligence officers and frontline killing machines now show further versatility by becoming engineers and cleaners, engulfing and removing debris from the battlefield. The civilian cellular population attempts to regenerate the structures that previously occupied the war zone. However, full resolution is often not possible and the fibroblast civilian engineers/builders attempt to provide some sort of workable repair in the form of fibrosis. Preservation of the infrastructure can be vital in determining how good this recovery is. Badly damaged roads (blood vessels) or deficient reserves of raw materials (nutrition, hypoxia) deprive the cells of the resources they need to achieve good repair.

Discipline, rules and regulations help to control the army and prevent it from running amok, but occasionally the system can go awry. Rogue officers misidentify specific elements of the civilian cellular population as the enemy and launch their weapons against them, yielding autoimmune disease.

General pathology

A comparison of cell division (mitosis versus meiosis)

Mitosis

Prometaphase: All chromosomes separate, become tightly coiled and replicate their DNA: new and old strands are linked by the centromere

Metaphase: nuclear membrane dissolves, centrioles move to opposite poles of the cell

Diagram showing replication of a maternal chromosome

Centriole

Original maternal chromosome	Original paternal chromosome	Replicated DNA mirrors the original

Anaphase: replicated chromosomes align along the mitotic spindle

Telophase: centromere divides, chromatids move apart along the spindle. The cell starts to constrict

Nuclear membrane re-forms, chromosomes become less tightly coiled and soon cease to be individually distinguishable

The 2 **daughter** cells are exact **diploid** replicas of the original

Meiosis

Recombination: In meiosis, unlike mitosis, before replication occurs there is cross-over of some genes between maternal and paternal chromosomes

Original maternal and paternal chromosomes cross-over: some genes from each are swapped		Replicated DNA contains a mixture of genes

Then the first meiotic division occurs in a similar fashion to mitosis, yielding 2 diploid daughter cells

First meiotic division

The daughter cells are **diploid** but the chromosomes are not exact replicas of the original, due to the chromatin exchange. Genes are not split by this exchange and certain genes always move together ('gene linkage')

Second meiotic division

Chromosomes align along the spindle and separate without further replication, giving four haploid daughter cells. In females, 3 atrophy, leaving 1 ovum, whereas in males all 4 become spermatozoa. The 2nd division occurs soon after the 1st in males, but is delayed by many years in females

Germline versus somatic mutation

Germline mutation:
The inherited genetic diseases caused by gene mutation belong in this group

Mutant gene in parental germ cell

Mutant gene in child's own germ cells; can be passed to future generations

Mutant gene inherited by child

Germline mutation: all somatic (body) cells carry the mutant gene(s)

Somatic mutation:
Diseases acquired by sporadic mutations are mainly related to the development of cancer

Genes in parental germ cell are normal

Normal genes inherited by child

Genes in child's own germ cells are normal; subsequent generations will be normal

Somatic mutation: often due to exogenous stimulus, e.g. radiation, viral infection. Only one tissue cell need develop the mutated gene since all its progeny, if viable, will carry the mutation. Only some tissue cells are affected

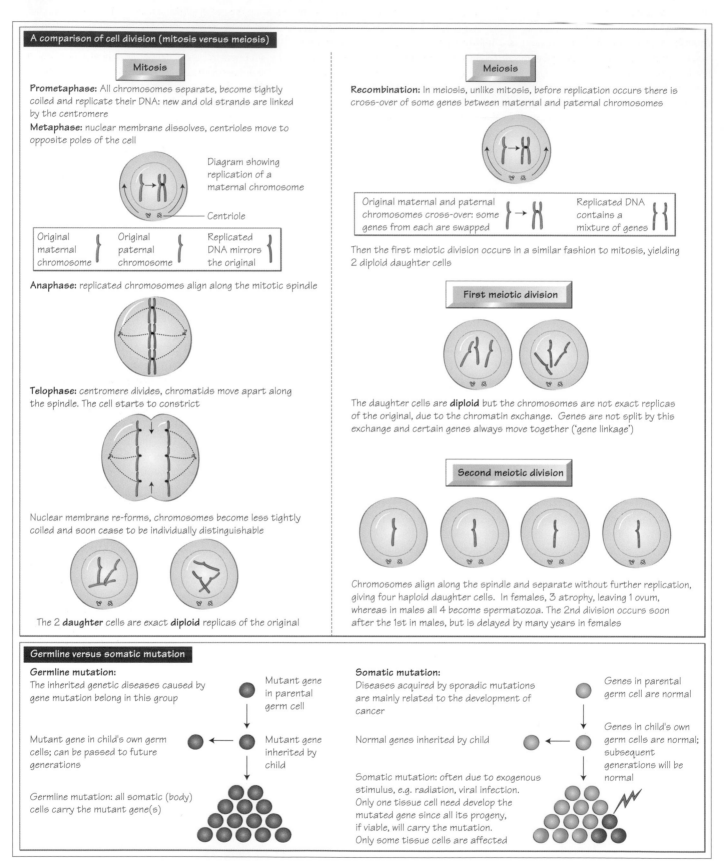

The human cell nucleus contains 23 pairs of chromosomes, of which 22 are autosomes and one is the sex chromosome. This paired arrangement is referred to as diploid. Each pair of chromosomes contains one of maternal origin and one of paternal origin. The chromosomal make-up of an individual is the karyotype. Chromosomes are composed of DNA and are inherited in Mendelian fashion, described first by the priest Gregor Mendel, who experimented with pea plants with different coloured flowers and realised that the inheritance of gene expression influenced flower colour in daughter plants.

DNA consists of a series of paired bases and is divided into introns and exons. The exons are responsible for encoding protein products; introns are 'silent' areas of DNA, which may be there to stabilise the chromosome. Introns are removed from transcribed DNA in order to form messenger RNA (mRNA), which takes the 'recipe' to the ribosomes, which assemble proteins in accordance with the template.

Mitosis

- When a cell divides, each chromosome replicates its DNA (prophase) – the original and new strands (chromatids) are linked by a centromere. Once this is done, the nuclear membrane dissolves and the centrioles move to opposite poles of the cell.
- The now duplicated chromosomes coil tightly to assume the traditional X shape. Their centromeres are linked to the centrioles by a 'spindle' and are at first aligned across the middle of the cell (metaphase).
- The centromere divides and each pair of chromatids moves apart by travelling in opposite directions along the spindle towards the centriole (anaphase).
- Once they have divided, the nuclear membrane is reformed, the cytoplasm begins to pinch off and the cell divides into two equal daughter cells, each with 46 chromosomes.
- Telomeres are the genetic sequences at the ends of each arm of the chromosomes. These are composed of repeat sequences of DNA that are essential for cell division as they provide a binding site for the DNA replicating enzymes. With each cell division, the telomeres shorten because the DNA synthase cannot replicate the base pairs that it is already using to anchor itself to the DNA strand. This has implications for senescence: some of the changes observed in old age, such as the increased frequency of genetic mutation, may be attributable to telomere shortening.

Meiosis

- This occurs in germ cells. The object of meiosis is to create a gamete (ovum or spermatid) with only 23 unpaired chromosomes (haploid), which will pair with another gamete during sexual reproduction.
- Replication of chromosomes begins in the same way as mitosis: each chromosome replicates and the two chromatids are linked at the centromere.
- At this stage, each chromosome lines up with its partner (i.e. maternal and paternal chromosomes pair off), and often there is an overlap between arms, which results in a crossover of genetic material. Thus the gamete will inherit chromosomes that differ slightly from the original paternal and maternal chromosomes, because some will contain a mixture.
- These chromosomes then align along the spindle and pull apart (anaphase of the first meiotic division). They divide into two daughter cells, each with 46 chromosomes, as in mitosis.
- The second meiotic division then takes place – in this the chromosomes do not replicate, but simply align along the spindle and the cell divides. This division is much delayed in women, who inherit their entire complement of germ cells at birth. Four cells are formed as the end product of meiotic division, each with 23 chromosomes. These form spermatozoa in the male. In the female, three cells atrophy, leaving just one haploid ovum.
- When we talk about cells having 'germline mutations' we mean that the mutation has occurred prior to this point, and that the gamete is carrying the mutation. 'Somatic mutations' take place during mitotic divisions that happen after fertilisation.

Terminology

The shorter arm of a chromosome is the 'p' arm, the longer is the 'q' arm. A locus encoding a particular protein or set of proteins is a gene. An allele is the term given for one gene: alleles are therefore paired – one of paternal and one of maternal origin and each occupy a specific part of a particular chromosome (the gene locus).

A dominant gene is one that by itself determines the corresponding phenotype and supersedes the effects of the paired gene. A recessive gene is one that will not show phenotypic expression unless it is paired with another recessive gene. For example, brown eyes are dominant over blue. In other words, only one copy of a dominant gene is necessary to generate the corresponding phenotype, whereas a recessive gene has to be present as both alleles.

Lyonisation of gene expression is the process whereby one X chromosome is inactived early (around day 16) during the development of an embryo with an XX karyotype, though whether it is the maternal or paternal chromosome varies in each cell. Every cell produced by subsequent division of these cells has the same phenotype thereafter. The inactivated chromosome is extruded from the nucleus to form a Barr body. The resulting organism is a mosaic, composed of two sets of cells that differ in their composition of active chromosomes. Lyonisation does not occur in normal males as they have only one X chromosome. Lyonisation is necessary to stop the female from having double the expression of all X chromosome proteins in her cells, where such overexpression would be harmful and very likely fatal.

General pathology

Autosomal dominant disorder: 50% of offspring will inherit the abnormal gene and will manifest the disease
Example: Marfan syndrome

X-linked disorder:
◆ Males donate their X chromosome to their daughters, so can only pass on the disease to them
◆ Females can transmit an X-linked disease to either sex offspring
◆ X-linked disease is often recessive, as shown here, i.e. an individual only expresses the disease if there is no normal X chromosome present
Example: Haemophilia

Autosomal recessive disorder: 50% of offspring will inherit the abnormal gene, but will only manifest the disease if another abnormal gene is inherited from the other parent. Recessive disorders are therefore much rarer than dominant disorders
The chance of inheriting a recessive disorder is increased if there is consanguinous marriage, e.g. between cousins. Alternatively a mutation in a gene may be reasonably prevalent if its effects vary in severity and do not result in the extinguishing of individuals with the trait before they have reproduced
Example: Cystic fibrosis

✳ Disease expression	◖ Female heterozygote	▣ Male heterozygote
	● Female homozygote	☐ Male normal

Clinical features of cystic fibrosis, an autosomal recessive disease:

● Hypertonic sweat, previously a useful diagnostic test in the neonate

● Repeated lung infections, bronchiectasis and abscess formation

● Gastrointestinal obstruction by inspissated (dried out) mucin

● Pancreatic duct obstruction by viscid mucin, with malabsorption

(See also chapter 43)

Clinical features of Marfan syndrome, an autosomal dominant inherited disease

● Very tall individuals with a wide arm-span and arachnodactyly

● Connective tissue in ciliary apparatus abnormal – recurrent lens dislocation common

● High-arched palate

● Lax ligaments ('double-jointed')

● Propensity to aortic root dilatation, aortic dissection and rupture, particularly in pregnant females

● Mitral valve prolapse

Clinical features of haemophilia-A, an X-linked recessive disorder causing factor VIII deficiency

● Variable clinical manifestation, depending on disease penetrance and expression

● Bleeding into soft tissue and joints after minor trauma; the latter can cause progressively marked joint damage

● Clinical tests show a normal prothrombin time and platelet count, but a prolonged partial thromboplastin time, indicating the presence of a defect in the intrinsic coagulation pathway

Clinical features of Down syndrome, a chromosomal disorder involving acquisition of an extra autosomal chromosome (trisomy 21)

● Severely reduced IQ (80%)

● Congenital heart defects (40%)

● Other congenital malformations (e.g. oesophageal atresia)

● Acute myeloblastic leukaemia (10-20x increased risk)

● Predisposition to bacterial infection

● Predisposition to autoimmune disease

● Dementia (Alzheimer protein excess accumulates in brain) – almost 100% with increasing age

Typical facies (also have single palmar crease)

While neoplasia can be claimed to be a genetic disease, the term is usually reserved for those conditions that are due to genetic defects which are present at birth. These defects are either inherited from the parents, or occur spontaneously very early in the germline. Several basic categories exist.

Chromosomal disorders

Chromosomal disorders affect an entire chromosome or a large part of it and are in the form of either duplication or deletion. Cells that do not have 23 paired chromosomes are referred to as aneuploid.

The usual cause of aneuploidy is non-disjunction (non-separation) of chromatids, or parts of chromatids, during meiosis. Non-disjunction is a feature particularly of older women, whose germ cells have waited many years before completing the second meiotic division. Hence disorders caused by non-disjunction are more commonly inherited from the mother. Spermatozoa are produced continually during adulthood and spontaneous mutations involving small segments of DNA are more likely than non-disjunction.

Occasionally, non-disjunction occurs post fertilisation during mitosis, resulting in mosaicism – some cells are affected and others are not.

Examples of chromosomal disorders include trisomy 21 (Down syndrome) in which there is an extra chrosome 21, Kleinfelter syndrome (47 XXY) due to an extra X chromosome and Turner syndrome (45 X0) where a second sex chromosome is lacking. Aneuploidy is often seen in malignant tumours.

Autosomal disorders

Autosomal disorders are due to mutations in a single gene that is inherited on one of the 22 autosomes. Dominant conditions require the presence of only one defective allele for the disease to manifest. Recessive disorders need both alleles to be defective.
• Autosomal dominant disorders tend to affect structural proteins. The cell cannot assemble structures properly if half the building bricks are defective e.g. Marfan syndrome.
• Autosomal recessive diseases tend to affect enzymes. Most enzymes are extremely efficient and even half normal levels permit adequate function e.g. cystic fibrosis.

Marfan syndrome

Marfan syndrome is an autosomal dominant disease due to a mutation in one of the fibrillin genes, most of which are on chromosome 15q. The prevalence is estimated at one per 5000. Fibrillins are important extracellular matrix components. The features of Marfan syndrome parallel the distribution of microfibrils in connective tissue.

Affected patients are strikingly tall, usually thin, with a wide arm-span, arachnodactyly (long fingers and toes) and a high arched palate. There is a susceptibility to aortic root dilatation and dissection at a relatively young adult age. Floppy mitral valve disease, causing prolapse and incompetence, is common. They also suffer from intermittent lens dislocation and retinal detachment.

Aortic dissection is a particular problem for Marfanoid females during pregnancy, when their hyperdynamic circulation causes increased aortic root pressure.

People with Marfan syndrome can undergo regular echocardiographic monitoring of the aortic root and be offered aortic root grafting when significant dilatation is detected.

Cystic fibrosis

Cystic fibrosis (CF) is an autosomal recessive disease. The cystic fibrosis transmembrane conductance regulator (CFTR) gene on chromosome 7q is mutated. The prevalence is one in 2000 live births. Around one in 25 of people of European descent are heterozygous.

The CFTR protein encodes a chloride ion channel that occurs in various epithelial types and allows chloride to enter or leave cells. The function of this channel can be modified by cyclic adenosine monophosphate (cAMP). It plays an important role in determining water secretion and/or reabsorption as water movement across these epithelia passively follows an osmotic gradient to which chloride movement contributes. In addition, the epithelial sodium channel (ENaC) requires normal CFTR protein to function properly. In cystic fibrosis, ENaC activity is decreased so sodium transport becomes defective. Impaired CFTR function can also affect bicarbonate movement.

Overall, the common functional problem is the production of abnormally thick mucus because the mucin-producing epithelia of affected organs (lungs, intestines and pancreas) secrete insufficient chloride ions into their lumens to draw in adequate water to dilute the mucus. This leads to the following problems:
• Neonatal small intestinal obstruction by thick mucus (meconium ileus).
• Bronchial occlusion leading to repeated infections and bronchiectasis. *Pseudomonas aeruginosa* is a common organism in this situation.
• Obstruction of the main pancreatic duct causes malabsorption, at first due to the pancreatic enzymes being unable to reach the small bowel, then later due to chronic pancreatitis.
• Bile duct obstruction can cause localised hepatic scarring.
• The vas deferens is fibrotic in males (only 2–3% are fertile).
• Sweat contains more sodium and chloride than normal (sweat gland ion channels respond differently to CFTR protein than ion channels elsewhere and fail to resorb sodium from sweat).

Around 800 different CF mutations have been identified, explaining the variable spectrum of the disease phenotypes. The most common mutation is the F508 deletion, where a phenylalanine molecule is omitted from the protein, resulting in misfolding. Some homozygotes have almost no manifestations of the disease if they have inherited mutations with only mild effects. The mildest form features only the absence of the vas deferens, without other abnormalities.

X-linked disorders

These conditions are inherited on the X chromosome. Almost all are recessive so usually only males are affected. Partial expression in females reflects unusual dominance of the defective allele after lyonisation. Examples include haemophilia A and colour blindness.

Other than hairy ears, no Y-linked conditions have been described, although the Y chromosome is essential for the male phenotype to develop.

Mitochondrial disorders

Although most of the mitochondrial proteins are encoded in the nucleus, a minority are produced by the mitochondrion, which has its own DNA and ribosomal apparatus. All of the mitochondria in a zygote are acquired from the mother. Therefore, mitochondrial diseases can only be passed from a mother to her children. They cannot be inherited from the father.

Mitochondria are especially important in neurological tissues and skeletal muscle, so mitochondrial diseases, such as Leber's hereditary optic neuropathy and some myopathies, tend to affect these tissues.

23 Disordered cell growth

Disorders of cell growth

Developmental disorders

- **Atresia**, e.g. congenital oesophageal atresia

- **Heterotopia/ectopia**: mature tissue at an inappropriate site, e.g. gastric mucosa may cause peptic ulcer in Meckel's diverticulum

- **Hamartoma** haphazardly arranged mature tissue appropriate to the site and incapable of normal functional activity, e.g. bronchial hamartoma

- **Aplasia/agenesis**: failure of development of an organ or tissue, e.g. congenital renal agenesis

Non-neoplastic disorders

- **Hyperplasia**: almost always found in the context of endocrine organ function: excess stimulus causes **an increase in cell number within an organ**. Example: Graves' disease causing hyperthyroidism

- **Hypoplasia**: a decrease in tissue/organ size due to **a loss of cells**, often in response to a decrease in stimulation. Example: post menopausal uterine and ovarian shrinkage

- **Hypertrophy**: an increase in organ or tissue size due to **an increase in cell size** – e.g. bladder muscle hypertrophy in response to urethral outflow obstruction by an enlarged prostate

- **Atrophy** (usually results from **decrease in cell size and loss of cells**) – occurs in many tissues deprived of a stimulus to work, e.g. thenar muscle atrophy following median nerve severance

- **Metaplasia: substitution of one mature tissue type for another** in response to a noxious stimulus, which is **reversible** if the stimulus is removed, e.g. Barrett's oesophagus

- **Dysplasia: premalignant change** in a tissue caused by mutation. The cells have many characteristics of malignant cells but do not invade or metastasise. Lower grades of dysplasia may regress. Progression to frank malignancy is likely, the higher the grade of the dysplasia, but it is not inevitable, e.g. cervix

Developmental disorders

Atresia: This is failure of luminal development, e.g. oesophageal atresia, which may present as a blind-ended oesophagus or a tracheo-oesophageal fistula.

Heterotopia/ectopia: This is well-developed tissue or organ at the wrong site, e.g. gastric or pancreatic heterotopia within a Meckel's diverticulum (a persistent vitellointestinal duct remnant).

Hamartoma: Hamartomas are tumour-like masses of tissue appropriate to a site, but haphazardly arranged. For example, a bronchial hamartoma – a benign lesion that may present as a coin-shaped shadow on a routine chest X-ray – is composed of islands of cartilage and respiratory epithelium embedded in smooth muscle and fibrous tissue.

Aplasia/agenesis: This is a failure to form an organ or tissue, e.g. unilateral renal agenesis. Spina bifida/meningomyelocoele/anencephaly result from the failure of closure of the neural tube; this leads to failure of development of the vertebral column/cranial bones (depending on severity) and associated neural tissue.

(Note that bone marrow aplasia is a commonly used misnomer. It is an example of hypoplasia, with little-to-no demonstrable haemopoietic tissue detectable in bone marrow biopsies in patients with previously normal bone marrow. This can be due to an idiosyncratic reaction to a drug (e.g. chloramphenicol) or secondary to viral infection.)

Non-tumorous growth disorders

Cells try to maintain their internal environment but external factors may induce different responses that relate to the site of the organ involved or its normal function. The cell has a limited range of responses:

- Stimuli that increase demand result in hyperplasia and/or hypertrophy.
- Lack of stimulation or work results in hypoplasia or atrophy.
- The changes may be reversible if the cause is corrected.

Hyperplasia

This is reversible if the stimulus is removed. It is an increase in tissue or organ size due to an increase in cell numbers, often driven by a hormonal stimulus. It typically affects glandular tissue as a normal physiological event, e.g. breast hyperplasia at puberty or pregnancy and endometrial hyperplasia during the menstrual cycle.

Pathological hyperplasia: This is often driven by a distant hormone-secreting tumour (e.g. pituitary) or is autoimmune (e.g. Graves' disease, Cushing syndrome), where the stimulus is not subject to the usual negative feedback mechanisms.

Hypertrophy

Hypertrophy is potentially reversible and involves the enlargement of an organ or tissue because of an increase in cell size in response to a stimulus. This is typically seen in muscle, responding to increased work requirement. Physiological examples are skeletal muscle hypertrophy with exercise, or myometrial hypertrophy in pregnancy.

Pathological hypertrophy: This may occur when an abnormal and prolonged increase in load is placed on an organ or tissue, e.g. left ventricular hypertrophy in hypertension.

Hypertrophy and hyperplasia: Hypertrophy and hyperplasia may occur in combination, e.g. prostatic glandular hyperplasia and fibromuscular hypertrophy, mainly in response to androgenic stimulation.

Hypoplasia

This is a failure of an organ or tissue to attain its expected size. Pathological examples are seen in a variety of congenital syndromes.

Atrophy

This is potentially reversible, but only if corrected early, and involves shrinkage of a tissue or organ due to loss of cells and a decrease in cell size. A physiological example is thymic atrophy at puberty.

Pathological atrophy:

- Disuse, e.g. muscle wasting in an immobilized fracture or following nerve severance.
- Response to pressure, e.g. renal atrophy in hydronephrosis due to ureteric obstruction, or cerebral atrophy secondary to raised intracranial pressure from hydrocephalus.

Metaplasia

Metaplasia is potentially reversible and is the replacement of one mature tissue type by another in response to altered environmental circumstances. Physiological example: squamous metaplasia of columnar-lined endocervix when the canal everts at puberty.

Pathological metaplasia:

- Squamous metaplasia of the normal bronchial ciliated pseudostratified columnar epithelium, in response to heat damage by smoking.
- Barrett's epithelium in gastro-oesophageal reflux disease (GORD, Chapter 51).
- Intestinal metaplasia of gastric mucosa in *Helicobacter*-infected stomach – *Helicobacter* cannot attach to the intestinal mucosa.
- Osseus metaplasia – this can occur in foci of dystrophic calcification, often an age-related phenomenon within the bronchial cartilage or due to precipitation of calcium in the necrotic core of an atheromatous deposit in an arterial wall.

Dysplasia

This term is still used in two different contexts – historically it has been used to describe abnormal development (as in 'cystic renal dysplasia'), characterised by disordered development of an organ or tissue: it is better to use the term 'dysgenesis' for this.

The preferred usage of the term is for a premalignant state (as in cervical dysplasia), characterised by disordered maturation of cells within an epithelium. Although the cells may look malignant, dysplasia cannot metastasise. There is some evidence that dysplasia may be reversible, particularly in the early stages. The alternative term, intraepithelial neoplasia is preferred to dysplasia in some organs (such as the cervix and prostate).

Typical sites at which dysplasia is found are frequently (but not exclusively) sites of previous metaplasia:

- Squamous mucosa in the bronchus of smokers.
- Squamous epithelium of the cervical transformation zone in patients with human papilloma virus (HPV) infection.
- Barrett's epithelium in GORD patients.
- Intestinal epithelium in *Helicobacter pylori* gastritis.

Characteristics of dysplasia include increased mitoses, disordered differentiation and atypical nuclear features.

Terminology – premalignancy versus predisposition to malignancy: Dysplasia is a premalignant condition. Some inherited mutations may confer an increased risk of developing malignancy, i.e. a predisposition to malignancy (e.g. familial polyposis coli).

24 Basic concepts in neoplasia

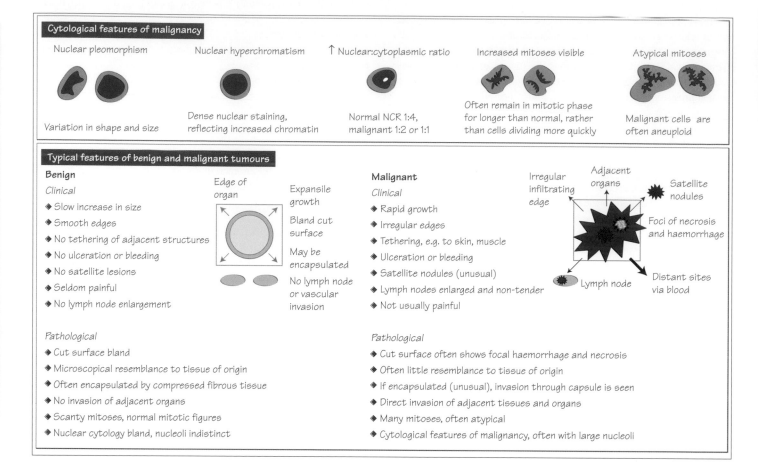

Cytological features of malignancy

Nuclear pleomorphism

Variation in shape and size

Nuclear hyperchromatism

Dense nuclear staining, reflecting increased chromatin

↑ Nuclear:cytoplasmic ratio

Normal NCR 1:4, malignant 1:2 or 1:1

Increased mitoses visible

Often remain in mitotic phase for longer than normal, rather than cells dividing more quickly

Atypical mitoses

Malignant cells are often aneuploid

Typical features of benign and malignant tumours

Benign

Clinical
- Slow increase in size
- Smooth edges
- No tethering of adjacent structures
- No ulceration or bleeding
- No satellite lesions
- Seldom painful
- No lymph node enlargement

Edge of organ

Expansile growth

Bland cut surface

May be encapsulated

No lymph node or vascular invasion

Pathological
- Cut surface bland
- Microscopical resemblance to tissue of origin
- Often encapsulated by compressed fibrous tissue
- No invasion of adjacent organs
- Scanty mitoses, normal mitotic figures
- Nuclear cytology bland, nucleoli indistinct

Malignant

Clinical
- Rapid growth
- Irregular edges
- Tethering, e.g. to skin, muscle
- Ulceration or bleeding
- Satellite nodules (unusual)
- Lymph nodes enlarged and non-tender
- Not usually painful

Irregular infiltrating edge

Adjacent organs

Satellite nodules

Foci of necrosis and haemorrhage

Lymph node

Distant sites via blood

Pathological
- Cut surface often shows focal haemorrhage and necrosis
- Often little resemblance to tissue of origin
- If encapsulated (unusual), invasion through capsule is seen
- Direct invasion of adjacent tissues and organs
- Many mitoses, often atypical
- Cytological features of malignancy, often with large nucleoli

Table 24.1 Tumour classification by histological subtype.

	Benign	Malignant
Epithelial tumours	*-oma*	*-carcinoma*
Epithelial		
Squamous or glandular	Squamous papilloma, adenoma	Squamous cell carcinoma, adenocarcinoma
Transitional (urothelium)	Papilloma (in UK this is not accepted as benign)	Transitional cell carcinoma
Mesothelium		Mesothelioma
Neuroectodermal		
Melanocytic	Melanocytic naevus (many do not consider this a neoplasm)	Malignant melanoma
Neuroendocrine tumour (NET)	Benign NET (rare)	Well or poorly differentiated NET (latter = small cell Ca)
Non-epithelial tumours (Note that many malignant connective tissue tumours show either no differentiation or show features of several different lineages)	*-oma*	*-sarcoma*
Connective tissue		
Fibrous, adipose, nerve	Fibroma, lipoma, neurofibroma	Fibrosarcoma, liposarcoma, neurofibrosarcoma
Cartilage, bone, blood vessels	Chondroma, osteoma, angioma	Chondrosarcoma, osteosarcoma, angiosarcoma
Smooth muscle, striated muscle	Leiomyoma, rhabdomyoma	Leiomyosarcoma, rhabdomyosarcoma
Glial	No benign gliomas	Gliomas (all malignant), e.g. astrocytoma
Lymphohaemopoeitic		
Lymphoid tissue	No benign lymphohaemopoeitic tumours	Multiple myeloma, Hodgkin and Non-Hodgkin lymphoma
Haemopoeitic cells		Leukaemias, e.g. AML, ALL, CLL, CML
Germ cell		
Ovary, testis	Mature teratoma (dermoid cyst)	Immature teratoma dysgerminoma (ovary) = seminoma (testis)
Embryonal		
Neuronal tissue	Ganglioneuroma	Neuroblastoma, PNET
Kidney		Nephroblastoma (Wilm's tumour)
Muscle		Embryonal rhabdomyoblastoma
Placenta	Hydatidiform mole	Choriocarcinoma (this can also develop *de novo* in ovary or testis)

In literal terms, a neoplasm is a new growth and is commonly referred to as a tumour. A neoplasm is produced when a cell escapes the usual mechanisms that regulate cell division and replicates outside their control. The resulting tumour is essentially composed solely of this cell type, although many tumours also possess a supporting connective tissue stroma which is induced by the growth of the tumour.

The most important division of tumour types is into benign and malignant. While there are many features that help to distinguish them, the key, defining property of malignant tumours that is not shown by benign neoplasms is that malignant neoplasms invade beyond their tissue of origin and spread to distant organs. For example, a tubular adenoma of the colon remains confined to the colonic epithelium. By contrast, a colonic adenocarcinoma invades through the colonic wall and if left unchecked will spread to other organs.

Nomenclature

The suffix -oma, seen in almost all tumour names, technically means nothing more than 'tumour', but its application is inconsistent such that it is used for benign tumours in some circumstances and malignant ones in others. Hence an adenoma is a benign tumour of glands whereas a melanoma is a malignant tumour of melanocytes and a lymphoma is a malignant tumour of lymphocytes.

The terms carcinoma and sarcoma add precision. A carcinoma is a malignant tumour of epithelial tissues. A sarcoma is a malignant tumour of connective tissue. The use of prefixes indicates the tissue type. Thus, an *adeno*carcinoma is a malignant tumour of glandular epithelium. A *leiomyo*sarcoma is a malignant tumour of smooth muscle. An adenoma and a leiomyoma are the benign counterparts.

Benign tumours

Benign tumours neither invade nor spread beyond their tissue of origin. They are typically well circumscribed, grow relatively slowly, closely resemble their tissue of derivation, have bland nuclear features and tend not to be necrotic. While they typically cause much less serious clinical problems than a malignant tumour, they are not without the potential to wreak havoc. A benign tumour still forms a mass and if that mass is in a sensitive region, serious complications can occur. For example, a benign posterior cranial fossa tumour, e.g. meningioma, may cause compression of the brainstem and death.

Malignant tumours

A malignant tumour is one that can invade and metastasise. A primary malignant tumour is a tumour that is still in its organ of origin. A secondary tumour is a metastatic deposit in a distant organ. Thus, a lung adenocarcinoma that has metastasised to the brain is a secondary tumour of the brain.

Invasion describes the process whereby a tumour spreads beyond its tissue of origin but retains direct continuity with the original tumour mass. For example, a squamous cell carcinoma of the skin starts in the epidermis but invades into the dermis and beyond.

Metastasis is the phenomenon in which deposits of the tumour develop in other organs, where those deposits are anatomically discontinuous from the primary tumour. Metastasis is a complex process and demands numerous properties of the tumour:

- The ability to move (autocrine motility factor).
- The ability to detach from adjacent cells (loss of cell–cell adhesion molecules).
- The ability to invade, requiring breakdown of basement membranes and the extracellular matrix (includes acquisition of synthesis of collagenases, metallomatrix proteases and plasminogen activator).
- The ability to survive outside the support of its normal environment.
- The ability to induce angiogenesis to provide a vascular supply (includes synthesis of VEGF, FGF or tumour growth factor β (TGFβ)).
- The ability to avoid elimination by the immune system (includes altered expression of MHC molecules).
- The ability to enter lymphatic and blood vessels.
- The ability to survive in the lymphovascular system.
- The ability to attach to endothelial cells and exit the vessel.
- The ability to infiltrate foreign tissue and survive in an alien cellular environment and resume angiogenesis.

These properties are in addition to those that confer autonomous cell division on the malignancy.

Vogelstein proposed the 'multi-hit hypothesis' of cancer development, which suggests that most cancers show several mutations that affect different cellular properties. This would concord with the need for a malignant tumour to have acquired numerous new properties.

Malignant tumours tend to have irregular borders, grow more rapidly, have abnormal cell nuclei and may show necrosis.

Grade

The grade of a tumour denotes how closely it resembles its tissue of origin. Grading systems are typically three tier: well differentiated, indicating a tumour that is very similar in appearance to its originating tissue; poorly differentiated, showing little resemblance; and moderately differentiated lie in between. Tumour-specific systems exist (such as the Bloom and Richardson scoring for breast carcinomas).

Stage

The stage of a tumour is an indication of how far it has spread beyond its tissue of origin. Various sorts of spread are possible:

- Direct spread into adjacent tissues.
- Via lymphatics (common in carcinomas).
- Via blood vessels (later in most carcinomas, early in some such as renal; common in sarcomas).
- Along nerves in the perineural space (e.g. pancreas, prostate).
- Across coelomic cavities (e.g. stomach to ovary, appendix to peritoneum).

Paraneoplastic phenomena

These are manifestations of a malignant tumour that are not secondary to the mass effect of the tumour but instead are caused by the synthesis of humoral mediators by the tumour. Small cell carcinoma of the lung is the best example and is associated with numerous paraneoplastic phenomena, such as ectopic adrenocorticotrophic hormone or Eaton–Lambert syndrome.

25 Tumorigenesis and oncogenesis

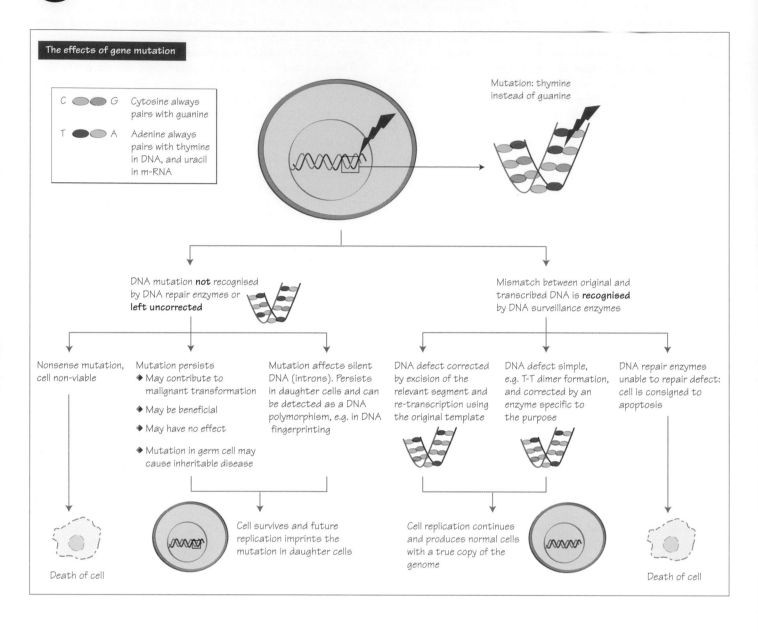

The effects of gene mutation

C ⬭⬭ G — Cytosine always pairs with guanine

T ⬭⬭ A — Adenine always pairs with thymine in DNA, and uracil in m-RNA

Mutation: thymine instead of guanine

DNA mutation **not** recognised by DNA repair enzymes or **left uncorrected**

Mismatch between original and transcribed DNA is **recognised** by DNA surveillance enzymes

Nonsense mutation, cell non-viable

Mutation persists
◆ May contribute to malignant transformation
◆ May be beneficial
◆ May have no effect
◆ Mutation in germ cell may cause inheritable disease

Mutation affects silent DNA (introns). Persists in daughter cells and can be detected as a DNA polymorphism, e.g. in DNA fingerprinting

DNA defect corrected by excision of the relevant segment and re-transcription using the original template

DNA defect simple, e.g. T-T dimer formation, and corrected by an enzyme specific to the purpose

DNA repair enzymes unable to repair defect: cell is consigned to apoptosis

Death of cell

Cell survives and future replication imprints the mutation in daughter cells

Cell replication continues and produces normal cells with a true copy of the genome

Death of cell

Tumorigenesis refers to the mechanisms by which a tumour arises. Oncogenesis pertains to malignant tumours specifically. Both benign and malignant tumours arise due to disordered cell growth and this implies nuclear dysfunction. Furthermore, the various abilities that a malignant tumour requires in order to behave as such (see Chapter 24) require aberrant protein expression and are again intimately connected with the cell nucleus.

The basic pathological process that produces this nuclear dysfunction is DNA mutation. This can have various consequences:
• A mutation in an intron will have no effect.
• The mutation may be incompatible with cell function, causing cell death.
• A point mutation of a single base causes the replacement of the correct amino acid with a new one that alters protein function.
• The mutation produces an inappropriate stop codon. The protein is shorter than normal and functions differently.
• The function of promoter and inhibitor regions of DNA can become impaired, leading to over- or underexpression of an otherwise functionally normal protein.
• Parts of two genes become fused, creating either a hybrid protein, or placing one gene under the control of another's promoter. This is especially important in many B cell lymphomas in which genes that control cell replication become aberrantly regulated by promoter regions that govern immunoglobulin production. These promoter regions are usually highly active in B lymphocytes, whereas those that should control cell division are much quieter. Hence, the cell division genes are overexpressed.

Assorted forms of mutation may allow a cell to activate a gene that it would not normally express and this is a phenomenon that is desirable to a cell with oncogenic aspirations.

More complex mutations, often occurring due to defective mitosis, cause deletion or duplication of part or all of a chromosome.

DNA protection
Huge numbers of base pairs are replicated during cell division. Errors are inevitable in this process, which is nevertheless remarkably accurate. Furthermore, various agents can damage DNA and given the core role of DNA in cell function, mechanisms that can repair damaged DNA, or detect mutations, are advantageous. Cells are equipped with assorted enzymes and other proteins that assist in this function. Some exist to detect base pair mismatch (the mutated pairing binds aberrantly, distorting the shape of the DNA molecule) or more general DNA damage. Some can attempt to repair damaged DNA, or initiate measures that prevent the cell from dividing until the damage can be repaired. If repair cannot be achieved, these proteins initiate apoptosis. Apoptosis sacrifices the cell, but prevents a potentially carcinogenic mutation from being passed on to daughter cells, aborting the tumour at inception.

The DNA protection system is itself encoded by DNA. Therefore, any mechanism that induces mutation can disrupt this system. Loss of the apoptotic cascades renders the cell resistant to various killing mechanisms, including those of T cells. Loss of DNA repair and mutation detection renders the cell susceptible to a myriad of further unchecked mutations, ideal for the creation of a cancer.

Control of cell division
Cell division is a significant event that must occur purposefully for an organ and organism to survive. Therefore, it is highly regulated. Assorted proteins in the nucleus act as gatekeepers either to entry into the cell cycle itself, or progression through the phases of the cycle. Predictably, mutations of these proteins are common across many phenotypically disparate tumours, both benign and malignant. Growth factor receptors are also vital in normal cell division. Tumour cells that can constitutively activate these receptors, for example by mutation of their adenylate cyclase subunit, can autonomously stimulate themselves to divide and thereby escape normal regulation.

Mutation of these proteins does not confer actual malignancy as they do not bestow those abilities given in Chapter 24. However, because these proteins are well characterised, they are frequently seen in schemes and theories of oncogenesis.

Target cells
Two main theories about the origins of cancer exist. One is that tumours consist of differentiated cells that have undergone mutation and regressed to an earlier developmental stage (de-differentiation). The newer theory is that mutated stem cells proliferate to form tumours exhibiting varying degrees of differentiation (hence their resemblance to the tissue of origin) and also form a small population of self-renewing cells that are protected against destruction by mechanisms that reflect the normal function of the originating stem cells.

Causes of mutation
Assorted agents can induce mutation:
• Ionising radiation.
• Free radicals.
• Chemicals.
• Some viruses (hepatitis B virus, Epstein–Barr virus, human papilloma virus) integrate their DNA into the nucleus, subverting its function. As viruses require massive synthesis of their nuclear material, enzymes and other proteins, an effect of these nuclear reprogramming mechanisms on other nuclear genes is possible.
• Inherited mutations in cell cycle, growth factor and DNA repair proteins.

The two purines have closely related chemical structures, as do the two pyrimidine bases, such that high energy subatomic particles, molecules bearing unpaired electrons and some chemicals can interconvert them, yielding mutations.

Numerous mutagenic chemical agents are known and include the following:
• Tobacco smoke – tars are the best known but many others exist (Chapter 6).
• Alcohol.
• Chemotherapy drugs – the very nature of these drugs is to damage DNA.
• Industrial chemicals.

Promoting and inducing agents
An inducing agent is one that directly causes a mutation (e.g. polycyclic hydrocarbons). A promoter is one that facilitates circumstances in which an inducer can work, or in which the consequences will be replicated (e.g. bile salt metabolites in Barrett's oesophagus and colorectal carcinoma). Promoters do not directly mutate DNA.

26 Oncogenes and tumour suppressor genes

Effects of oncogenes

('dominant' mutation, i.e. only one allele mutated to produce the effect)

◆ **Secreted products – e.g. growth factors:**
Increased growth factor (autocrine or paracrine effects) or abnormal growth factor production (e.g. c-sis encodes FGF). Many other growth factor mutations are linked to tumours, e.g. PDGF, EGF

◆ **Cell surface – e.g. growth factor receptors:**
Increased growth factor receptor expression or abnormal growth factor receptors (e.g. Her-2-neu encodes EGFR – gene amplification due to mutation indicates that the drug Herceptin will be clinicallly effective)

◆ **Signal transduction pathways:**
Permanent activation of intracellular signalling mechanisms causes continuous signal transduction (e.g. v-src encodes a protein tyrosine kinase, c-ras encodes a membrane-associated G-protein receptor). Ras gene point mutations are the commonest oncogene mutations, e.g. colon, breast and lung cancers

◆ **Nuclear proteins:**
Mutations of the messenger molecules which initiate DNA transcription produce oncoproteins which continually stimulate cell division. Translocation of c-myc to lie beside the Ig gene occurs in Burkitt's lymphoma (t8:14); amplification of myc is seen in breast and lung cancer

◆ **Resistance to apoptosis**
(e.g. BCl-2 mutation prevents caspase activation)

Sites of action of oncogene products

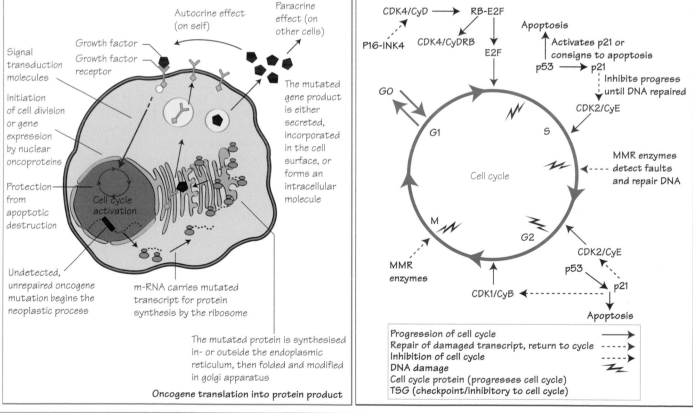

Oncogene translation into protein product

Effects of tumour suppressor genes

('recessive' mutation, i.e. both alleles must be mutated)
Some TSG act on intermediate messengers, e.g. beta-catenin, in the cytoplasm, on microtubules or cell-cell adhesion mechanisms (e.g. APC acts at all these points)

TSGs affecting the cell cycle

◆ **p53, p21, p16-INK4:**
P53 – a 'caretaker gene'. P53 protein is produced if there is DNA damage. If DNA repair is possible, p53 activates transcription of p21 protein. This inhibits CDK, arresting the cell cycle while DNA repair enzymes work. If repair is impossible the cell is consigned to apoptotic death. P53 mutation permits further mutations to occur

◆ **Retinoblastoma gene (RB):**
RB binds transcription factor E2F, preventing it from driving the cell cycle from G1 to S phase. Phosphorylation of RB by CDK causes it to dissociate from E2F. E2F activates DNA transcription genes, allowing progression from G1 to S phase. P16-INK4 binds CDK4/CyD, preventing phosphorylation of RB, this inhibiting progression

◆ **Cyclin kinases (e.g. CyB, D, E) and cyclin dependent kinases (e.g. CDK1, 2, 4):**
They are suppressed by p53, p21 or p16, or non-phosphorylated RB protein

◆ **DNA mismatch repair enzymes (e.g. MLH-1, MSH-2):**
MMR remove mismatched DNA segments and install accurate replacements. These genes protect against spontaneous replicative errors during mitosis

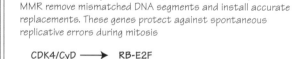

The mechanisms introduced in the preceding chapter are controlled by genes, mutations in which contribute to the development of cancer. These are referred to by the global term 'oncogenes'. The term oncogene has now come to mean a 'dominant' gene whose effects will be felt if only one allele is mutated. These effects usually increase the activity of the gene product (a 'gain of function mutation'), whereas a tumour suppressor gene behaves in a 'recessive' fashion so both alleles must be mutated (a 'loss of function mutation').

Oncogenes

An oncogene arises by mutation of a proto-oncogene. The term is clumsy as proto-oncogenes do not exist to generate oncogenes – they are genes that encode proteins which contribute to normal cell function but if mutated can assist in carcinogenesis. Unlike tumour suppressor genes, most proto-oncogenes require mutation of only one allele to exert their effect.

Subversion of growth factor pathways provides a mechanism by which a neoplastic cell may escape the normal regulation of cell replication. Numerous growth factors exist and influence different tissues. With the exception of steroid hormones, which penetrate the cell membrane to enter the nucleus directly and bind to a nuclear receptor, they tend to share a common pathway: a cell surface receptor signals to the nucleus via a second messenger to effect gene transcription. Mutations in this pathway allow aberrant activation of the signal to initiate replication.

The ras family of oncogenes falls within this category. The ras proteins are activated by binding guanosine triphosphate (GTP). Normally the GTP is rapidly hydrolysed to guanosine diphosphate (GDP), deactivating the ras protein. Mutated ras proteins resist hydrolysis of GTP and remain activated.

Cell surface tyrosine kinases are a second category of growth factor oncogenes. An example is the c-kit oncogene that is encountered in chronic myeloid leukaemia and gastrointestinal stromal tumours. Mutated c-kit is so important to the tumour cells that monoclonal antibodies directed against c-kit provide an effective treatment for both these conditions.

Proteins that promote cell division are another example. Their synthesis is tightly regulated but mutations may affect their transcription or function. For example, in Burkitt's lymphoma, the promoter regions for the immunoglobulin heavy chain gene become fused with the expression sequence for myc, a 'fusion gene' that contributes to the initiation of cell division. This new gene expresses aberrantly high levels of c-myc and the affected cells divide at a very high rate.

An abnormal fusion gene also occurs in follicular lymphoma. A t(14;18)(q32;q21) translocation causes the immunoglobulin heavy chain gene promoter to regulate bcl-2 expression. Bcl-2 is an anti-apoptotic protein and an abnormally high expression of it provides the cell with resistance to apoptosis, a useful property for a tumour cell. Expression of bcl-2 happens in many other B cell lymphomas and many non-haematoreticular tumours.

Another important fusion gene is the Philadelphia chromosome, a t(9;22)(q34;q11) translocation that creates the bcr-abl fusion protein.

It is encountered in chronic myeloblastic leukaemia (CML), but may also be found in some acute leukaemias. It is of considerable diagnostic importance in CML and in monitoring patients for relapse.

Tumour suppressor genes

Tumour suppressor genes (TSGs) encompass those genes that act to detect or repair damaged DNA, or eliminate the affected cell if repair fails. For them to contribute to carcinogenesis, both alleles must be mutated. This is Knudson's 'two hit' hypothesis, epitomised by inherited retinoblastoma (see Chapter 78). The affected protein is encoded by the retinoblastoma 1 (RB-1) gene, a cell cycle regulator that is mutated in a variety of tumours.

Inactivation of RB-1 requires both alleles to be defective (two hits). In inherited retinoblastoma, a germline mutation means that the patient is born with one allele already defective. Therefore, only one somatic mutation is required, whereas a normal individual would need two or

Most familial tumours involve germline TSG mutations in one allele. A later 'sporadic' second mutation affects the remaining allele. Such genes are often rich in cytosine–guanine pairs, which are easily inactivated by methylation. Examples include RB-1, p16 and the APC gene. Other inactivating mutations may involve the deletion of large segments of DNA, which by chance include the TSG.

One of the most important and studied tumour suppressor genes is p53. This versatile protein is upregulated in situations of DNA damage and can both activate the transcription of DNA repair genes and halt the cell cycle pending successful DNA repair. Should the repair processes fail, apoptosis is initiated. The Li–Fraumeni syndrome is a very rare inherited disease in which p53 is mutated; patients develop a variety of tumours.

The DNA mismatch repair enzymes, e.g. MLH-1 and MSH-2 remove mismatched segments and install accurate replacements. These genes protect best against spontaneous replicative errors during mitosis. Inherited defects in them lead to microsatellite instability, seen by the accumulation of multiple small, silent, mutations. Ultimately, some of the mutations are not silent, but the microsatellite instability provides a means for screening for the defect. The hereditary non-polyposis colorectal carcinoma (HNPCC) syndrome is due to mutation of this system.

Apoptosis is a complex biological pathway that has many components, both pro- and anti-apoptotic; the former are in the tumour suppressor category. They include receptors for tumour necrosis factor, the Fas ligand receptor and caspases.

The precise mechanisms of some TSGs, e.g. BRCA1 (inherited breast cancer) and the neurofibromatosis 1 (NF-1) gene is not yet clear.

Telomerases

Telomerases are found in stem cells and some tumour cells. They sustain the telomeres at the end of chromosomal DNA and confer on a cell the ability to replicate an indefinite number of times. Normally, they are only expressed by male germ cells, lymphoid cells and stem cells.

General pathology

The 20 most commonly diagnosed cancers (excluding non-melanoma skin cancers)

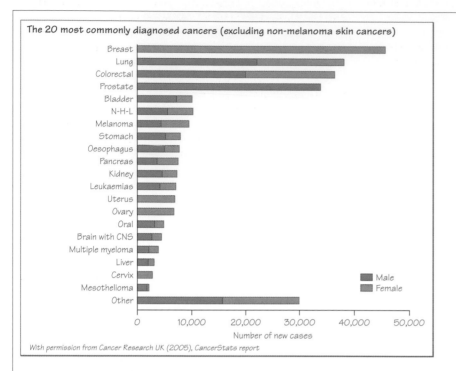

Breast
Lung
Colorectal
Prostate
Bladder
N-H-L
Melanoma
Stomach
Oesophagus
Pancreas
Kidney
Leukaemias
Uterus
Ovary
Oral
Brain with CNS
Multiple myeloma
Liver
Cervix
Mesothelioma
Other

■ Male
■ Female

0   10,000   20,000   30,000   40,000   50,000
Number of new cases

With permission from Cancer Research UK (2005), CancerStats report

The 20 most common causes of death from cancer

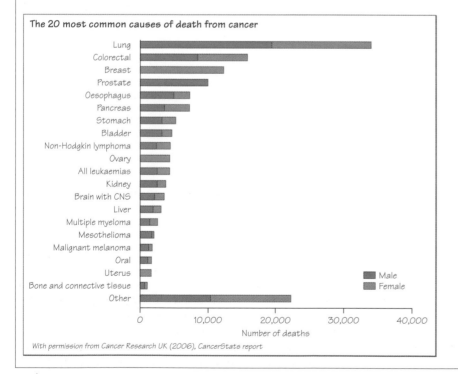

Lung
Colorectal
Breast
Prostate
Oesophagus
Pancreas
Stomach
Bladder
Non-Hodgkin lymphoma
Ovary
All leukaemias
Kidney
Brain with CNS
Liver
Multiple myeloma
Mesothelioma
Malignant melanoma
Oral
Uterus
Bone and connective tissue
Other

■ Male
■ Female

0   10,000   20,000   30,000   40,000
Number of deaths

With permission from Cancer Research UK (2006), CancerStats report

Normal bowel (x40): compare this with colonic adenocarcinoma, below

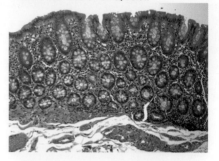

Adenocarcinoma (x40): poorly-formed glands haphazardly infiltrate the tissue

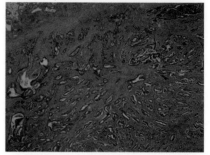

Small cell carcinoma (x200): pleomorphic tumour with smudged dark blue nuclei

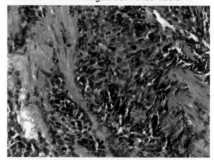

Squamous cell carcinoma (x200): sheets and nests of tumour with pink cytoplasm and focal keratin (arrow)

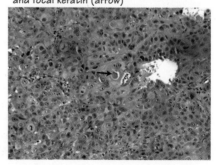

Carcinomas are far more common than sarcomas. The tumours discussed here are the major types of carcinoma. While any of these tumours when seen in a particular organ may exhibit specific nuances, they share generic properties and if these are learnt it is possible to describe a considerable amount of the pathology of the common carcinomas, regardless of the organ of origin.

A carcinoma has some resemblance to the tissue from which it is derived, but displays differences that identify it as malignant. These can be divided into architectural and cytological.

Architectural: By definition, a carcinoma is a malignant tumour of the epithelium and therefore invades the underlying tissue rather than being confined to the epithelium (the semantics of the term carcinoma *in situ* are not addressed here). The carcinoma possesses architectural features that resemble those of the originating tissue, but these are disorganised and less well formed.

Cytological: Carcinoma cells tend to share several nuclear features (these are also common to many non-epithelial malignant tumours):
- Pleomorphism
- Hyperchromatism.
- Nucleolation.
- High nuclear : cytoplasmic ratio.
- Mitotically active.

All of these features reflect the abnormalities in the DNA that underlie the malignant nature of the cell. The increased proliferative activity is seen as an increased number of mitoses, some of which will be abnormally formed due to aneuploidy. The nucleoli reflect active DNA transcription and can therefore be prominent in a carcinoma. Hyperchromatism similarly reflects increased quantities of DNA. The elevated nuclear activity increases the size of the nucleus relative to the cytoplasm. Pleomorphism is a further feature of the abnormal genetic constitution of the tumour (Chapter 24).

Specific carcinomas

The three most common types of carcinoma are described and illustrated in this chapter. Other specific tumour types, e.g. transitional cell carcinoma (TCC), sarcomas, etc., are described in the relevant organ systems later in the book.

Adenocarcinoma

Adenocarcinoma is a malignant tumour of glandular epithelium and is a common tumour type in a wide variety of organs, including the gastrointestinal and hepatobiliary tracts, lung and ovaries.

By definition an adenocarcinomatous tumour must exhibit glandular differentiation. This is usually discerned by the presence of glands. Mucin production is also a feature of an adenocarcinoma, but only occasionally – in poorly differentiated tumours – is it the sole marker of glandular differentiation, without accompanying glandular structures.

Adenocarcinomas are common in a variety of sites and frequently metastasise to the same target organs (lung and liver), thus the ability to distinguish the primary site for metastatic tumours can be helpful given that different primaries require different chemotherapy. Pathognomonic features do not yet exist, but useful markers include the cytokeratin subtypes CK7 and CK20, TTF-1 (thyroid transcription factor 1, found in thyroid but also many lung adenocarcinomas) and CA-125 (ovarian tumours, among others).

Squamous cell carcinoma

Squamous cell carcinoma is a malignant tumour of squamous epithelium. Squamous cell carcinomas can be encountered in a variety of organs and are a common type in the skin, oesophagus, oropharynx, lung, cervix and anus. Other organs, such as the bladder, can develop primary squamous cell carcinomas, but they constitute only a minority of the carcinomas in these regions.

Squamous cell carcinomas have the defining characteristics of keratinisation and the presence of intercellular bridges or prickles. The latter are a fixation artefact in which the intercellular desmosomes are accentuated. The keratinisation may either be in the form of extracellular aggregates or more subtle intracellular keratinisation. In addition, the squamous cells are often particularly large and polyhedral. The nuclear : cytoplasmic ratio is increased, as is the size of the cell, but the absolute quantity of cytoplasm may still be substantial.

Small cell carcinoma

Small cell carcinoma is a high grade malignant tumour that is derived from epithelial neuroendocrine cells. The lung is the main site, but many organs can manifest primary small cell carcinoma, albeit rarely.

The term small cell is not ideal, as the cells are actually 2–3 times the size of a lymphocyte. The designation 'small' refers more to the relative size of the cell compared to other carcinomas. The cells have a very high nuclear : cytoplasmic ratio. Importantly, the cells lack nucleoli, to the extent that the presence of nucleoli warrants reconsideration of the diagnosis. Instead, the cells have finely granular chromatin (often referred to as salt and pepper). Pleomorphism is also a feature that is not marked. The high DNA content of the cells and limited cytoplasm makes them susceptible to deformation. This leads to the phenomenon of moulding, whereby the cells mould their contours to fit and tessellate with their neighbours. An extension of this process is the Azzopardi effect in which the fragility of the cells causes leakage of DNA, which accumulates in blood vessel walls.

Example generic descriptions

Pathology reports tend to read as follows. Try to see the features described here in the photographs opposite.

Adenocarcinoma (colon to illustrate): 'The colon is invaded by a tumour that is composed of irregular glands which vary in shape and size and have complex luminal contours. The glands are lined by hyperchromatic, pleomorphic cells that possess prominent nucleoli. Frequent mitoses are present and include abnormal forms. Nuclear crowding and stratification are present.'

Squamous cell carcinoma (skin to illustrate): 'The skin exhibits invasion by a tumour that is formed of irregular sheets and islands of enlarged, polyhedral cells that have hyperchromatic, pleomorphic, mitotically active nuclei. The nuclear : cytoplasmic ratio is increased. The tumour produces extracellular whorls of keratin and intercellular bridges are observed.'

Small cell carcinoma (lung to illustrate): 'The bronchial biopsy displays invasion by sheets of cells that have a high nuclear : cytoplasmic ratio. The cells possess granular chromatin and show nuclear moulding. Nucleoli are not seen. Frequent mitoses are present. An included blood vessel features the Azzopardi effect (nuclear smearing).'

28 Tumour prognosis and treatment

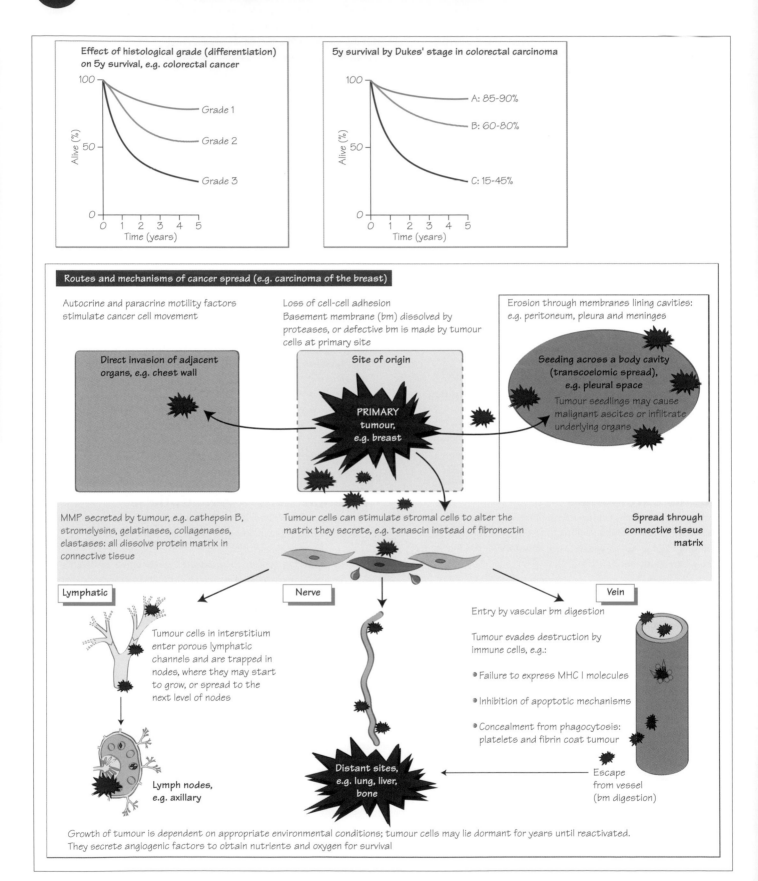

Effect of histological grade (differentiation) on 5y survival, e.g. colorectal cancer

Alive (%) — Time (years)
- Grade 1
- Grade 2
- Grade 3

5y survival by Dukes' stage in colorectal carcinoma

Alive (%) — Time (years)
- A: 85-90%
- B: 60-80%
- C: 15-45%

Routes and mechanisms of cancer spread (e.g. carcinoma of the breast)

Autocrine and paracrine motility factors stimulate cancer cell movement

Loss of cell-cell adhesion
Basement membrane (bm) dissolved by proteases, or defective bm is made by tumour cells at primary site

Erosion through membranes lining cavities: e.g. peritoneum, pleura and meninges

Direct invasion of adjacent organs, e.g. chest wall

Site of origin

PRIMARY tumour, e.g. breast

Seeding across a body cavity (transcoelomic spread), e.g. pleural space
Tumour seedlings may cause malignant ascites or infiltrate underlying organs

MMP secreted by tumour, e.g. cathepsin B, stromelysins, gelatinases, collagenases, elastases: all dissolve protein matrix in connective tissue

Tumour cells can stimulate stromal cells to alter the matrix they secrete, e.g. tenascin instead of fibronectin

Spread through connective tissue matrix

Lymphatic

Tumour cells in interstitium enter porous lymphatic channels and are trapped in nodes, where they may start to grow, or spread to the next level of nodes

Lymph nodes, e.g. axillary

Nerve

Distant sites, e.g. lung, liver, bone

Vein

Entry by vascular bm digestion

Tumour evades destruction by immune cells, e.g.:

- Failure to express MHC I molecules
- Inhibition of apoptotic mechanisms
- Concealment from phagocytosis: platelets and fibrin coat tumour

Escape from vessel (bm digestion)

Growth of tumour is dependent on appropriate environmental conditions; tumour cells may lie dormant for years until reactivated. They secrete angiogenic factors to obtain nutrients and oxygen for survival

Prognosis

Various factors determine tumour prognosis.

Stage

This is the most important parameter and is an assessment of the extent of the primary tumour and its spread, gauged by a combination of clinical evaluation, imaging and pathological examination of specimens.

Various staging systems exist. Many cancers are staged by the TNM system (tumour, nodes, metastases) in which the primary tumour, regional lymph nodes and distant metastases are assessed independently and assigned a score. The nodal parameter reflects the tendency of many carcinomas to spread initially to local lymph nodes, prior to distant metastases. Where necessary, the TNM assessment can be converted to an equivalent clinical stage between 1 and 4. Different stages and TNM scores prompt certain treatment decisions.

Two other important staging systems are the Dukes' classification of colorectal carcinoma and the Ann Arbor system for lymphoma.

Different tumours have different patterns of spread. The reasons are varied and not entirely understood, but include the anatomy of the lymphovascular and venous drainage of the organ (e.g. GI tumours tend to spread to the liver). The type of tumour may influence which organs are a more conducive metastatic environment, while, conversely, some organs seem to have a resistance to metastases (the kidney is affected by surprisingly few metastases given its high blood flow).

Grade

High grade (3) tumours are more aggressive than low grade (1) tumours.

Other factors

- Tumour subtype.
- Suitability of the organ for surgical resection.
- Expression of receptor molecules that can be targeted by drugs (e.g. oestrogen receptors in breast cancer).
- Immunosuppression.
- Cachexia

Treatment

Treatment can be curative or palliative. The same modalities may be used in both, but differ in their intensity. The treatment options are:
- Surgery.
- Radiotherapy.
- Cytotoxic chemotherapy.
- Targeted molecular therapy.

Both chemotherapy and radiotherapy work on the premise that more cancer cells than normal cells are in the proliferative phase and are therefore vulnerable to DNA damage. Normal cells are not immune, but treatment aims to kill more cancer cells than normal cells, achieved by fractionating the dose.

Future options may include:
- Targeting tumour cell gene products.
- Induction of differentiation to non-proliferative mature tissues.
- Gene therapy.
- Stem cell transplantation.

Palliative therapy attempts to alleviate symptoms in patients in whom cure is not possible.

Cure and tumour-free survival

Previously, survival for 5 years after cancer diagnosis was considered to denote cure. With improved treatments many people survive for 5 years with a residual tumour burden so the terminology has become 'disease-free survival'. However, it remains a convenient way of comparing outcomes and is supplemented by survival curves that plot the percentage of patients still alive against the time post diagnosis.

For any given tumour, stage greatly affects the 5-year survival. As a general rule of thumb, 5-year survival rates (5YSR) by stages are:
- Stage 1: 80–90%.
- Stage 2: 60%.
- Stage 3: 40%.
- Stage 4: 0–20%.

This is very approximate. Hodgkin's lymphoma is a notable exception, as even stage 4 disease has a 5YSR of around 50%.

Tumours that have a poor 5YSR do so for two main reasons. Tumours with a poor prognosis may be intrinsically aggressive and/or resistant to treatment. However, the tumour's behaviour may be such that it tends to present with late stage disease, by which point curative options are dwindling; yet if the tumour was detected at stage 1, the 5YSR might be very good (e.g. ovarian carcinoma).

Tumours with a very poor 5YSR include stomach (9%), lung (5%), oesophagus (5%) and pancreas (2.4%).

Prevention

Screening

Screening aims to detect a cancer either at a preinvasive stage or, failing that, at stage 1. Certain properties must apply for a screening programme to be successful:

1 Tumour behaviour can be predicted sufficiently for intervention to be successful, ideally by identifying non-invasive disease.
2 Treatment is available.
3 The target population has enough people at risk to justify the expense of a screening campaign (either national or specific subgroups).
4 There is a cost-effective and reliable screening tool.
5 The tool is acceptable to the screenable population.
6 A diagnostic test is available to follow up a positive screening test.
7 Repetition of screening is feasible if necessary.

In the UK, cervical cancer and breast cancer screening occur and piloting of colorectal cancer screening has recently commenced.

Breast cancer screening provokes debate. Some suggest that it has revealed small in situ carcinomas that may never have manifested invasive disease during life and only cause worry, surgery and expense. Others suggest that early identification of these tumours has greatly reduced the long-term risk of death from breast cancer.

Colorectal cancer screening employs the faecal occult blood (FOB) test, followed by colonoscopy in FOB-positive people. The FOB is notorious for false positives and some colorectal cancers do not bleed. Faecal screening for mutated genes, like ras, may supersede FOB.

Certain industries, like the rubber and dye industries, involve carcinogenic chemicals such that targeted screening of workers becomes viable.

The Japanese incidence of gastric carcinoma is high enough to justify screening. The Japanese regularly identify early gastric carcinoma, which has a 95% 5YSR, compared with the 9% 5YSR for gastric carcinoma as a whole.

Vaccination

Virally induced cancers (human papilloma virus (HPV) and cervical carcinoma, hepatitis B virus (HBV) and hepatocellular carcinoma) can be prevented if infection never occurs. Effective vaccines for HBV and HPV exist.

Systems pathology

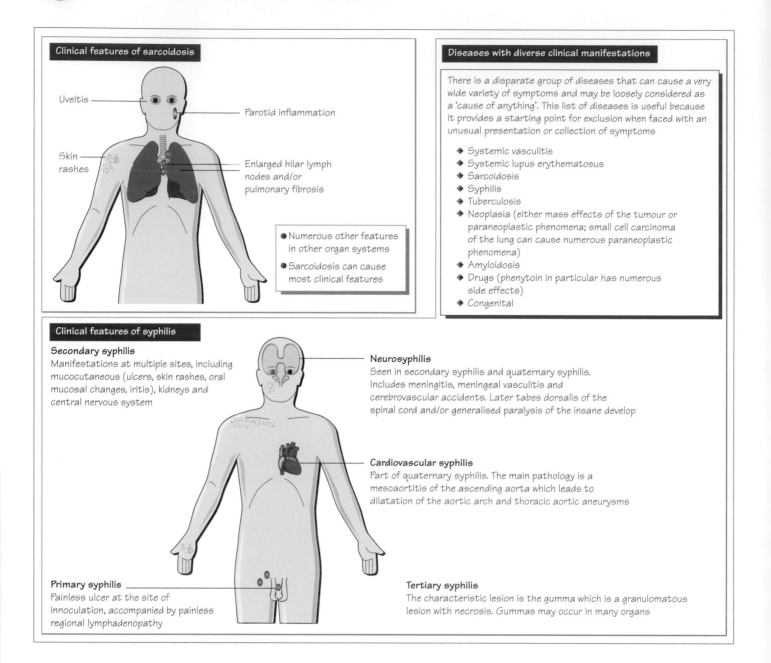

Clinical features of sarcoidosis

Uveitis

Parotid inflammation

Skin rashes

Enlarged hilar lymph nodes and/or pulmonary fibrosis

- Numerous other features in other organ systems
- Sarcoidosis can cause most clinical features

Diseases with diverse clinical manifestations

There is a disparate group of diseases that can cause a very wide variety of symptoms and may be loosely considered as a 'cause of anything'. This list of diseases is useful because it provides a starting point for exclusion when faced with an unusual presentation or collection of symptoms

- ◆ Systemic vasculitis
- ◆ Systemic lupus erythematosus
- ◆ Sarcoidosis
- ◆ Syphilis
- ◆ Tuberculosis
- ◆ Neoplasia (either mass effects of the tumour or paraneoplastic phenomena; small cell carcinoma of the lung can cause numerous paraneoplastic phenomena)
- ◆ Amyloidosis
- ◆ Drugs (phenytoin in particular has numerous side effects)
- ◆ Congenital

Clinical features of syphilis

Secondary syphilis
Manifestations at multiple sites, including mucocutaneous (ulcers, skin rashes, oral mucosal changes, iritis), kidneys and central nervous system

Neurosyphilis
Seen in secondary syphilis and quaternary syphilis. Includes meningitis, meningeal vasculitis and cerebrovascular accidents. Later tabes dorsalis of the spinal cord and/or generalised paralysis of the insane develop

Cardiovascular syphilis
Part of quaternary syphilis. The main pathology is a mesoaortitis of the ascending aorta which leads to dilatation of the aortic arch and thoracic aortic aneurysms

Primary syphilis
Painless ulcer at the site of innoculation, accompanied by painless regional lymphadenopathy

Tertiary syphilis
The characteristic lesion is the gumma which is a granulomatous lesion with necrosis. Gummas may occur in many organs

Sarcoidosis

Definition

Sarcoidosis is a chronic, multisystem granulomatous disease of uncertain aetiology.

Epidemiology

The prevalence is 10–40 per 100 000. The presentation is usually between 20 and 40 years and the disease is slightly more common in females. The condition is found worldwide, but the highest incidence is in Scandinavia. Afro-Caribbeans have a higher incidence.

Pathology

The disease is characterised by the presence of non-caseating granulomas that can develop in a wide variety of organs. Fibrosis may accompany the granulomatous response.

The granulomas are typically described as 'naked' in that there is little associated lymphocytic infiltrate. The macrophages within the granulomas may also include concretions known as asteroid bodies and Schaumann bodies. However, none of these features, either alone or in combination, is diagnostic of sarcoidosis. Furthermore, it is possible for the granulomas to show necrosis. Therefore, histology alone cannot offer an unequivocal diagnosis. Instead, the histology must be considered in the overall clinical context.

The cause of the granulomas is unknown. Atypical mycobacteria have been postulated, but this hypothesis has not been proven.

As well as the granulomatous and fibrotic process, a vasculitic element to the disease may be encountered, particularly in the lung.

While sarcoid can affect any organ system in the body, the lungs are one of the principal sites. Pulmonary disease can either take the form of hilar lymphadenopathy alone, hilar lymphadenopathy and pulmonary fibrosis, or pulmonary fibrosis alone, or rarely a necrotising granulomatous vasculitis. Lymph nodes outside the mediastinum are also frequently involved in sarcoidosis.

- The skin is affected in 25%.
- Ocular involvement is found in 25% and is usually in the form of uveitis.
- Arthralgia or arthritis occurs in up to 50%.
- Other organs are affected less frequently, although parotid involvement, when combined with uveitis is characteristic.

Clinical correlations

Simply knowing that sarcoidosis is a multisystem granulomatous disease makes remembering many of the potential clinical features easier, although the typical distribution still has to be learnt.

Hypercalcaemia can develop in one in 10 patients with sarcoidosis and is due to the presence of the 1α vitamin D hydroxylase enzyme within the macrophages of the sarcoid granulomas. The activity of this enzyme leads to excess activated vitamin D, which raises blood calcium.

Prognosis

Many patients do very well in the long term, either recovering spontaneously, or after treatment with glucocorticoids.

Syphilis

Definition

Syphilis is a sexually transmitted infection that is caused by the spirochaete *Treponema pallidum*.

Epidemiology

Until recently, the incidence of syphilis in the UK was under 1000 cases per year for the entire population, but the disease may be making a small resurgence. The disease is found worldwide, although it has been suggested that dissemination of the organism to all parts of the globe was a consequence of migration and exploration.

Pathology

Treponema pallidum is a spirochaete that does not stain with normal methods, instead requiring specialised techniques such as Young's stain. Infection is via the mucosal membranes, usually by sexual transmission. The immune response to syphilis is granulomatous and this brings with it fibrosis. Vasculitis also occurs at certain stages and in certain organs.

Infection with *Treponema pallidum* is chronic and can persist for decades. Four stages are described:

1 Primary syphilis is the initial infection and presents around 2 weeks after infection. The characteristic lesion is a painless ulcer on the affected organ, usually the penis, vulva or vagina, that is associated with painless lymphadenopathy.

2 Secondary syphilis occurs approximately 6–8 weeks after the primary infection and has a myriad of features that include a skin rash (which can affect the palms and soles), mouth ulcers and other oral mucosal lesions, lymphadenopathy, fever, iritis, hepatitis and glomerulonephritis.

3 Tertiary syphilis develops at least 3 years after the primary infection and is characterised by the gumma, which consists of a collection of granulomas that surround a central region of necrosis. Many organs can be affected, although bowing of the tibia is characteristic.

4 Quaternary syphilis encompasses cardiovascular syphilis and neurosyphilis. Cardiovascular syphilis arises after 10–40 years and is a mesoaortitis of the thoracic aorta. This affects the vasa vasorum of the aorta, leading to damage to the tunica media and elastic laminae. Although fibrosis takes place, the aortic wall is structurally compromised and aneurysm develops.

Neurosyphilis is complex and features various stages that span the more general divisions of syphilis. Meningeal neurosyphilis is seen in the first 2 years and presents with a headache, cranial nerve palsies, seizures or confusion.

Meningovascular syphilis presents around 6–7 years. The pathological process is inflammation of the pia and arachnoid mater in association with vasculitis. The vasculitis can cause a cerebrovascular accident. The spinal cord may be affected as well as the brain.

Generalised paralysis of the insane and tabes dorsalis occur around 15–20 years after the initial infection and fall into the quaternary stage. The former shows meningeal fibrosis and cerebral atrophy, with ongoing chronic inflammation around the blood vessels. Assorted focal neurological defects that would correspond to a focal cerebral lesion can be seen, as well as dementia. Tabes dorsalis is produced by demyelination of the posterior columns, dorsal roots and dorsal root ganglia of the spinal cord. Hence, the features are those that would be expected from a loss of fine touch and conscious proprioception, together with a more panmodality sensory impairment due to damage to the sensory information contained within the dorsal roots.

Systems pathology

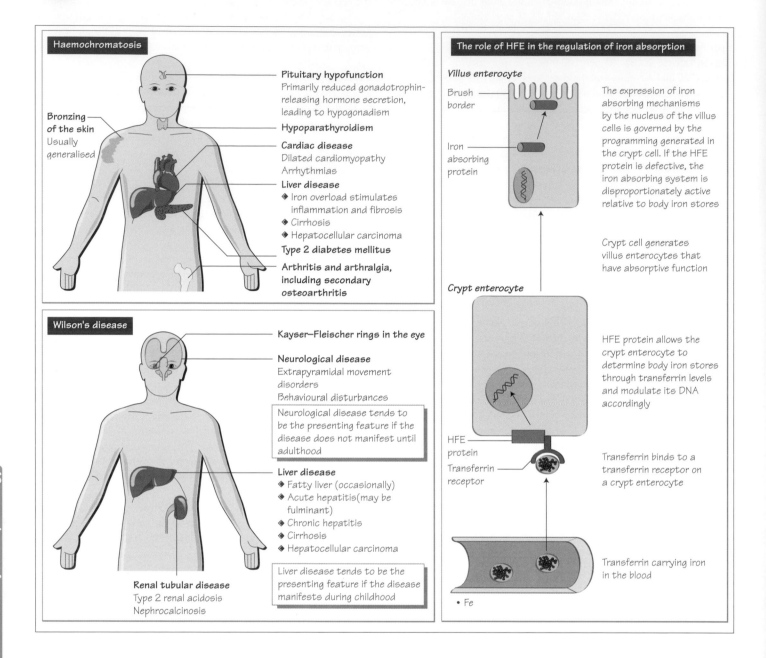

Haemochromatosis

Pituitary hypofunction
Primarily reduced gonadotrophin-releasing hormone secretion, leading to hypogonadism

Hypoparathyroidism

Cardiac disease
Dilated cardiomyopathy
Arrhythmias

Liver disease
◆ Iron overload stimulates inflammation and fibrosis
◆ Cirrhosis
◆ Hepatocellular carcinoma

Type 2 diabetes mellitus

Arthritis and arthralgia, including secondary osteoarthritis

Bronzing of the skin
Usually generalised

Wilson's disease

Kayser–Fleischer rings in the eye

Neurological disease
Extrapyramidal movement disorders
Behavioural disturbances

Neurological disease tends to be the presenting feature if the disease does not manifest until adulthood

Liver disease
◆ Fatty liver (occasionally)
◆ Acute hepatitis(may be fulminant)
◆ Chronic hepatitis
◆ Cirrhosis
◆ Hepatocellular carcinoma

Liver disease tends to be the presenting feature if the disease manifests during childhood

Renal tubular disease
Type 2 renal acidosis
Nephrocalcinosis

The role of HFE in the regulation of iron absorption

Villus enterocyte

Brush border

Iron absorbing protein

The expression of iron absorbing mechanisms by the nucleus of the villus cells is governed by the programming generated in the crypt cell. If the HFE protein is defective, the iron absorbing system is disproportionately active relative to body iron stores

Crypt cell generates villus enterocytes that have absorptive function

Crypt enterocyte

HFE protein allows the crypt enterocyte to determine body iron stores through transferrin levels and modulate its DNA accordingly

HFE protein
Transferrin receptor

Transferrin binds to a transferrin receptor on a crypt enterocyte

Transferrin carrying iron in the blood

• Fe

72 *Pathology at a Glance.* By C.J. Finlayson and B.A.T. Newell. Published 2009 by Blackwell Publishing. ISBN: 978-1-4051-3650-1

Wilson's disease

Definition
Wilson's disease is an autosomal recessive inherited condition in which there is impaired hepatic secretion of copper that results in toxic accumulation of copper.

Epidemiology
Wilson's disease is rare and has a prevalence of 30 per 1 000 000. The male : female ratio is equal. The disease usually presents between 5 and 30 years.

Pathology
The gene is located on chromosome 13q14.3–21.1 and codes for an ATPase protein (ATP7B) that is necessary for the excretion of copper in the bile. Impairment of this gene interferes with the excretion of excess copper.

Copper is an essential mineral that is normally present in the body as a prosthetic component of proteins such as cytochrome oxidase, superoxide dismutase and tyrosinase, or stored in carrier proteins, such as caeruloplasmin. Free copper is toxic and induces damage via the generation of oxygen free radicals (which is interesting given copper's role as part of superoxide dismutase in protecting against free radicals).

The accumulation of copper occurs throughout the body but the organs that characteristically show effects are the liver, brain, eye and, to a lesser publicised extent, the kidney.
- In the liver, the initial changes are the deposition of fat and glycogen in the mitochondria. This progresses to hepatocyte necrosis and attendant inflammation. When chronic, such processes are the basis of chronic hepatitis and cirrhosis.
- Although copper gathers in the entire brain, the basal ganglia first bear the brunt of the damage. Neuronal loss occurs, myelinated fibres degenerate and there is a proliferation of astrocytes. Macroscopic changes may be seen in the lenticular nuclei, which are shrunken and discoloured brown.
- Accumulation of copper in the iris causes the characteristic Kayser–Fleischer ring. This is highly suggestive of Wilson's disease. Sunflower cataracts can also occur.
- The failure of the liver to deal with the copper excretory load places an excessive burden on the kidney. The renal tubules react badly to the strain and damage to them yields type II renal tubular acidosis (in which there is proteinuria, aminoaciduria, glycosuria, hypercalcuria and bicarbonate wasting).

Clinical correlations
Wilson's disease can produce the gamut of liver disorders, ranging from steatosis or acute hepatitis (which may be fulminant) through chronic hepatitis to cirrhosis and hepatocellular carcinoma. The cirrhosis is typically macronodular.

Neurological disease is centred around extrapyramidal movement disorders, which on occasion may resemble Parkinson's disease and in general encompass dyskinesia and akinetic-rigid syndromes. There are typically also behavioural disturbances.

For reasons that are not clearly understood, there is usually a marked reduction in the blood levels of caeruloplasmin, the protein that carries copper in the blood.

Prognosis
Treatment with copper chelating agents such as penicillamine, coupled with dietary measures, are very effective.

Haemochromatosis

Definition
Haemochromatosis is an autosomal recessive disease in which there is excessive absorption of iron from the small intestine, leading to iron overload.

Epidemiology
The prevalence of homozygotes is 3000 per 1 000 000. Presentation is generally between 40 and 60 years. The male : female ratio is 5–10 : 1 due to the protective effective of menstruation, which provides an alternative mechanism for the elimination of excess iron.

Pathology
The gene is situated on chromosome 6p21.3, although alternative loci have been described for variants of the disease. The protein is designated HFE. There is a linkage with the human leucocyte antigen (HLA) types A3 and B14.

The HFE protein is found on duodenal crypt enterocytes and is associated with the transferrin receptor. It is believed to be involved in enabling the crypt and villus to determine body iron stores and adjust the degree of iron absorption accordingly. Perturbation of this mechanism in haemochromatosis results in inappropriately elevated absorption of iron.

Like free copper, free iron causes tissue damage by increasing oxidative injury. However, the range of organs that are affected is different.
- The liver shows haemosiderosis, chronic hepatitis, fibrosis and/or cirrhosis. Hepatocellular carcinoma complicates 30% of these cases of cirrhosis.
- Deposition of iron and melanin in the dermis yields a characteristic bronzing of the skin.
- Diabetes mellitus occurs, although exocrine pancreatic dysfunction is rare. It has been suggested that the cause of the diabetes mellitus may be in part related to disrupted handling of chromium, given that chromium is essential for the normal function of insulin and competes with iron to be bound by transferrin.
- The pituitary is often affected, usually in the form of defective gonadotrophin release, which leads to hypogonadism.
- Other endocrine organs are often involved, e.g. thyroid.
- The iron is also toxic to the heart and can produce a dilated cardiomyopathy, as well as assorted arrhythmias due to damage to the conducting system.
- An arthropathy is found in 25–50% and characteristically involves the second and third metacarpals. Secondary osteoarthritis can develop.

Clinical correlations
Most of the clinical features are predictable from an understanding of the pathology. This extends to the biochemical features. Serum iron, hepatic iron content and urinary iron content are all increased due to the elevated absorption of iron and raised iron load. Ferritin increases. Transferrin saturation is high due to the large amount of iron present to occupy the binding sites. Therefore, the remaining total iron binding capacity is low as it is already largely employed.

Prognosis
Venesection removes the excess iron and can result in improvements in most of the affected organs.

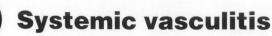

Systems pathology

Clinical features of Wegener's granulomatosis

- Upper respiratory tract disease such as epistaxis, nasal septum destruction, laryngeal damage
- Pulmonary disease including cavitating lung lesions
- Glomerulonephritis

- Numerous other clinical features can develop in any organ systems
- As with polyarteritis nodosa and microscopic polyarteritis, Wegener's granulomatosis can present with almost any clinical feature

Typical distribution of different types of vasculitis

Wegener's granulomatosis

- Necrotising granulomatous vasculitis. cANCA +
  M= F
  Usually middle-aged
- Nose
- Lung
- Kidney

Churg-Strauss

- Rare granulomatous vasculitis affecting any small/medium sized vessels
- Marked eosinophil infiltrate present
- Patients usually appear asthmatic due to lung vessel involvement. cANCA+

Buerger's

- Young male smokers
- Develop severe atheroma in arteries of lower leg

Giant cell arteritis

- F:M = 2:1 Usually >50 years
- Superficial temporal artery biopsied for diagnosis, risk is from damage to retinal and cerebral arteries
- >50% have granulomas

Takayasu's

- Young Far Eastern females
- Aortic arch and branches
- <50% have granulomas

Henoch–Schönlein purpura (HSP)

- Affects small blood vessels in skin and gut
- Children. IgA complexes. Good prognosis

Polyarteritis nodosa (PAN) and microscopic polyarteritis (MPA)

- Very variable in their distribution and have a wide age range
- In PAN medium-sized arteries and veins are involved
  F:M 2:1
- MPA is a necrotising vasculitis of small vessels which is pANCA –ve
  M = F

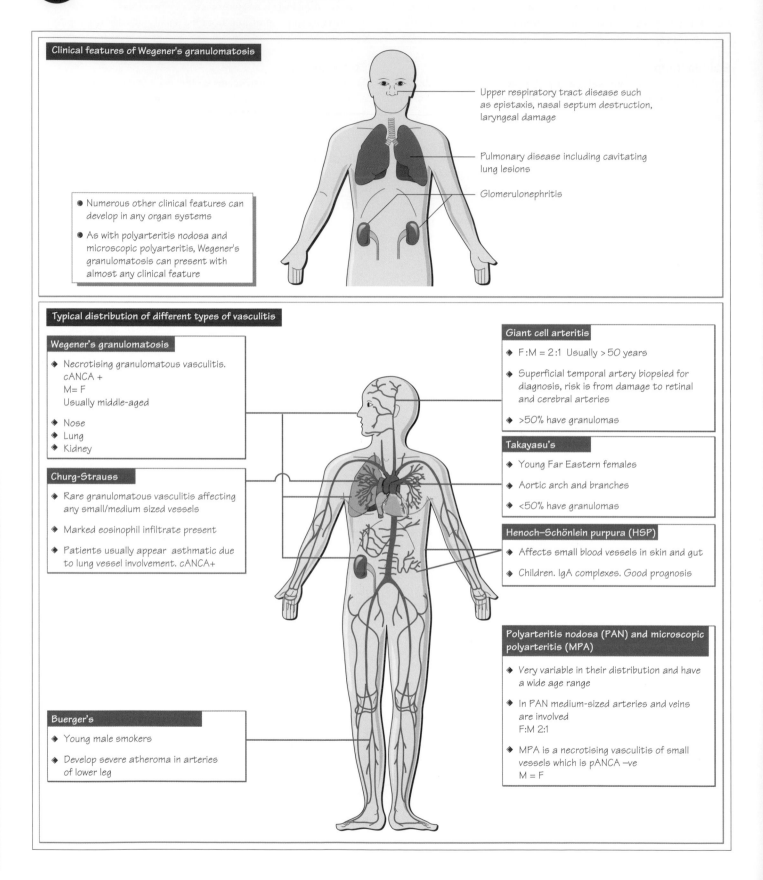

The systemic vasculitides are a group of conditions that are characterised by inflammation of blood vessels throughout multiple organ systems. Each type of vasculitis has specific elements to its pathology and clinical presentation, but there are common elements.

Common pathology

Inflammation of the blood vessel is seen as an infiltrate of one or more types of inflammatory cells into the wall of the vessel. This is often associated with fibrinoid necrosis of the wall of the vessel. The inflammation and damage to the wall of the blood vessel can result in ischaemia of the tissue supplied by the vessel, thrombosis and haemorrhage.

With the capacity to cause ischaemia, vasculitic diseases can produce a myriad of clinical features given that almost all organs in the body are vascularised. The pattern of features seen in the different types of vasculitis reflects the organs that are particularly affected and the size of the vessels that are involved.

Wegener's granulomatosis

Wegener's granulomatosis is a necrotising, granulomatous vasculitis that can affect a wide range of ages but tends to present around 40 years. The prevalence is 10 per 1 000 000. The male to female ratio is equal. The disease is rare in Afro-Caribbeans.

Pathology

The disease affects small arteries and veins and is characterised by a necrotising granulomatous inflammatory infiltrate.

The upper and lower respiratory tract and kidney are the two characteristic sites of involvement. The upper respiratory tract includes the nose and paranasal sinuses and involvement in these locations can present as epistaxis, nasal septal perforation or nasal bridge collapse. Renal involvement is in the form of glomerulonephritis that can be crescentic. Renal involvement, as with other organs, may not necessarily include the presence of granulomas.

While the respiratory tract and glomerulonephritis sites may be the classical distribution, any organ can be affected, including the eye and nervous system. As with other vasculitides, neurological disease may include a mononeuritis multiplex.

There are antineutrophil cytoplasmic antibodies that are targeted against proteinase-3 of the neutrophil antibodies. This variant of ANCAs is known as c-ANCA (c denoting cytoplasmic) and, while very suggestive of Wegener's granulomatosis, is not pathogmonic.

Microscopic polyarteritis

Microscopic polyarteritis affects small arteries and veins in numerous organ systems. The prevalence is approximately 6–7 per 1 000 000. The age range is wide and the male to female ratio is equal. Renal disease is particularly common. ANCAs are present, but tend to be of the p-ANCA type (p signifying perinuclear), directed against myeloperoxidase.

Polyarteritis nodosa

Polyarteritis nodosa is another necrotising vasculitis, but unlike Wegener's granulomatosis the affected vessels are small and medium sized. The prevalence is 2–3 per 1 000 000. The age range is wide. The male : female ratio is 2 : 1. There is associated hepatitis B virus infection in 20–30%.

Pathology

In the early stages, the inflammatory infiltrate in an involved vessel is composed of neutrophils and eosinophils. Fibrinoid necrosis is present. The process is transmural and may extend into the surrounding tissues. The whole circumference is inflamed in small vessels, whereas the distribution may be segmental in larger vessels. Rupture of the vessel can occur.

Later, the inflammatory response switches to chronic inflammatory cells. The wall exhibits fibrosis and there can be aneurysms.

Most organs can be affected, although the pulmonary arteries are typically spared.

Churg–Strauss syndrome

Churg–Strauss syndrome is a very rare, necrotising granulomatous vasculitis that involves small blood vessels. It is characterised by peripheral blood eosinophilia and pulmonary involvement that resembles asthma. Clinical features can also be present in multiple other organ systems.

Giant cell arteritis

This disease is also known as temporal arteritis and is a granulomatous vasculitis of medium to large vessels, mainly those of the head. It is rare before 50 years, but has an incidence of 15–20 per 100 000 per year over the age of 50. The male : female ratio is 1 : 2. There is an association with polymyalgia rheumatica.

Pathology

The artery shows chronic inflammation that features granulomas. The inflammation is often discontinuous, such that an afflicted artery may nevertheless have normal regions. This can cause problems in determining the significance of a normal temporal artery biopsy. Disruption of the integrity of the internal elastic lamina by inflammation is seen, or the lamina may be reduplicated.

In addition to the headache associated with disease in the temporal artery, there can also be retinal ischaemia causing blindness, claudication of the jaw and tongue and cerebrovascular accidents. Rarely, the aortic arch is involved.

Takayasu's arteritis

Takayasu's arteritis occurs in medium-sized and large vessels, typically the aortic arch and its branches. It is rare and is most frequently encountered in the Far East. Patients tend to be young and female.

Pathology

The inflammation is initially located in the adventitia and vasa vasorum of the artery and progresses to fibrosis. The inflammation is composed of chronic inflammatory cells.

As well as the aortic arch, the carotid, subclavian, femoral and renal arteries can be affected and the clinical features reflect ischaemia in the territories of these vessels.

Systems pathology

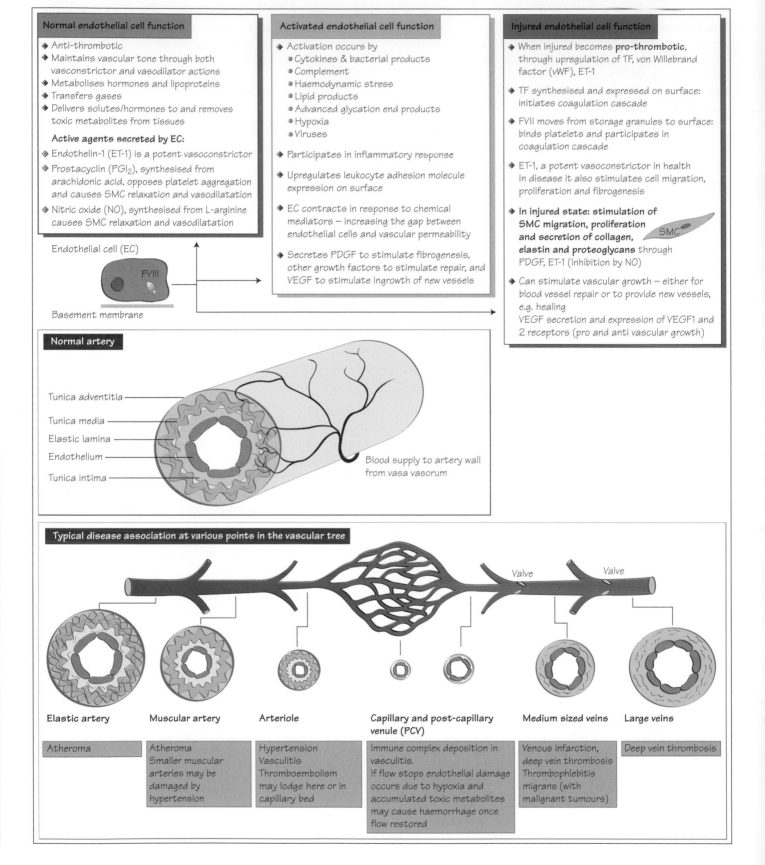

Normal endothelial cell function

◆ Anti-thrombotic
◆ Maintains vascular tone through both vasoconstrictor and vasodilator actions
◆ Metabolises hormones and lipoproteins
◆ Transfers gases
◆ Delivers solutes/hormones to and removes toxic metabolites from tissues

Active agents secreted by EC:
◆ Endothelin-1 (ET-1) is a potent vasoconstrictor
◆ Prostacyclin (PGI_2), synthesised from arachidonic acid, opposes platelet aggregation and causes SMC relaxation and vasodilatation
◆ Nitric oxide (NO), synthesised from L-arginine causes SMC relaxation and vasodilatation

Endothelial cell (EC)

FVIII

Basement membrane

Activated endothelial cell function

◆ Activation occurs by
  ● Cytokines & bacterial products
  ● Complement
  ● Haemodynamic stress
  ● Lipid products
  ● Advanced glycation end products
  ● Hypoxia
  ● Viruses
◆ Participates in inflammatory response
◆ Upregulates leukocyte adhesion molecule expression on surface
◆ EC contracts in response to chemical mediators – increasing the gap between endothelial cells and vascular permeability
◆ Secretes PDGF to stimulate fibrogenesis, other growth factors to stimulate repair, and VEGF to stimulate ingrowth of new vessels

Injured endothelial cell function

◆ When injured becomes **pro-thrombotic**, through upregulation of TF, von Willebrand factor (vWF), ET-1
◆ TF synthesised and expressed on surface: initiates coagulation cascade
◆ FVII moves from storage granules to surface: binds platelets and participates in coagulation cascade
◆ ET-1, a potent vasoconstrictor in health In disease it also stimulates cell migration, proliferation and fibrogenesis
◆ **In injured state: stimulation of SMC migration, proliferation and secretion of collagen, elastin and proteoglycans** through PDGF, ET-1 (Inhibition by NO)   SMC
◆ Can stimulate vascular growth – either for blood vessel repair or to provide new vessels, e.g. healing VEGF secretion and expression of VEGF1 and 2 receptors (pro and anti vascular growth)

Normal artery

Tunica adventitia
Tunica media
Elastic lamina
Endothelium
Tunica intima

Blood supply to artery wall from vasa vasorum

Typical disease association at various points in the vascular tree

Valve   Valve

Elastic artery	Muscular artery	Arteriole	Capillary and post-capillary venule (PCV)	Medium sized veins	Large veins
Atheroma	Atheroma Smaller muscular arteries may be damaged by hypertension	Hypertension Vasculitis Thromboembolism may lodge here or in capillary bed	Immune complex deposition in vasculitis. If flow stops endothelial damage occurs due to hypoxia and accumulated toxic metabolites may cause haemorrhage once flow restored	Venous infarction, deep vein thrombosis Thrombophlebitis migrans (with malignant tumours)	Deep vein thrombosis

76 *Pathology at a Glance*. By C.J. Finlayson and B.A.T. Newell. Published 2009 by Blackwell Publishing. ISBN: 978-1-4051-3650-1

The figure outlines the important features of arteries and veins of different calibre. The smaller muscular arteries and arterioles determine the mean arterial pressure and have a basal tone that is partially regulated by factors secreted by the endothelium, which acts on the vascular smooth muscle cells (SMCs), and partially by the autonomic nervous system. The SMCs are arranged around the lumen in a spiral fashion and the basal tone is a balance between vasodilatation and vasoconstriction. The sympathetic and parasympathetic nerves run in the tunica adventitia and can stimulate the SMCs directly or via endothelial cells.

Endothelium

This flattened cell type lines the entire vascular tree and is one of the most metabolically active cells. It develops from the embryonic mesoderm and is *not* a type of epithelium.

Endothelial cell properties vary along the vascular tree – e.g. larger vessels, more liable to endothelial damage by shearing forces, contain more vWF. At the capillary level, the endothelium is freely permeable to gases and allows movement of solutes and metabolites along concentration gradients, though less quickly and freely than gases.

Two of the most important of the many functions of unstimulated endothelium are the maintenance of peripheral vascular resistance and the prevention of thrombosis. Many different agents can activate endothelium. Activation induces new or increased gene expression of the following:
• Adhesion molecules.
• Cytokines.
• Growth factors.
• Vasoactive mediators.
• MHC molecules: MHC I molecules are constitutively expressed, but numbers increase with stimulation. MHC II molecules can occasionally be induced in endothelial cells.

Some endothelial changes are of rapid onset (minutes) – for instance the reversible vasodilatation and increase in vascular permeability associated with histamine release, or exposure of tissue factor (TF) on the cell surface – but new protein synthesis or alteration in gene expression requires hours or days.

Damaged endothelium loses its antithrombotic properties and its surface becomes thrombogenic and abnormally adhesive to inflammatory cells. Increased numbers of MHC I molecules are displayed on the cell surface. This is important in initiating thrombosis and in atherosclerosis.

The endothelial cell plays a key role in angiogenesis (important in healing and repair and neoplasia).

Capillary endothelial subtypes
• **Continuous**: typical of skin, muscle, lungs and, most importantly, the central nervous system, where the very tight cell–cell junctions protect the brain from the blood-borne entry of damaging agents (the 'blood–brain barrier'). The basement membrane layer is complete, sheathing the capillary and adding an extra layer of protection.
• **Fenestrated**: e.g. renal glomerulus or intestinal villi. There are gaps between endothelial cells through which fluid and solutes can pass freely, though larger molecules (e.g. albumin, other plasma proteins) and blood cells are retained. The basement membrane is intact and solutes and fluid must filter through this mesh of collagen and negatively charged glycoprotein to reach their destination.
• **Discontinuous**: e.g. liver or splenic sinusoids. Large gaps exist between endothelial cells with corresponding basement membrane

defects. Erythrocytes and plasma proteins pass freely through the gaps. The blood eventually drains back into the veins. Leukocytes can also pass through. Macrophages line the sinusoids and engulf bacteria and other particles, removing them from the circulation – particularly important in the spleen, where blood-borne pathogens can be presented to lymphoid tissue for an immune response.

(Lymphatic endothelium is discontinuous in the bulb-like sacs in which the lymph vessels originate and becomes continuous as the vessel calibre increases; a muscle layer develops in the walls of medium-sized and larger lymphatics.)

Vascular smooth muscle cells

SMCs can contract or relax in response to stimuli – either endothelial, catecholamines released by the sympathetic nervous system or angiotensin II. They can migrate to and proliferate in the intima after injury. SMCs also have fibroblast-like functions (synthesis of collagen, elastin and proteoglycans; growth factors and cytokines). This is important in the generation of the fibrous cap, which stabilises atheromatous plaques.

Aneursyms
• Aneurysms occur when there is severe erosion of the media.
• An aneurysm is a bulge in the wall of a blood vessel.
• Aneurysms occur in arteries and occasionally the left ventricle (post myocardial infarction) but are very rare in veins.
• Aneurysms occur at points of weakness:
  • usually due to atheroma;
  • sometimes due to inflammatory damage (e.g. syphilis);
  • occasionally connective tissue abnormalities (e.g. Marfan's);
  • sometimes following trauma, e.g. partial medial tear, often due to a traffic accident.

Types of aneurysm
• **Fusiform aneurysms**: most aneurysms are fusiform (spindle shaped) (typical of atheroma).
• **Saccular aneurysms**: these often occur after focal vessel damage, e.g. trauma or infection. Bacteria from the bloodstream may lodge in an atheromatous plaque – which can be seen following an operation on a bacteria-rich site like bowel – when there is often a transient bacteraemia. The roughened wall over an atheromatous plaque, often with overlying thrombus, provides a nidus for infection.
• **Berry aneurysm**: a berry aneurysm (congenital weakness in the media at the branching points of cerebral vessels) is not related to atheroma.
• **Aortic dissection** (previously called 'dissecting aneurysm'): this is only of partial thickness and is not a true aneurysm, but is usually considered with aneurysms. Dissection is typical of Marfan's syndrome but may occur in the elderly, in whom medial degeneration is not uncommon – a tear in the intima allows blood to track along a congenitally weak media. This may rupture back into the aorta ('double-barrelled aorta') or rupture through the adventitia, causing death by cardiac tamponade or exsanguination. It is unusual for aortic dissection to complicate atheroma.

Complications of aneurysms
• Rupture.
• Thrombosis.
• Thromboembolism.

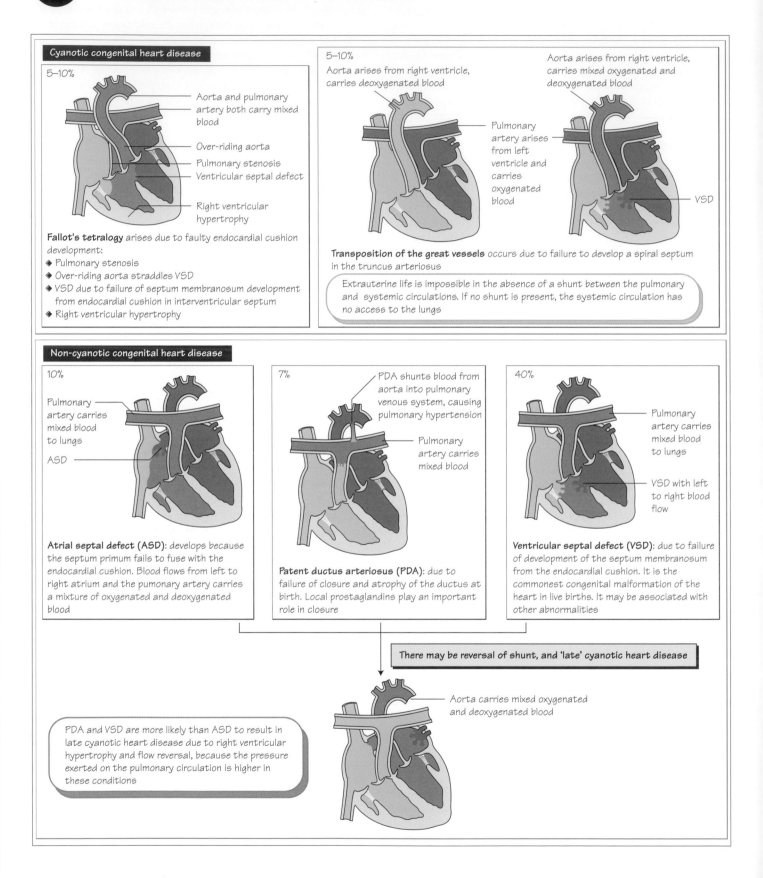

Cyanotic congenital heart disease

5–10%

Aorta and pulmonary artery both carry mixed blood

Over-riding aorta
Pulmonary stenosis
Ventricular septal defect

Right ventricular hypertrophy

Fallot's tetralogy arises due to faulty endocardial cushion development:
◆ Pulmonary stenosis
◆ Over-riding aorta straddles VSD
◆ VSD due to failure of septum membranosum development from endocardial cushion in interventricular septum
◆ Right ventricular hypertrophy

5–10%
Aorta arises from right ventricle, carries deoxygenated blood

Aorta arises from right ventricle, carries mixed oxygenated and deoxygenated blood

Pulmonary artery arises from left ventricle and carries oxygenated blood

VSD

Transposition of the great vessels occurs due to failure to develop a spiral septum in the truncus arteriosus

Extrauterine life is impossible in the absence of a shunt between the pulmonary and systemic circulations. If no shunt is present, the systemic circulation has no access to the lungs

Non-cyanotic congenital heart disease

10%

Pulmonary artery carries mixed blood to lungs

ASD

Atrial septal defect (ASD): develops because the septum primum fails to fuse with the endocardial cushion. Blood flows from left to right atrium and the pumonary artery carries a mixture of oxygenated and deoxygenated blood

7%

PDA shunts blood from aorta into pulmonary venous system, causing pulmonary hypertension

Pulmonary artery carries mixed blood

Patent ductus arteriosus (PDA): due to failure of closure and atrophy of the ductus at birth. Local prostaglandins play an important role in closure

40%

Pulmonary artery carries mixed blood to lungs

VSD with left to right blood flow

Ventricular septal defect (VSD): due to failure of development of the septum membranosum from the endocardial cushion. It is the commonest congenital malformation of the heart in live births. It may be associated with other abnormalities

There may be reversal of shunt, and 'late' cyanotic heart disease

PDA and VSD are more likely than ASD to result in late cyanotic heart disease due to right ventricular hypertrophy and flow reversal, because the pressure exerted on the pulmonary circulation is higher in these conditions

Aorta carries mixed oxygenated and deoxygenated blood

Systems pathology

The major development of the heart occurs during weeks 3–12 of pregnancy; by 4 weeks the primitive heart has begun to beat. Thus, the developing heart is particularly susceptible to teratogenic influences, such as maternal rubella infection, during this period of gestation. Congenital cardiac defects may also be sporadic, or associated with an underlying disease, such as Down syndrome or Edward syndrome.

The primitive heart is a single tubular structure. This tube must fold and partition itself into a left and right side, with each side being subdivided into an atrium, ventricle and outflow tract artery. All four chambers must also be appropriately connected to the relevant blood vessels and equipped with valves. Many congenital cardiac defects reflect disruption of the processes of folding and partition.

The endocardial cushions are a particularly important structure in the development of the heart. They form the valve ring, the valves, interatrial septum and the upper (membranous) part of the interventricular septum. Therefore, if their behaviour is aberrant, defects in these components of the heart result.

Congenital heart disease is divided into acyanotic and cyanotic forms. In acyanotic disease, the blood in the systemic circulation is adequately oxygenated. In cyanotic conditions, the defect disrupts the flow of blood to the extent that the systemic blood is inadequately oxygenated and cyanosis results. Cyanotic disease usually presents a more serious and immediate problem for the neonate than acyanotic disease.

Acyanotic congenital heart disease
Ventricular septal defect
With the exception of the bicuspid aortic valve, this is the commonest congenital cardiac defect (approximately 40%). The defect is situated in the membranous part of the interventricular septum. It permits a left-to-right shunt of a proportion of the oxygenated blood in the left ventricle into the right ventricle. The right ventricle then has to re-pump this blood through the lungs.

A ventricular septal defect (VSD) may progress in one of three ways. In 50% there is spontaneous closure, usually in early childhood. Alternatively, the defect can remain the same absolute size, but becomes relatively smaller as the heart grows and therefore its effect on cardiac dynamics decreases. However, with larger defects, the volume of blood shunted back into the right ventricle overloads the right ventricle and pulmonary circulation. Right ventricular hypertrophy and pulmonary hypertension result. These can ultimately produce reversal of the shunt once the pressure in the pulmonary system exceeds that in the left ventricle. Once this process occurs, the right-to-left shunt means that deoxygenated blood bypasses the lungs and enters the systemic circulation, yielding cyanosis. This overall phenomenon is known as Eisenmeiger's syndrome and is a serious complication.

Small VSDs may produce no symptoms and may be discovered incidentally.

Atrial septal defect
This is the atrial counterpart of a VSD and accounts for around 10% of congenital heart disease. The defect arises most commonly in the ostium secundum and is located in the region of the fossa ovalis. Ostium primum defects are situated near the atrioventricular valves and are associated with Down syndrome. Sinus venosus defects develop near the entry of the superior vena cava.

The changes to cardiac blood flow are similar to those of a VSD and are initially those of a left-to-right shunt. Many patients are asymptomatic and do not present until adulthood.

Patent ductus arteriosus
The ductus arteriosus connects the pulmonary artery to the aortic arch. It functions *in utero* to shunt blood away from the lungs to the systemic circulation. This is important because the non-aerated lungs have a relatively high vascular resistance against which the right heart needs to be protected. Shortly after birth, the ductus arteriosus closes and normal circulation is established. However, in some individuals, it remains open, allowing oxygenated blood from the aorta to re-enter the pulmonary circulation. Thus, the left ventricle pumps a fraction of its output straight back to itself. The pulmonary circulation is also exposed to the systemic pressures generated by the left ventricle and pulmonary hypertension can result.

Coarctation of the aorta
This is a narrowing of the aorta that accounts for 7% of congenital heart disease. The coarctation is usually near the ductus arteriosus, distal to the left subclavian artery. The increased peripheral resistance induces left ventricular hypertrophy and collateral vessels can develop to try to bypass the obstructed aorta.

Cyanotic congenital heart disease
Tetralogy of Fallot
This is the commonest cyanotic defect and accounts for 5–10% of all congenital heart defects. It is associated with Down syndrome and is an endocardial cushion defect. The four components of the tetralogy are a VSD, a malplaced aorta that overrides the defect, a stenotic pulmonary outflow tract and a hypertrophied right ventricle. The overriding aorta, in combination with a VSD and hypertrophic right ventricle, allows deoxygenated blood to enter the systemic circulation, producing cyanosis.

Transposition of the great vessels
This contributes to 5–10% of congenital heart defects and occurs when the septum that partitions the original single outflow tract of the primitive cardiac tube fails to follow the proper spiral pathway. This causes the aorta to arise from the right ventricle and the pulmonary artery from the left ventricle. As the vena cavae and pulmonary veins are appropriately sited, two independent circulations develop, with the blood in the systemic arteries circling round and round a system that does not incorporate the lungs, thereby giving cyanosis. The condition is fatal post delivery unless the ductus arteriosus and/or foramen ovale remain patent and provide some form of connection between the two circulations. Even then, marked cyanosis persists and surgical correction is essential.

Systems pathology

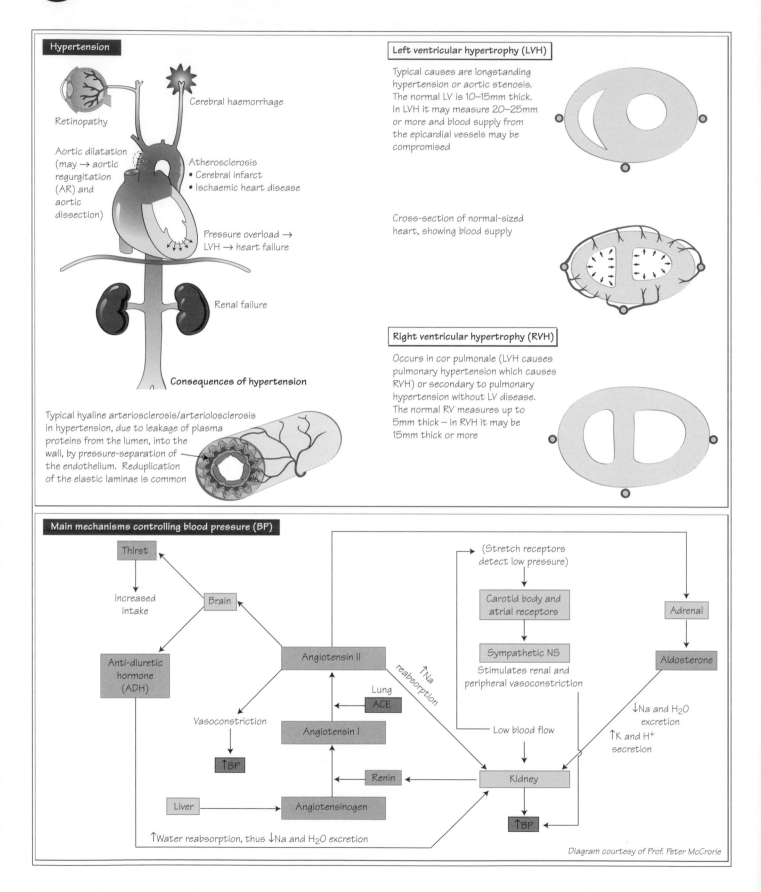

Hypertension

Retinopathy

Cerebral haemorrhage

Aortic dilatation (may → aortic regurgitation (AR) and aortic dissection)

Atherosclerosis
• Cerebral infarct
• Ischaemic heart disease

Pressure overload → LVH → heart failure

Renal failure

Consequences of hypertension

Typical hyaline arteriosclerosis/arteriolosclerosis in hypertension, due to leakage of plasma proteins from the lumen, into the wall, by pressure-separation of the endothelium. Reduplication of the elastic laminae is common

Left ventricular hypertrophy (LVH)

Typical causes are longstanding hypertension or aortic stenosis. The normal LV is 10–15mm thick. In LVH it may measure 20–25mm or more and blood supply from the epicardial vessels may be compromised

Cross-section of normal-sized heart, showing blood supply

Right ventricular hypertrophy (RVH)

Occurs in cor pulmonale (LVH causes pulmonary hypertension which causes RVH) or secondary to pulmonary hypertension without LV disease. The normal RV measures up to 5mm thick – in RVH it may be 15mm thick or more

Main mechanisms controlling blood pressure (BP)

Thirst

Increased intake

Brain

(Stretch receptors detect low pressure)

Carotid body and atrial receptors

Adrenal

Anti-diuretic hormone (ADH)

Angiotensin II

$\uparrow$Na reabsorption

Sympathetic NS

Aldosterone

Stimulates renal and peripheral vasoconstriction

Vasoconstriction

Lung ACE

$\downarrow$Na and H_2O excretion

Angiotensin I

$\uparrow$K and H^+ secretion

$\uparrow$BP

Low blood flow

Renin

Kidney

Liver

Angiotensinogen

$\uparrow$BP

$\uparrow$Water reabsorption, thus $\downarrow$Na and H_2O excretion

Diagram courtesy of Prof. Peter McCrorie

 Pathology at a Glance. By C.J. Finlayson and B.A.T. Newell. Published 2009 by Blackwell Publishing. ISBN: 978-1-4051-3650-1

Systemic hypertension is defined in terms of either the systolic or diastolic blood pressure and is considered to be present if there is a sustained systolic pressure of over 140 mmHg and/or a sustained diastolic pressure greater than 90 mmHg. These figures reflect the levels of blood pressure at which treatment becomes prudent to prevent complications.

Control of blood pressure

Blood pressure is the product of the cardiac output and the peripheral vascular resistance. Cardiac output itself is dependent on the heart rate and stroke volume and the available circulating volume.

Central to the regulation of cardiac contractility and peripheral vascular resistance is the sympathetic nervous system. Increased sympathetic activity produces a positive inotropic and chronotrophic effect on the heart, thereby elevating stroke volume. At a systemic level, increased sympathetic tone causes vasoconstriction, thereby raising peripheral vascular resistance. However, the process is more sophisticated than blanket vasoconstriction in all vascular beds such that skeletal muscle, which requires an elevated blood flow during exercise, tends to show vasodilatation, due to the balance of α- and β-adrenoreceptors within its vessels and the superimposed factor of local autoregulation.

Baroreceptors within the aortic arch and carotid bodies sense blood pressure and relay this information back to the brainstem where it is integrated with other parameters to modify autonomic tone. While the sympathetic nervous system is the main effector arm in controlling blood pressure, the parasympathetic nervous system can have a role in reducing blood pressure by slowing the heart.

Working alongside the sympathetic nervous system are hormones that operate to increase the circulating volume. As the kidney is integral to the body's regulation of its sodium and water balance, many of these hormones act through the kidney, or are generated by it.

Renin is released by the kidney through a complex response at the juxtaglomerular apparatus that detects decreased renal blood flow. Renin catalyses the conversion of angiotensinogen (produced by the liver) to angiotensin I. This is in turn converted to angiotensin II, the active form, by angiotensin converting enzyme (ACE). ACE is expressed on endothelial cells, especially those within the lung. Angiotensin II has vasoconstrictor effects and also stimulates the adrenal to release aldosterone, which promotes sodium and water retention by the kidney, thereby increasing the volume of fluid in the circulation. Furthermore, aldosterone can directly promote sodium and water retention by the kidney by altering blood flow between glomeruli. Operating in conjunction with the renin–angiotensin–aldosterone system is that of antidiuretic hormone and thirst/drinking.

Understanding the normal control of blood pressure enables treatments to be devised and their mechanism of action appreciated.

Causes

In 95% of cases, hypertension is primary and lacks a cause. The secondary causes are as follows:

1 Renal:
- Renal artery stenosis.
- Glomerulonephritis.
- Polycystic kidneys.
- Renin-producing tumour.
- Scleroderma.

2 Endocrine:
- Cushing's syndrome.
- Acromegaly.
- Phaeochromocytoma.
- Hyperaldosteronism.

3 Miscellaneous:
- Aortic coarctation.
- Pregnancy.

Complications of hypertension

Atherosclerosis: Hypertension is one of the risk factors for the development of atherosclerosis. The elevated pressure can damage the endothelium, thereby rendering it susceptible to atherosclerosis.

Arteriosclerosis: The endothelium of smaller arteries and arterioles is also damaged by the increased pressure and this permits a leakage of proteins into the vessel wall, which produces narrowing and downstream ischaemia.

Left ventricular hypertrophy: The elevated afterload placed on the ventricle by the increased systemic pressure induces hypertrophy of the left ventricle. Once the hypertrophy reaches a critical level, around a ventricular thickness of 15 mm, the penetration of branches of the coronary arteries through the ventricle becomes compromised in terms of providing adequate blood flow, and ischaemia can occur. This ischaemia may precipitate arrhythmias.

Aortic dilatation: As well as placing a stress on the heart, hypertension also increases the load on the aortic arch, which bears the brunt of the initial force. Dilatation can distort the aortic root, leading to aortic regurgitation, or culminate in a dissecting aneurysm.

Haemorrhagic stroke: In addition to being a risk factor for ischaemic stroke via atherosclerosis, hypertension can cause haemorrhagic cerebrovascular accidents (CVAs). This is believed to reflect the development of microaneurysms in the cerebral circulation secondary to the increased stress on the vessel wall. Rupture of these aneurysms produces a haemorrhagic CVA.

Retinopathy: Hypertension may induce changes in the retinal blood vessels. These can result in patches of oedema and haemorrhage.

Nephropathy: Hyaline arteriosclerosis in the kidney can disrupt the blood supply to the glomeruli, causing ischaemic atrophy and necrosis. The affected glomeruli are sclerotic and non-functional. If a sufficient number of glomeruli are damaged, renal impairment results.

Accelerated hypertension

This is also known as malignant hypertension and is a serious, life-threatening condition in which there is severe, uncontrolled hypertension that is associated with headache, confusion and a high risk of end organ damage such as haemorrhagic CVA, retinal haemorrhage and renal failure.

Systems pathology

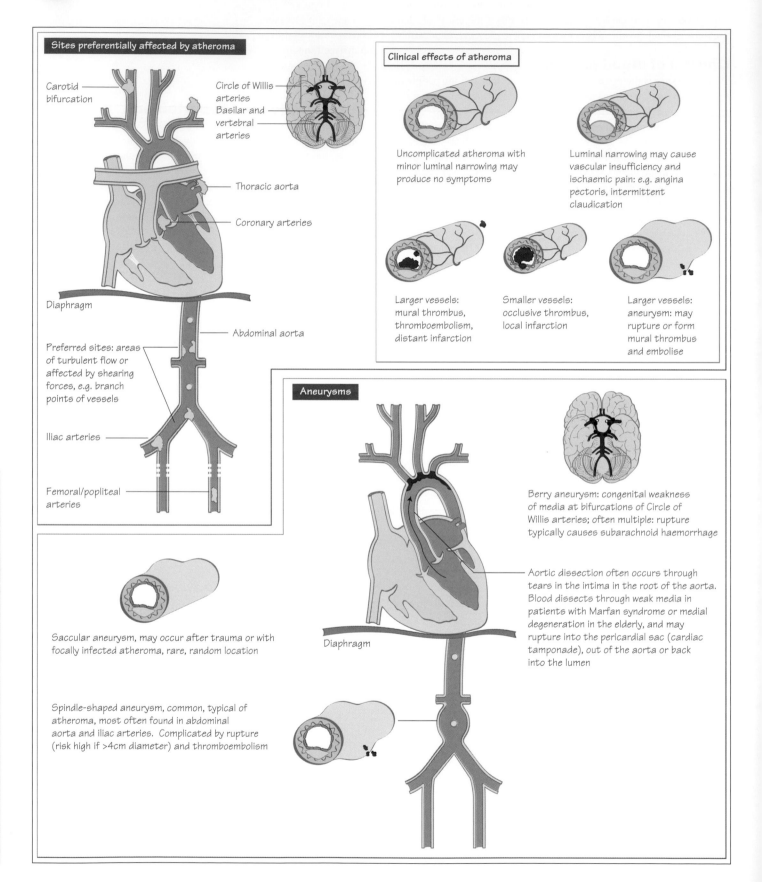

Sites preferentially affected by atheroma

Carotid bifurcation

Circle of Willis arteries

Basilar and vertebral arteries

Thoracic aorta

Coronary arteries

Diaphragm

Abdominal aorta

Preferred sites: areas of turbulent flow or affected by shearing forces, e.g. branch points of vessels

Iliac arteries

Femoral/popliteal arteries

Clinical effects of atheroma

Uncomplicated atheroma with minor luminal narrowing may produce no symptoms

Luminal narrowing may cause vascular insufficiency and ischaemic pain: e.g. angina pectoris, intermittent claudication

Larger vessels: mural thrombus, thromboembolism, distant infarction

Smaller vessels: occlusive thrombus, local infarction

Larger vessels: aneurysm: may rupture or form mural thrombus and embolise

Aneurysms

Berry aneurysm: congenital weakness of media at bifurcations of Circle of Willis arteries; often multiple: rupture typically causes subarachnoid haemorrhage

Aortic dissection often occurs through tears in the intima in the root of the aorta. Blood dissects through weak media in patients with Marfan syndrome or medial degeneration in the elderly, and may rupture into the pericardial sac (cardiac tamponade), out of the aorta or back into the lumen

Diaphragm

Saccular aneurysm, may occur after trauma or with focally infected atheroma, rare, random location

Spindle-shaped aneurysm, common, typical of atheroma, most often found in abdominal aorta and iliac arteries. Complicated by rupture (risk high if >4cm diameter) and thromboembolism

Atherosclerosis and arteriosclerosis

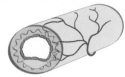

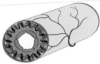

Atherosclerosis – hardening of arteries due to atheroma

Fibrosis and calcification of the plaque reduce distensibility of the artery and cause hardening

This does not cause hypertension as the vessels which determine peripheral resistance (smaller muscular arteries and arterioles) are not affected

Arteriosclerosis – hardening of arterioles

The usual cause is hypertension, which affects the arterioles, the vessels mainly responsible for peripheral resistance (BP= COxPR)

The high pressure leads to duplication of elastic laminae and an increase in the smooth muscle component of the wall, which narrow the lumen and thicken the wall

Plasma proteins are forced into the wall of the artery, where they form an amorphous eosinophilic layer, called 'hyaline change' within the wall, causing stiffness ('sclerosis')

Evolution of an atheromatous plaque

Expression of endothelial adhesion molecules is induced by:
Cholesterol
Cytokines
Oxidative stress
Shear stress
Lipoprotein A
Advanced glycosylation end-products (increased in diabetes)

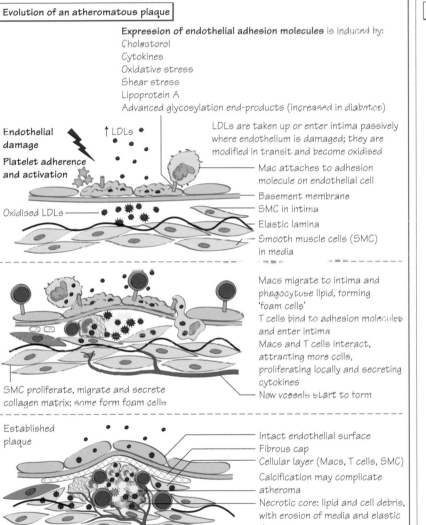

Endothelial damage

Platelet adherence and activation

↑LDLs

Oxidised LDLs

LDLs are taken up or enter intima passively where endothelium is damaged; they are modified in transit and become oxidised

Mac attaches to adhesion molecule on endothelial cell
Basement membrane
SMC in intima
Elastic lamina
Smooth muscle cells (SMC) in media

Macs migrate to intima and phagocytose lipid, forming 'foam cells'
T cells bind to adhesion molecules and enter intima
Macs and T cells interact, attracting more cells, proliferating locally and secreting cytokines
New vessels start to form

SMC proliferate, migrate and secrete collagen matrix; some form foam cells

Established plaque

Intact endothelial surface
Fibrous cap
Cellular layer (Macs, T cells, SMC)
Calcification may complicate atheroma
Necrotic core: lipid and cell debris, with erosion of media and elastic damage
New blood vessels proliferate

Complications of atheroma

Thrombosis may complicate atheroma, due to endothelial cell damage

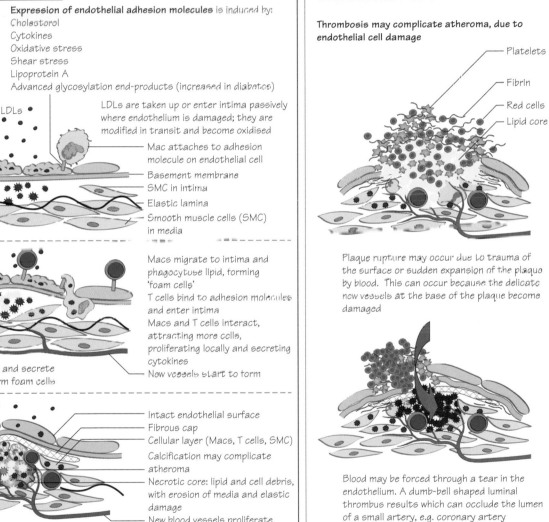

Platelets
Fibrin
Red cells
Lipid core

Plaque rupture may occur due to trauma of the surface or sudden expansion of the plaque by blood. This can occur because the delicate new vessels at the base of the plaque become damaged

Blood may be forced through a tear in the endothelium. A dumb-bell shaped luminal thrombus results which can occlude the lumen of a small artery, e.g. coronary artery

Definition

Atheroma is a gruel-like accumulation of fat, cells, collagen and matrix proteins which develops at sites of damage to the endothelium of arteries.

Typical sites affected are the branches of major arteries (particularly the carotid bifurcation, the iliac and femoral vessels) and the circle of Willis, the coronary arteries and the abdominal aorta.

Aetiology

The underlying aetoiological factor is endothelial damage, which may be due to a variety of causes:

• Cigarette smoke (via free radical formation, carbon monoxide or direct chemical effects).

• Haemodynamic forces (shearing forces): turbulent blood flow at the branch points of arteries may damage the intima. Once atheromatous plaques have formed, they deform the surface and create turbulence, exacerbating the problem.

• Hyperlipidaemia, which may be genetic or secondary.

• Immune mechanisms, either infective agents or circulating antibody–antigen complexes.

• Viral and other antigens: experimental models and human studies have supported a role for infection in the promotion of atherosclerosis. Although no one infective agent has been found to cause atheroma, patients with severe disease often show seropositivity to several bacterial and viral agents.

• Irradiation: inclusion of major arteries in a field irradiated for carcinoma (theoretical, not a common cause of atheroma).

In terms of taking a history and managing a patient, the key factors are smoking, diabetes mellitus, family history, hypertension and hyperlipidaemia.

Precursor lesion

Two candidates exist and both may be important:

1 The 'fatty streak': a deposit of lipid within the wall of an artery without a significant inflammatory response, found in young adults, often within pulmonary arteries or other vessels where atheroma seldom occurs. Thus the distribution does not mirror atheroma, but the mechanism of insudation of lipid into the intima may be similar.

2 The 'intimal cushion': these lesions are seen in very young children and mirror the distribution of atheroma, at the ostia of vessels. Degeneration is seen in the connective tissue in these areas, and there may be intimal smooth muscle cells present.

Pathogenesis

In terms of a basic overview, lipid from the blood seeps into the vessel wall and an inflammatory response is initiated and sustained by cytokines released by the inflammatory cells. If atheroma becomes 'complicated' by rupture and thrombosis or calcification, sequelae such as ischaemic heart disease, stroke, gangrene or aneurysm formation may follow.

Patients with severe atheroma often have increased circulating inflammatory markers such as C-reactive protein, fibrinogen and interleukins. These markers can be useful in detecting patients with unstable atheromatous plaques.

Mechanism

Damage to the endothelium permits low density lipoproteins (LDLs), which are rich in cholesterol, to enter the tunica intima of the artery, either passively or by active uptake. During this entry process, the lipid becomes oxidised. The endothelial cell damage also causes the endothelium to upregulate various cell surface adhesion molecules.

The presence of lipid in the intima excites a macrophage inflammatory response. The macrophages phagocytose the lipid to become foam cells.

The upregulated adhesion molecules on the endothelium allow T cells to bind and enter the intima where they interact with the macrophages to boost the inflammatory response and recruit more cells. As part of this process, cytokines are released that promote smooth muscle proliferation. The smooth muscle cells migrate to the intima and synthesise collagen. The generation of new, small blood vessels is also induced by the cytokines. These new vessels are fragile.

The culmination of these events is the generation of an atherosclerotic plaque. This is based in the tunica intima and is covered by an intact endothelium beneath which is a fibrous cap. Under the cap is a cellular layer of macrophages and T lymphocytes, which overlies the lipid-rich necrotic core of the plaque. This necrotic core damages the internal elastic lamina and the tunica media.

Complications

Arterial thrombosis is closely linked to atherosclerosis. An atherosclerotic plaque can trigger thrombosis when its endothelial cell cover is damaged, resulting in exposure of the basement membrane or the lipid-rich necrotic core of the plaque. Various complications can then occur.

Endothelial denudation: Shearing forces may tear the endothelium off the basement membrane. Exposure of collagen or von Willebrand factor prompts the activation of the coagulation cascade and of platelets.

Plaque rupture: This follows sudden haemorrhagic expansion of the plaque. Softer plaques, with more foam cells, are more likely to rupture than others. The dynamic balance between the formation of the fibrous cap and its degradation by macrophage enzymes (or by smooth muscle cell inhibition by tumour necrois factor) is important. The highly thrombogenic, friable and easily dislodged lipid-laden core is exposed to the lumen of the artery. Likely sequelae are:

• **Thromboemboli** from larger vessels, often containing cholesterol crystals, may flick off into the circulation and impact in a small arteriole or capillary bed, causing ischaemic damage.

• **Vascular occlusion** of smaller vessels, e.g. coronary artery thrombosis and myocardial infarction.

Treatment
Preventative

Dietary changes or the use of statins, which lower the level of LDLs, and the cessation of smoking are probably the simplest preventative measures. Hypertension and diabetes must be controlled.

Treatment of established atheroma and its sequelae

• Stenting of stenosed vessels.

• By-passing of occluded or stenotic arterial segments.

• Removal of gangrenous tissue (thromboembolism), e.g. toes

• Specific disease, e.g. myocardial infarction, stroke.

Ischaemic heart disease

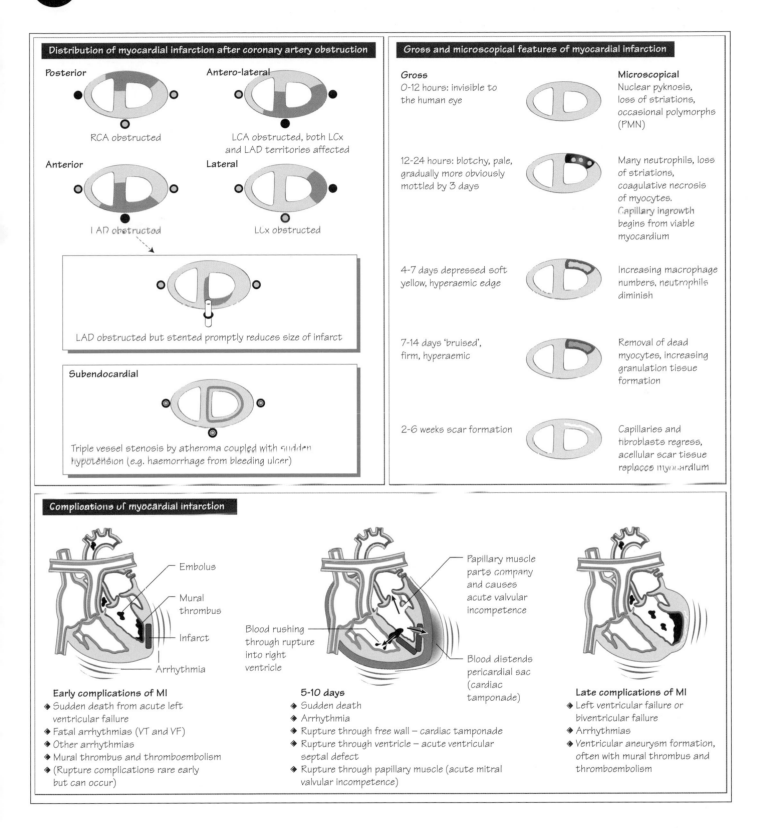

Distribution of myocardial infarction after coronary artery obstruction

Posterior

RCA obstructed

Antero-lateral

LCA obstructed, both LCx and LAD territories affected

Anterior

LAD obstructed

Lateral

LCx obstructed

LAD obstructed but stented promptly reduces size of infarct

Subendocardial

Triple vessel stenosis by atheroma coupled with sudden hypotension (e.g. haemorrhage from bleeding ulcer)

Gross and microscopical features of myocardial infarction

Gross	Microscopical
0-12 hours: invisible to the human eye	Nuclear pyknosis, loss of striations, occasional polymorphs (PMN)
12-24 hours: blotchy, pale, gradually more obviously mottled by 3 days	Many neutrophils, loss of striations, coagulative necrosis of myocytes. Capillary ingrowth begins from viable myocardium
4-7 days depressed soft yellow, hyperaemic edge	Increasing macrophage numbers, neutrophils diminish
7-14 days 'bruised', firm, hyperaemic	Removal of dead myocytes, increasing granulation tissue formation
2-6 weeks scar formation	Capillaries and fibroblasts regress, acellular scar tissue replaces myocardium

Complications of myocardial infarction

Embolus

Mural thrombus

Infarct

Arrhythmia

Early complications of MI
- Sudden death from acute left ventricular failure
- Fatal arrhythmias (VT and VF)
- Other arrhythmias
- Mural thrombus and thromboembolism
- (Rupture complications rare early but can occur)

Blood rushing through rupture into right ventricle

Papillary muscle parts company and causes acute valvular incompetence

Blood distends pericardial sac (cardiac tamponade)

5-10 days
- Sudden death
- Arrhythmia
- Rupture through free wall – cardiac tamponade
- Rupture through ventricle – acute ventricular septal defect
- Rupture through papillary muscle (acute mitral valvular incompetence)

Late complications of MI
- Left ventricular failure or biventricular failure
- Arrhythmias
- Ventricular aneurysm formation, often with mural thrombus and thromboembolism

Systems pathology

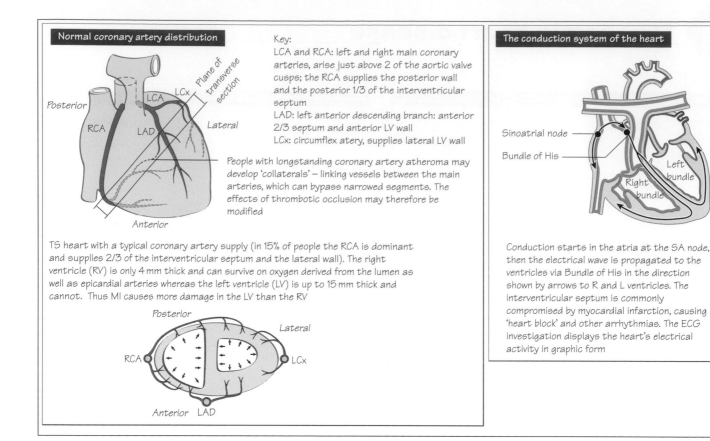

Normal coronary artery distribution

Posterior

Plane of transverse section

RCA
LCA
LCx
LAD
Lateral

Anterior

Key:
LCA and RCA: left and right main coronary arteries, arise just above 2 of the aortic valve cusps; the RCA supplies the posterior wall and the posterior 1/3 of the interventricular septum
LAD: left anterior descending branch: anterior 2/3 septum and anterior LV wall
LCx: circumflex atery, supplies lateral LV wall

People with longstanding coronary artery atheroma may develop 'collaterals' – linking vessels between the main arteries, which can bypass narrowed segments. The effects of thrombotic occlusion may therefore be modified

TS heart with a typical coronary artery supply (in 15% of people the RCA is dominant and supplies 2/3 of the interventricular septum and the lateral wall). The right ventricle (RV) is only 4 mm thick and can survive on oxygen derived from the lumen as well as epicardial arteries whereas the left ventricle (LV) is up to 15 mm thick and cannot. Thus MI causes more damage in the LV than the RV

Posterior

Lateral

RCA
LCx

Anterior LAD

The conduction system of the heart

Sinoatrial node
Bundle of His
Left bundle
Right bundle

Conduction starts in the atria at the SA node, then the electrical wave is propagated to the ventricles via Bundle of His in the direction shown by arrows to R and L ventricles. The interventricular septum is commonly compromised by myocardial infarction, causing 'heart block' and other arrhythmias. The ECG investigation displays the heart's electrical activity in graphic form

Definition

Ischaemic heart disease is the collective term used for angina pectoris, myocardial infarction (MI) and ischaemic chronic cardiac failure, all of which share ischaemia of the myocardium secondary to atherosclerosis of the coronary arteries as their underlying cause.

Angina pectoris

Angina pectoris is cardiac pain that results from myocardial ischaemia secondary to inadequate blood flow. In stable angina, this ischaemia is precipitated by exercise, whereby the myocardial oxygen demand increases beyond that which can be supplied by the atherosclerotically narrowed coronary arteries. The onset of the angina is predictable and can be relieved with sublingual glyceryl trinitrate (GTN).

Unstable angina occurs at rest or on minimal exertion. There is underlying severe coronary artery atherosclerosis. The angina is precipitated by a sudden change in the plaque that nevertheless falls short of that necessary to occlude the artery completely. The pain lasts for longer than stable angina and is less responsive to GTN. Unstable angina indicates a significant risk of an MI in the near future.

Prinzmetal angina is a variant that is more common in women and is due to vasospasm of the coronary arteries, which may reflect adrenergic stimulation, local release of platelet granules or an imbalance between endothelial-derived nitric oxide (NO; vasodilatation) and endothelin 1 (ET-1; vasoconstriction).

Myocardial infarction
Definition

Myocardial infarction is irreversible necrosis of (part of) the myocardium due to inadequate blood flow.

Epidemiology

The UK incidence is approximately one per 250 per year and rises with age. The risk factors follow those for atherosclerosis, of which the principal ones are smoking, hypercholesterolaemia, diabetes mellitus, hypertension, family history, male gender and previous/known ischaemic heart disease or atherosclerosis.

While MIs are common in both men and women, in the absence of an underlying cause of accelerated atherosclerosis, MIs are unusual in premenopausal women.

Pathology

Almost all MIs are due to *in situ* thrombosis of a coronary artery that is caused by rupture of an atherosclerotic plaque. In 75%, the plaque fissures rather than manifesting superficial ulceration.

In 90% of cases, an MI is transmural and follows complete occlusion of a single coronary artery. The necrosis involves the whole thickness of the infarcted region of myocardium. The figure shows the regions of the heart that are affected by occlusion of specific coronary arteries.

The remaining 10% of MIs are subendocardial and reflect severe triple vessel coronary artery atherosclerosis, typically coupled with a sudden drop in blood pressure. Coronary artery blood flow falls dramatically, but complete occlusion does not occur. This fall produces ischaemia in the most vulnerable part of the myocardium, which is the subendocardial myocardium. This susceptibility of the subendocardial myocardium reflects the fact that the coronary arteries lie on the outside of the heart and have to penetrate through to the subendocardial region. Clinically subendocardial MIs present as non-q wave infarcts or non-ST elevation infarcts.

Table 36.1 Characteristic features of occlusion of major arteries.

Artery	Territory	ECG leads	Particular complications
Left anterior descending (LAD)	Interventricular septum and much of the anterior left ventricle, part of adjacent right ventricle	V1–V6, particularly V3 and V4	Cardiac failure, rupture events, pulmonary oedema Heart block implies a large volume of damaged myocardium as a LAD infarct can only cause this by infarcting much of the bundle of His
Circumflex	Lateral wall of left ventricle	I, aVL, V5 and V6	No specific complications
Left main stem	LAD and circumflex combined	LAD and circumflex combined	Normally fatal due to massive myocardial loss
Right coronary artery	Inferior aspect of left ventricle, part of right ventricle. SA and AV nodes	II, III and aVF	Even small infarcts can damage the SA and AV nodes, leading to heart block
Branches of right coronary artery	Right ventricle, known as 'true posterior infarct' Rare	Place chest leads on right side of chest to see ST elevation Dominant R in V1	Right heart failure giving massive peripheral oedema without pulmonary oedema

Once the vascular event has occurred, the process within the myocardium is one of ischaemic coagulative necrosis. This has a characteristic time course for both the macroscopic and microscopic features that is useful at autopsy and is popular with examiners. The figure gives details of the changes, and in summary they are those of coagulative necrosis, acute neutrophilic inflammation, a macrophage clean-up operation and fibroblastic repair. If an MI is fatal in the first few hours, the only change that might be encountered at autopsy is the causative occlusive thrombus.

Complications

Numerous complications can follow an MI. These tend to have characteristic times of onset. With the exceptions of mural thrombosis and Dressler's syndrome (which is thought to be an autoimmune response secondary to myocardial damage), the complications reflect either cellular malfunction due to ischaemia and hypoxia or weakness of the myocardium due to necrosis (Table 36.1).

Ischaemia of cardiac myocytes impairs the function of the $Na^+/K^+/$ATPase system, which disrupts the cell's ability to maintain its resting membrane potential. This can lead to depolarisation of the cell and, in turn, this can provide a focus for the generation of an arrhythmia. Ventricular fibrillation and pulseless ventricular tachycardia are two fatal arrhythmias that require very prompt defibrillation if sinus rhythm and cardiac output are to be restored and death averted.

Infarction of the conducting system can lead to various degrees of heart block. The right coronary artery supplies both the sinoatrial (SA) node and atrioventricular (AV) node and even relatively small infarctions in the right coronary artery territory can produce life-threatening heart blocks if they involve these small structures. By contrast, if a left coronary artery is to induce complete heart block, it is likely to have done so by infarcting the whole of the bundle of His complex. This will be accompanied by a similarly large volume of infarcted myocardium and the patient is likely to have serious left ventricular failure.

The contractile function of ischaemic cells is also impaired, leading to acute cardiac failure. Once the ischaemia has progressed to necrosis the loss of muscle bulk can also cause cardiac failure. Necrotic muscle may rupture under the stress of continued cardiac activity, yielding rupture of the interventricular septum, rupture of the free wall of the left ventricle or rupture of a papillary muscle.

In the longer term, the fibrous scar that remains after healing of the infarction can be weak and may deform, resulting in a ventricular aneurysm. The aneurysm can distort the conducting system and produce an arrhythmia. In addition, thrombus can form within the aneurysm and act as a source of emboli.

Prognosis

Even with current thrombolytic therapy, approximately 40% of MIs are fatal and a significant proportion of these are fatal within the first few minutes.

Thrombolysis can limit the extent of the myocardial damage. Paradoxically, re-opening the coronary artery can cause reperfusion injury, in which restoration of blood flow induces tissue damage. This process can reflect downstream carriage of toxic intracellular metabolites that are released during the period of ischaemia, as well as free radical-mediated damage that results when oxygen delivery is restored to injured tissues. Nevertheless, the benefits of thrombolysis considerably outweigh those posed by this phenomenon.

While thrombolysis may be the most dramatic therapy, the more simple aspirin has a similar effect on mortality through its antiplatelet effects. Beta-blockers are also valuable agents as they have a calming effect on myocardial contractility (thereby limiting rupture-related complications) and myocardial electrical excitability. ACE inhibitors may prevent the harmful left ventricular remodelling that can occur after an anterior MI.

Stenting within the first 3 hours is effective in limiting the extent of an MI. Ideally, reperfusion should be achieved within 30 minutes of the acute event.

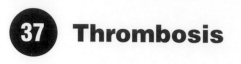

37 Thrombosis

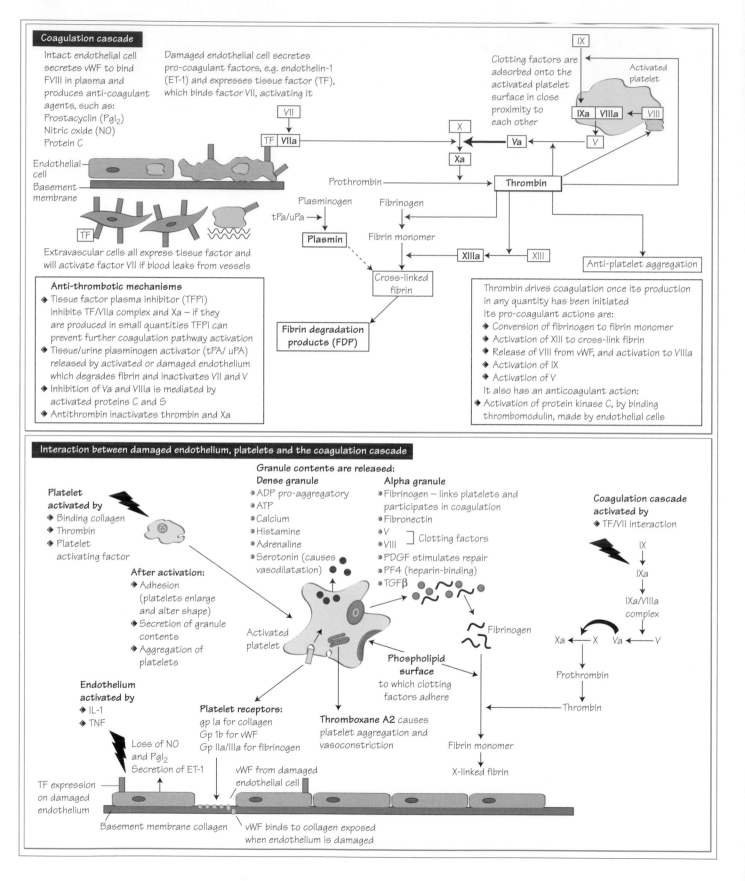

Coagulation cascade

Intact endothelial cell secretes vWF to bind FVIII in plasma and produces anti-coagulant agents, such as:
Prostacyclin (PgI$_2$)
Nitric oxide (NO)
Protein C

Endothelial cell
Basement membrane

Extravascular cells all express tissue factor and will activate factor VII if blood leaks from vessels

TF

Damaged endothelial cell secretes pro-coagulant factors, e.g. endothelin-1 (ET-1) and expresses tissue factor (TF), which binds factor VII, activating it

VII
TF VIIa

Clotting factors are adsorbed onto the activated platelet surface in close proximity to each other

Activated platelet

IX
IXa VIIIa
VIII

X
Va
V

Xa

Prothrombin — Thrombin

Plasminogen   Fibrinogen
tPa/uPa →
Plasmin   Fibrin monomer

XIIIa ← XIII

Anti-platelet aggregation

Cross-linked fibrin

Fibrin degradation products (FDP)

Anti-thrombotic mechanisms
◆ Tissue factor plasma inhibitor (TFPi) inhibits TF/VIIa complex and Xa – if they are produced in small quantities TFPi can prevent further coagulation pathway activation
◆ Tissue/urine plasminogen activator (tPA/ uPA) released by activated or damaged endothelium which degrades fibrin and inactivates VII and V
◆ Inhibition of Va and VIIIa is mediated by activated proteins C and S
◆ Antithrombin inactivates thrombin and Xa

Thrombin drives coagulation once its production in any quantity has been initiated
Its pro-coagulant actions are:
◆ Conversion of fibrinogen to fibrin monomer
◆ Activation of XIII to cross-link fibrin
◆ Release of VIII from vWF, and activation to VIIIa
◆ Activation of IX
◆ Activation of V
It also has an anticoagulant action:
◆ Activation of protein kinase C, by binding thrombomodulin, made by endothelial cells

Interaction between damaged endothelium, platelets and the coagulation cascade

Platelet activated by
◆ Binding collagen
◆ Thrombin
◆ Platelet activating factor

After activation:
◆ Adhesion (platelets enlarge and alter shape)
◆ Secretion of granule contents
◆ Aggregation of platelets

Granule contents are released:
Dense granule
● ADP pro-aggregatory
● ATP
● Calcium
● Histamine
● Adrenaline
● Serotonin (causes vasodilatation)

Alpha granule
● Fibrinogen – links platelets and participates in coagulation
● Fibronectin
● V
● VIII] Clotting factors
● PDGF stimulates repair
● PF4 (heparin-binding)
● TGFβ

Activated platelet

Fibrinogen

Phospholipid surface
to which clotting factors adhere

Coagulation cascade activated by
◆ TF/VII interaction

IX
IXa
IXa/VIIIa complex
Xa ← X ← Va ← V
Prothrombin
Thrombin

Endothelium activated by
◆ IL-1
◆ TNF

Platelet receptors:
gp Ia for collagen
Gp Ib for vWF
Gp IIa/IIIa for fibrinogen

Thromboxane A2 causes platelet aggregation and vasoconstriction

Fibrin monomer
X-linked fibrin

Loss of NO and PgI$_2$
Secretion of ET-1

TF expression on damaged endothelium

vWF from damaged endothelial cell

Basement membrane collagen   vWF binds to collagen exposed when endothelium is damaged

Systems pathology

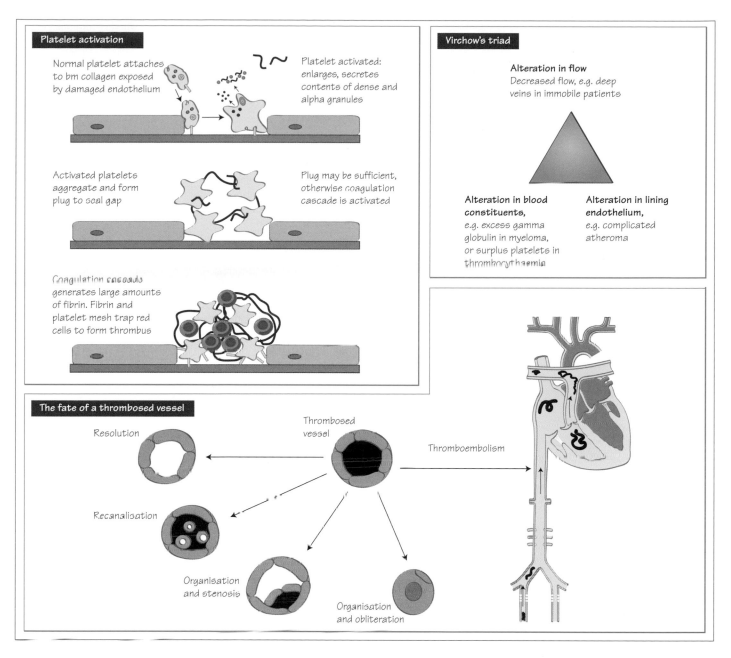

Platelet activation

Normal platelet attaches to bm collagen exposed by damaged endothelium

Platelet activated: enlarges, secretes contents of dense and alpha granules

Activated platelets aggregate and form plug to seal gap

Plug may be sufficient, otherwise coagulation cascade is activated

Coagulation cascade generates large amounts of fibrin. Fibrin and platelet mesh trap red cells to form thrombus

Virchow's triad

Alteration in flow
Decreased flow, e.g. deep veins in immobile patients

Alteration in blood constituents,
e.g. excess gamma globulin in myeloma, or surplus platelets in thrombocythaemia

Alteration in lining endothelium,
e.g. complicated atheroma

The fate of a thrombosed vessel

Resolution

Thrombosed vessel

Thromboembolism

Recanalisation

Organisation and stenosis

Organisation and obliteration

A thrombus is a mass that is formed from and by the constituents of the coagulation system within the vascular tree. Thrombosis is the term given to the process that generates a thrombus. A haematoma is a blood clot within the tissues.

The purpose of thrombosis is to seal breaches in the vasculature in order to prevent blood loss and exsanguination. The thrombotic system therefore needs to be configured to respond to events that signal loss of continuity of the vascular system, but also to remain dormant until these incidents occur. Inappropriate thrombosis in a healthy blood vessel can occlude that vessel and cause infarction.

In the 1890s, Rudolf Virchow described the three factors crucial to triggering thrombosis: alterations to the constituents of the blood, the vessel wall and the blood flow (Virchow's triad). Similarly, the thrombotic system possesses three components: endothelial cells, platelets and the coagulation cascade.

Other than trauma, the factors that dominate in initiating pathological thrombosis vary between the vessels and the clinical situation.

In arteries, endothelial damage and flow alterations due to distortion by atheroma and aneurysms are the most important factors. Veins rely on the skeletal muscles to pump blood back to the heart so a decreased flow rate caused by venous stasis due to immobility is more important. In bed-bound, postoperative patients endothelial activation by acute inflammatory mediators is a significant factor.

Normal haemostasis

The function of normal haemostasis is to activate the clotting system where it is needed and to target its action to the breach. This is achieved by complex interactions between the endothelium, platelets and clotting cascade.

Endothelium

Endothelium in its resting state has an antithrombotic stance, due to secretion of the vasodilator and antiplatelet aggregation agent prostacyclin and the vasodilator nitric oxide (NO).

Once activated, endothelium secretes the vasoconstrictor endothelin-1 (ET-1), expresses tissue factor on its surface and secretes platelet activating factor (PAF).

Endothelial damage leads to the expression of von Willebrand factor (vWF) on the endothelial surface. If endothelial cells are so damaged that they tear away from the surface, the underlying basement membrane and collagen are exposed to the bloodstream and trigger haemostasis.

Platelets

Platelets normally circulate in an inactive state, but when activated they adhere to each other, damaged endothelium, exposed basement membrane and fibrin in order to form a plug. Platelets are activated by thrombin, contact with basement membrane and PAF.

Activated platelets display surface receptors that allow them to bind to vWF, to collagen or to TF/VIIa on endothelial cells, thereby causing them to anchor to the site of damage, each other and the fibrin framework of a clot.

Activation of platelets also precipitates the release of their granules. Thromboxane A2 is a potent vasoconstrictor that slows blood flow and enhances platelet aggregation. Activated platelets adsorb clotting factors onto their phospholipid surfaces, which brings them into close apposition, thereby facilitating the cascade.

Small breaches in the endothelium occur all the time and platelet plugs readily seal them while the endothelium regenerates.

Coagulation cascade

The role of the clotting cascade is to generate an insoluble mesh of cross-linked fibrin in which platelets, erythrocytes and leucocytes become trapped to yield a clot. The components of the cascade are the clotting factors, most of which are proteins that are made by the liver. They activate in sequence, thereby amplifying a small initial signal into the generation of a large quantity of fibrin.

The main precipitant for the cascade is activation of factor VII by tissue factor. Tissue factor is expressed on all cells except undamaged endothelium and the blood cells so will readily be exposed if the endothelium is disrupted. The cascade then spirals down until pro-thrombin is converted to thrombin. Thrombin in turn triggers the conversion of fibrinogen to fibrin.

The factor VII-mediated sequence is known as the extrinsic pathway. However, there is also an intrinsic pathway that is initiated by the activation of factor XI by thrombin or by activated factor IX/factor VIII complexes on platelets. The intrinsic pathway allows the platelets to feed into the cascade and also for the cascade to amplify itself.

Deficiencies in factors VIII and IX cause severe bleeding problems (haemophilia and Christmas disease); deficiencies in factor VII cause severe bleeding problems in embryonal life and deficient tissue factor is incompatible with life.

Pathologically significant locations of thrombus

Arterial thrombosis

Atheroma is the most common cause of arterial thrombosis; endothelial damage is the usual trigger. The consequences depend upon the calibre of the vessel: occlusion of a small artery causes tissue infarction (e.g.

myocardial infarction or thrombotic stroke), whereas thrombus on the wall of a large vessel will not be large enough to occlude the vessel but can embolise and produce distant infarction.

Cardiac thrombosis

This is usually secondary to stagnant flow, as may occur with an arrhythmia (e.g. atrial fibrillation), myocardial infarction or valvular disease.

Venous thrombosis

Thrombus tends to form in the valve cusps of medium-sized and large veins, where turbulent flow is most likely. As there is little endothelial cell damage, platelets form only a small attachment to the vein wall and downstream thrombus builds up gradually – like seaweed, waving gently in the flow. If the vein becomes occluded, more blood, carrying more platelets and clotting factors, arrives through tributaries and the thrombus is propagated, still with a relatively small attachment to the wall. The thrombus can attain a length of 20 cm or more.

Occlusion of the deep veins (deep venous thrombosis (DVT)) of the calf muscle or the popliteal vein may cause swelling, pain and dusky skin discoloration of the affected lower leg, but can also be asymptomatic. If untreated, a DVT may resolve without any complications, but there can be local long-term disturbances of the venous drainage. More significant is the acute complication of a pulmonary embolism in which part of the venous thrombus breaks off and impacts in the pulmonary circulation (see Chapter 41).

The classic test for DVT (Homan's sign – abrupt dorsiflexion of the foot elicits pain in the calf muscles) is no longer advised as it is feared it might precipitate a pulmonary embolism and has been superseded by more sensitive imaging techniques.

Thrombolysis

Once a thrombus has been generated, a process needs to exist that can remove that thrombus when the damage to the vessel has been repaired. The thrombolytic system functions to break down thrombi and remove them. It also opposes the initiation of clotting in the first place and ensures that haemostasis only occurs when the precipitating signal is of appropriate magnitude to warrant this activation.

Sequelae following thrombosis

- **Embolisation**: all or part of the thrombus detaches and is carried to another site by the blood flow. Effects vary according to the site of origin of the embolus.
- **Resolution**: the thrombus is cleared by normal antithrombotic mechanisms or by therapeutic drugs such as streptokinase.
- **Re-canalisation**: small endothelial-lined channels develop to bypass the thrombosed segment.
- **Repair**: as much thrombus as possible is removed by thrombolytic activity, then the remainder is organised and re-endothelialised to restore the integrity of the blood vessel. This causes a degree of luminal stenosis.
- **Fibrous obliteration**: organisation and fibrosis of the thrombosed segment causes fibrous obliteration of the lumen of the vessel.

Embolism and disseminated intravascular coagulation

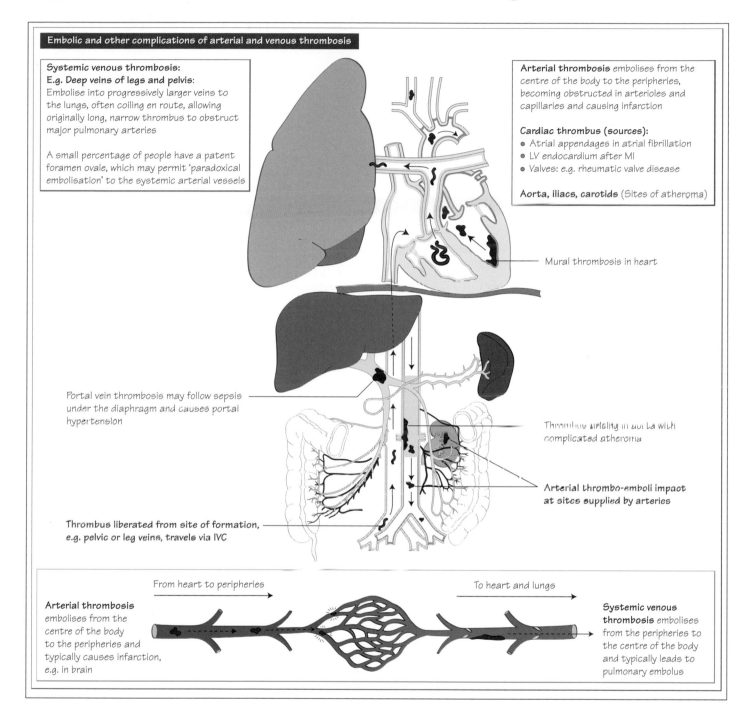

Embolic and other complications of arterial and venous thrombosis

Systemic venous thrombosis:
E.g. Deep veins of legs and pelvis:
Embolise into progressively larger veins to the lungs, often coiling en route, allowing originally long, narrow thrombus to obstruct major pulmonary arteries

A small percentage of people have a patent foramen ovale, which may permit 'paradoxical embolisation' to the systemic arterial vessels

Arterial thrombosis embolises from the centre of the body to the peripheries, becoming obstructed in arterioles and capillaries and causing infarction

Cardiac thrombus (sources):
- Atrial appendages in atrial fibrillation
- LV endocardium after MI
- Valves: e.g. rheumatic valve disease

Aorta, iliacs, carotids (Sites of atheroma)

Mural thrombosis in heart

Portal vein thrombosis may follow sepsis under the diaphragm and causes portal hypertension

Thrombus arising in aorta with complicated atheroma

Arterial thrombo-emboli impact at sites supplied by arteries

Thrombus liberated from site of formation, e.g. pelvic or leg veins, travels via IVC

From heart to peripheries

To heart and lungs

Arterial thrombosis embolises from the centre of the body to the peripheries and typically causes infarction, e.g. in brain

Systemic venous thrombosis embolises from the peripheries to the centre of the body and typically leads to pulmonary embolus

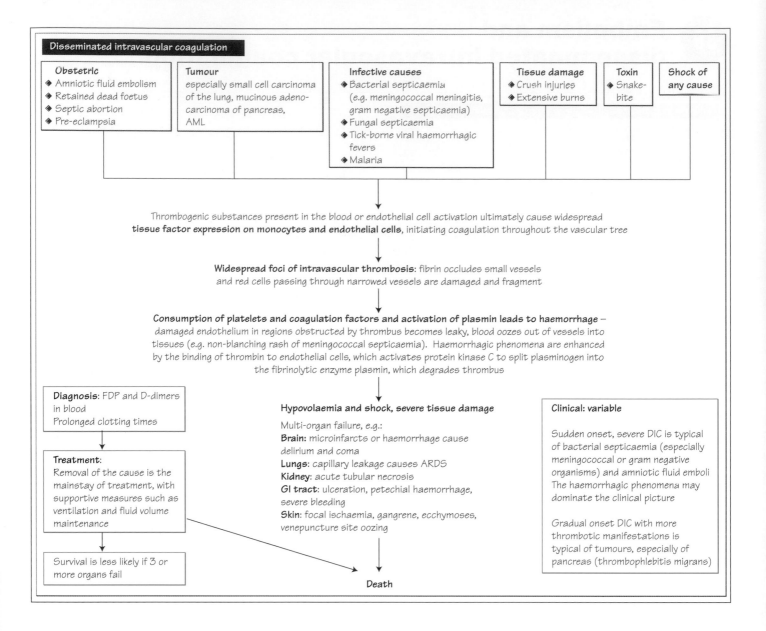

Disseminated intravascular coagulation

Obstetric	Tumour	Infective causes	Tissue damage	Toxin	Shock of
◆ Amniotic fluid embolism ◆ Retained dead foetus ◆ Septic abortion ◆ Pre-eclampsia	especially small cell carcinoma of the lung, mucinous adeno-carcinoma of pancreas, AML	◆ Bacterial septicaemia (e.g. meningococcal meningitis, gram negative septicaemia) ◆ Fungal septicaemia ◆ Tick-borne viral haemorrhagic fevers ◆ Malaria	◆ Crush injuries ◆ Extensive burns	◆ Snake-bite	any cause

Thrombogenic substances present in the blood or endothelial cell activation ultimately cause widespread **tissue factor expression on monocytes and endothelial cells**, initiating coagulation throughout the vascular tree

Widespread foci of intravascular thrombosis: fibrin occludes small vessels and red cells passing through narrowed vessels are damaged and fragment

Consumption of platelets and coagulation factors and activation of plasmin leads to haemorrhage – damaged endothelium in regions obstructed by thrombus becomes leaky, blood oozes out of vessels into tissues (e.g. non-blanching rash of meningococcal septicaemia). Haemorrhagic phenomena are enhanced by the binding of thrombin to endothelial cells, which activates protein kinase C to split plasminogen into the fibrinolytic enzyme plasmin, which degrades thrombus

Diagnosis: FDP and D-dimers in blood
Prolonged clotting times

Treatment:
Removal of the cause is the mainstay of treatment, with supportive measures such as ventilation and fluid volume maintenance

Survival is less likely if 3 or more organs fail

Hypovolaemia and shock, severe tissue damage

Multi-organ failure, e.g.:
Brain: microinfarcts or haemorrhage cause delirium and coma
Lungs: capillary leakage causes ARDS
Kidney: acute tubular necrosis
GI tract: ulceration, petechial haemorrhage, severe bleeding
Skin: focal ischaemia, gangrene, ecchymoses, venepuncture site oozing

Clinical: variable

Sudden onset, severe DIC is typical of bacterial septicaemia (especially meningococcal or gram negative organisms) and amniotic fluid emboli
The haemorrhagic phenomena may dominate the clinical picture

Gradual onset DIC with more thrombotic manifestations is typical of tumours, especially of pancreas (thrombophlebitis migrans)

Death

Embolism

An embolus is a substance carried in the blood that lodges in and obstructs vessels distant to the point of origin of the embolus.
• Ninety-nine per cent of emboli are formed of thrombus (thromboemboli), which can originate on either the arterial or venous side of the circulation. Portal vein thrombus seldom embolises, in part due to the low pressure within the system.
• Fat globules or chunks of bone marrow may embolise if mobilised into the circulation, e.g. through fracture of the long bones by trauma – larger pieces are seen in the lungs, but showers of fat globules may cause microcirculatory damage, particularly in the brain.
• Accidental introduction of air into the venous system may occur through faulty intravenous cannulation equipment – this is usually gradual and causes respiratory discomfort as bubbles form in small vessels, but can be remedied quickly without harm. Large air emboli (e.g. due to homicidal slitting of the jugular vein) can form a bolus that obstructs cardiac function, although 50–100 ml of air are required.
• Amniotic fluid may occasionally enter the maternal circulation, e.g. in unskilled instrumentation during 'back street' abortions. This is

highly thrombogenic and often causes disseminated intravascular coagulation (DIC).
• Nitrogen may come out of solution and form bubbles that obstruct the microvasculature of the brain, joints and other organs in divers who ascend to the surface too quickly (the 'bends').

The effects of thromboembolism are dictated by the direction of flow and the site of the originating thrombus.

Arterial thromboembolism

Blood flows from the aorta to the tissues, passing from larger to smaller arteries. Arterial emboli usually arise from an atheroma-associated thrombus on the wall of a large vessel or from thrombus in the heart. Emboli from theses sources cause distant infarction when they become impacted in a smaller artery (e.g. infarction of toes, segments of bowel, kidney). Sometimes cholesterol crystals can be seen in the thromboemboli on microscopic examination. Arterial infarcts tend to be wedge-shaped. These infarcts normally produce coagulative necrosis. Atherosclerosis at the carotid artery bifurcation is a common source of emboli to the brain and may produce narrowing that is audible as a bruit.

Cardiac thromboembolism

A cardiac mural thrombus can develop in atrial fibrillation, during an acute myocardial infarction (MI) or in a ventricular aneurysm. The vegetations of endocarditis can also serve as a source of emboli. The embolism can be to anywhere in the systemic arterial tree but is particularly likely to cause cerebrovascular complications, such as transient ischaemic attacks or ischaemic stroke.

Systemic venous thromboembolism

Venous blood drains towards the heart from the tissues. The first site of impaction is therefore the pulmonary circulation and a **pulmonary embolism** results. Small venous emboli can be dealt with efficiently by the fibrinolytic system and it is estimated that only 10% of pulmonary emboli become clinically apparent. Larger emboli may cause death due to shock and abrupt right heart failure. Medium-sized emboli or showers of small emboli that overwhelm the fibrinolytic system may cause breathlessness, pleuritic chest pain and haemoptysis.

Rarely, a venous embolism reaches a right atrium in which not only is an atrial septal defect present but a right-to-left shunt also exists. Under such circumstances, a venous embolus may enter the systemic circulation and thus a deep venous thrombosis may give rise to a paradoxical embolus affecting arterial territory.

Portal vein thrombosis

The portal vein may thrombose secondary to adjacent sepsis, which may occur if collections of infected material surround the porta hepatis, such as in perforation of a viscus. Portal vein thrombosis may occasionally complicate severe acute cholecystitis.

The thrombosis causes 'pre-hepatic' portal hypertension, in which the liver is normal. The effects in the portal circulation are similar to those of portal hypertension caused by cirrhosis: blood backs up along the splenic vein, causing splenic engorgement, and opening of portal–systemic anastamoses may occur.

Disseminated intravascular coagulation

This very serious deregulation of intravascular clotting mechanisms occurs when foci of thrombosis are simultaneously activated throughout the entire vascular tree. Many triggers are known, though ultimately most of these work by upregulating tissue factor expression on monocytes/macrophages and endothelial cells (which normally do not express this on their surfaces), which initiates the clotting cascade. In infective causes this is through the formation of a lipopolysaccharide/lipopolysaccharide binding protein complex, which binds CD14 on macrophages/monocytes leading to activation and tissue factor expression.

The formation and removal of multiple thrombi throughout the smaller blood vessels and capillary tree quickly exhausts the plasma supplies of both coagulation factors and antithrombotic factors. Depending on which element predominates, the clinical picture is either that of thrombosis or haemorrhage.

In haemorrhagic disease, the endothelial cell damage, which is often coincident and produced by the same stimulus that invoked the DIC, leads to bleeding and oozing. The overwhelmed coagulation cascade is unable to seal the small defects caused by endothelial cell drop-out. Marked blood volume depletion occurs and multiorgan failure develops. Organ failure occurs, with the kidneys and lungs tending to be first. If more than three organ systems fail, death is almost inevitable.

Clinically, DIC is apparent as widespread petechial haemorrhages within the skin and mucous membranes – at postmortem these petechiae are seen throughout the gut and the mucous membrane of the bronchial tree, and over the pericardial surface. At quite an early stage, the detection of fibrin degradation products in the blood indicates the onset of DIC. All clotting tests (international normalised ratio (INR), activated partial thromboplastin time (APTT) and thrombin time (TT)) are abnormal in DIC and there is thrombocytopenia.

Treatment involves removing the stimulus (e.g. septicaemia), replacing the lost blood and clotting factors and supporting failing organs.

39

Cardiac valvular disease

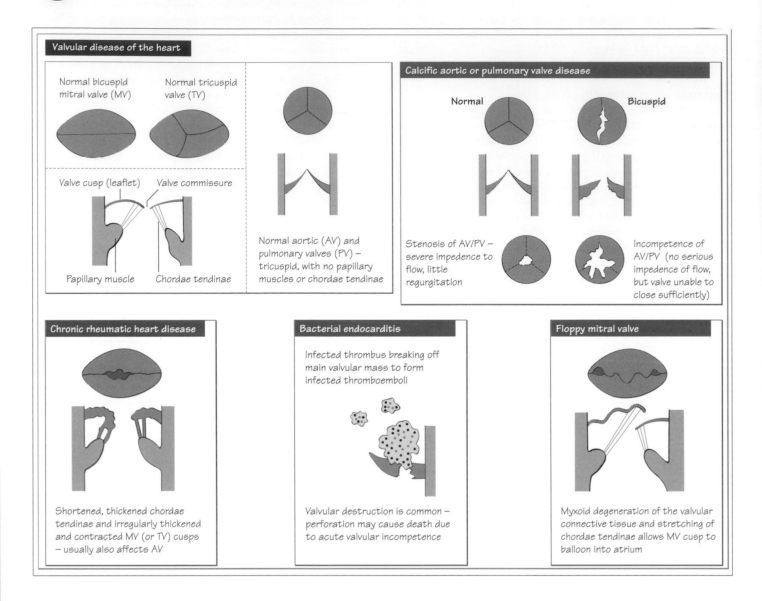

Valvular disease of the heart

Normal bicuspid mitral valve (MV)

Normal tricuspid valve (TV)

Valve cusp (leaflet) Valve commissure

Papillary muscle Chordae tendinae

Normal aortic (AV) and pulmonary valves (PV) – tricuspid, with no papillary muscles or chordae tendinae

Calcific aortic or pulmonary valve disease

Normal Bicuspid

Stenosis of AV/PV – severe impedence to flow, little regurgitation

Incompetence of AV/PV (no serious impedence of flow, but valve unable to close sufficiently)

Chronic rheumatic heart disease

Shortened, thickened chordae tendinae and irregularly thickened and contracted MV (or TV) cusps – usually also affects AV

Bacterial endocarditis

Infected thrombus breaking off main valvular mass to form infected thromboemboli

Valvular destruction is common – perforation may cause death due to acute valvular incompetence

Floppy mitral valve

Myxoid degeneration of the valvular connective tissue and stretching of chordae tendinae allows MV cusp to balloon into atrium

Systems pathology

 Pathology at a Glance. By C.J. Finlayson and B.A.T. Newell. Published 2009 by Blackwell Publishing. ISBN: 978-1-4051-3650-1

The heart valves are essential to ensure that the blood flow through the four cardiac chambers moves in the right direction and that the energy of cardiac contraction is devoted to achieving this without wastage. Defective cardiac valves are usually considered in terms of two functional abnormalities:
• A stenotic valve fails to open properly and therefore does not allow adequate blood flow across it.
• A regurgitant valve fails to close properly and therefore permits blood to be expelled in the wrong direction.
Sometimes a diseased valve will exhibit both stenotic and regurgitant behaviour.

Valve disease affects the left side of the heart far more often than the right. The aortic valve is involved more than the mitral valve. Valve dysfunction is typically associated with a murmur due to the resulting turbulent flow across the valve. Normal blood flow is laminar and therefore silent.

Aortic and pulmonary valves

Stenosis of the ventricular outflow valves increases the afterload on the affected ventricle. The ventricle responds by hypertrophy, in order to overcome the increased resistance. Although this is initially successful, the metabolic demands of the ventricle increase and blood flow across the thickened muscle becomes progressively impaired until the ventricle is at risk of ischaemia during vigorous activity. This can manifest as angina or even sudden death. Inadequate expulsion of blood from the ventricle due to the blockage posed by the stenotic valve can cause dyspnoea or exertional syncope. In severe aortic stenosis, the pressure gradient across the valve exceeds 100 mmHg, meaning that the left ventricle has to generate a pressure 100 mmHg above systolic blood pressure just to overcome the resistance of the valve. This massive effort can be felt as a heave.

Regurgitant valves increase the volume load on the ventricle. The main adaptive response is dilatation. Thus, unlike aortic stenosis, aortic regurgitation is associated with a displaced apex beat. Although the dilatation accommodates the greater volume of blood, Laplace's law means that to generate the same pressure, the wall tension and therefore cardiac exertion, is increased. While Starling's law of the heart initially allows the heart to adapt, a volume is reached at which the heart cannot adapt and the ventricle fails to deal with the preload.

Mitral and tricuspid valves

While the atrioventricular (AV) valves can also be affected by either stenosis or regurgitation, the atria tend to manifest the same pathological response to both, namely dilatation. The much thinner wall of the atrial myocardium seems unable to generate significant hypertrophy to counter stenosis without dilating.

Dilatation of the atria can disorganise the conducting system, leading to atrial fibrillation.

Stenotic AV valves prevent adequate ventricular filling and cardiac output can therefore be inadequate during exertion, leading to dyspnoea or syncope.

Causes of cardiac valvular disease

Various diseases can damage the heart valves, but there are two primary conditions of the valves that are particularly important.

Infective endocarditis

Infective endocarditis is caused by colonisation of the valves by microorganisms, typically bacteria. The resulting acute inflammatory process and proliferation of the bacteria destroy the valve tissue such that infective endocarditis tends to cause regurgitation, although stenosis can also result from neovascularisation and thickening of the cusps, as well as fusion and fibrotic healing of damaged cusps.

Most cases of infective endocarditis affect valves that are already damaged, such as by rheumatic fever, congenital malformations or degenerative change, or involve prosthetic valves. Less commonly, normal valves are infected during an episode of septicaemia.

Damaged valves are more at risk because the local turbulent blood flow can often generate small thrombi on their surface and these provide a foothold for bacteria that gain access to the bloodstream during a transient bacteraemia. Such bacteraemias can follow relatively trivial mucosal damage, such as dental work, and are normally dealt with by the immune system without incident. *Streptococcus* tends to be the genus that takes advantage of damaged valves, with enterococci and staphylococci comprising most of the remainder. Infective endocarditis of normal valves is usually caused by *Staphylococcus aureus*.

As well as destroying the valve, the infected vegetation is a shaggy, friable structure that can give rise to emboli, leading to complications of cerebrovascular accident, splenic and renal infarcts and splinter haemorrhages. Furthermore, the infection can spread to the underlying valve ring and myocardium. A small abscess can result and in the case of the aortic valve this is ideally placed to interfere with the AV conduction system. The response to the infection often leads to high levels of circulating immune complexes, so related immune complex deposition diseases such as glomerulonephritis can occur.

The right side of the heart is relatively protected from infective endocarditis by its status as a low pressure system. The turbulence and thrombosis vital in the pathogenesis of infective endocarditis are far more readily generated by the high pressure left ventricle. However, right-sided infective endocarditis can develop in intravenous drug abusers and is often caused by *Staph. aureus*.

Rheumatic fever

This is a multisystem condition of inflammatory aetiology that affects the heart, joints, skin and brain. It develops 2–3 weeks after infection with certain strains of Lancefield group A streptococci and is believed to be due to cross-reactivity between bacterial antigens and those in the affected organs. Although rare in the United Kingdom, it remains common in the Indian subcontinent, Africa and the Middle East. It usually affects children and young adults.

The characteristic lesion in the heart is the Aschoff body, which is a pale focus of eosinophilic hyaline material that is surrounded by lymphocytes and macrophages (Anitschkow cells). Aschoff bodies can affect any of the three layers of the heart. Involvement of the valves also incorporates acute inflammation, neovascularisation and focal fibrinoid necrosis. These changes are followed by fibrosis such that the affected valves become stiff and thickened with fusion of the cusps. The process can extend onto the chordae tendinae of the AV valves. The heart can also show myocarditis and a thick, shaggy, fibrinous pericarditis.

The condition also features arthritis, painful subcutaneous nodules, the characteristic rash of erythema marginatum and Sydenham's chorea.

The fibrotic tendency of the healing process in rheumatic fever means that the resulting valve lesions tend to be stenotic and rheumatic fever accounts for the vast majority of cases of mitral stenosis worldwide. Note that if the stenotic valve is sufficiently stiffened and deformed it is unable to close properly and is therefore also regurgitant.

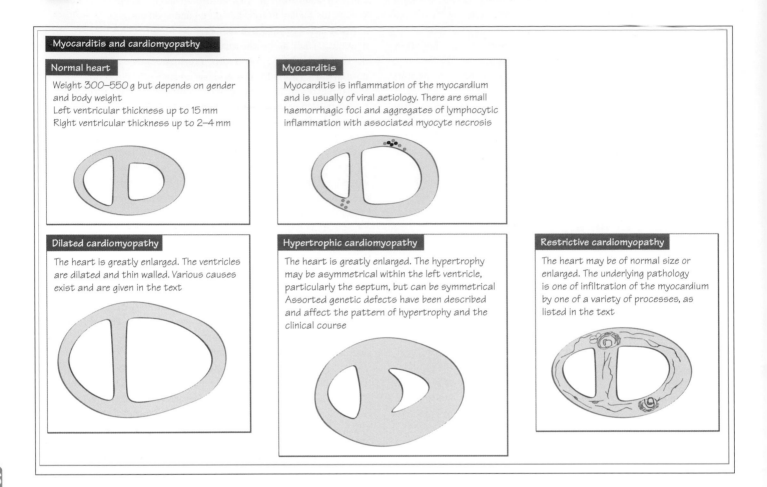

Myocarditis and cardiomyopathy

Normal heart

Weight 300–550 g but depends on gender and body weight
Left ventricular thickness up to 15 mm
Right ventricular thickness up to 2–4 mm

Myocarditis

Myocarditis is inflammation of the myocardium and is usually of viral aetiology. There are small haemorrhagic foci and aggregates of lymphocytic inflammation with associated myocyte necrosis

Dilated cardiomyopathy

The heart is greatly enlarged. The ventricles are dilated and thin walled. Various causes exist and are given in the text

Hypertrophic cardiomyopathy

The heart is greatly enlarged. The hypertrophy may be asymmetrical within the left ventricle, particularly the septum, but can be symmetrical Assorted genetic defects have been described and affect the pattern of hypertrophy and the clinical course

Restrictive cardiomyopathy

The heart may be of normal size or enlarged. The underlying pathology is one of infiltration of the myocardium by one of a variety of processes, as listed in the text

Hypertrophic cardiomyopathy

This is an autosomal dominant disease in which there is hypertrophy of the left ventricle in the absence of another cause. A significant number of cases develop as sporadic new mutations without a family history. A variety of mutations exists and tends to affect one of the contractile proteins, such as myosin or troponin. Different mutations are associated with different disease severities and clinical presentations.

Pathology

The typical macroscopic appearance is asymmetrical hypertrophy of the left ventricle, such that the ventricular septum in particular is disproportionately enlarged. However, variants exist in which the hypertrophy is uniform.

Microscopically, the cardiac myocytes are arranged in a disordered, whorled pattern. This disorganisation is recapitulated within the individual myocytes by their disarrayed myofibrils. The myocytes have enlarged nuclei and contain elevated quantities of glycogen. Accompanying the myocyte changes is interstitial fibrosis.

Functional implications

The hypertrophied myocardium is stiffer than usual and is less distensible. Therefore, diastolic filling is impaired. A fourth heart sound may occur because the atrium contracts forcefully to try to fill the ventricle.

Decreased ventricular filling reduces the amount of blood available for systolic ejection. In exercise, the increase in heart rate reduces the time available for diastolic filling and the filling defect is worsened.

The hypertrophy distorts the ventricle and this can sometimes distort the mitral valve ring, yielding mitral regurgitation. The papillary muscles can also be disturbed by the hypertrophy and become an independent cause of mitral regurgitation. Thus, a ventricle that is already filling poorly may also expel some of its reduced volume of available blood in the wrong direction.

The increased contractility of the left ventricle increases the velocity at which blood is ejected. By the Bernoulli principle, this is accompanied by a decrease in the pressure across the left ventricular outflow tract. As a consequence, the anterior leaflet of the mitral valve is drawn towards the interventricular septum. With the septum already hypertrophied, this yields a dynamic obstruction of the outflow tract. The positive inotropic effect encountered in exercise can exacerbate this problem.

The thickened, hypertrophic left ventricle has increased metabolic demands, but oxygen delivery becomes impaired with excessive degrees of ventricular hypertrophy. The elevated metabolic requirements of exercise place additional stress on this system.

Clinical correlations

Hypertrophic cardiomyopathy is the classic cause of sudden, unexpected death in a young athelete. The disease is notorious for remaining silent in this fashion. Death can result from a combination of inadequate ventricular filling – the ventricular outflow obstruction reducing cardiac output (including blood flow through the coronary arteries) and myocardial ischaemia.

Less dramatic presentations share similarities with aortic stenosis and for similar reasons. There is an obstructed, hypertrophic left ventricle that is at risk of ischaemia and cannot maintain adequate output in the face of exertion.

Dilated cardiomyopathy

This is by far the commonest cardiomyopathy and is characterised by dilatation and impaired contraction of one or both ventricles. By definition, primary dilated cardiomyopathy excludes the secondary causes of ischaemic heart disease, hypertension and valve disease. However, this leaves many other causes:

- Alcohol.
- Genetic.
- Viral.
- Rheumatic fever.
- Autoimmune.
- Drugs: anthracycline chemotherapy.
- Collagen vascular diseases: systemic lupus erythematosus (SLE), scleroderma, rheumatoid arthritis
- Inherited neurological disorders: muscular dystrophy, myotonic dystrophy, Friedreich's ataxia, Refsum's disease.
- Haemochromatosis.
- Thyrotoxicosis.
- Peripartum cardiomyopathy.
- Nutritional deficiencies: thiamine, selenium, phosphate.

Pathology

There is progressive dilatation of the ventricles and the myocardium is pale and flabby. If dilatation of the atrioventricular valve rings occurs, valvular regurgitation may result. The dilated ventricle can become susceptible to mural thrombus.

The dilated myocardium is functionally defective, so progressive cardiac failure results.

Restrictive cardiomyopathy

This is the rarest of the three cardiomyopathies and is due to an abnormality of the ventricle which renders it stiff and therefore impedes ventricular filling and reduces cardiac output. Most of the causes reflect some form of infiltrative process and include the following:

- Amyloidosis.
- Sarcoidosis.
- Haemochromatosis.
- Radiation damage.
- Glycogen storage disease.
- Scleroderma.
- Loeffler's eosinophilic endocarditis.
- Endomyocardial fibrosis.

Arrhythmogenic right ventricular dysplasia

This is a genetic disorder that is of fairly recent description and features in the list of causes of sudden death in young adults. The right ventricle is thinned, replaced by fat and prone to arrhythmias.

Myocarditis

Myocarditis is inflammation of the myocardium and is rare. It is typically of infective aetiology. A multitude of viruses can cause myocarditis, but coxsackie A and B and enteroviruses are the most common. More unusual causes include diphtheria, rheumatic fever and chloroquine.

The pathogenesis is most likely to be T cell-mediated attack against viral antigens expressed on the myocardial cell membrane. There is a chronic inflammatory cell infiltrate with destruction of cardiac myocytes.

Presentation can be dramatic with marked cardiac failure. A cardiac transplant may be necessary although many cases are far more mild.

Pericarditis

Several different types of pericarditis exist:

- Serous: e.g. rheumatic fever, SLE, scleroderma, tumours, uraemia.
- Fibrinous: this is the commonest and often occurs during acute myocardial infarction (MI). Dressler's syndrome occurs several weeks after an MI.
- Purulent/suppurative: usually infective in aetiology.
- Haemorrhagic: may be seen with metastatic tumour.
- Tuberculous.
- Chronic: small adhesions, often seen at postmortem, of little significance.

Pericarditis often has the appearances of two buttered slices of bread that have been pressed together, then pulled apart ('bread and butter pericarditis').

Constrictive pericarditis

In this condition the pericardium becomes thickened and non-expansile. This interferes with ventricular filling, leading to reduced cardiac output. Many of the clinical features therefore overlap with those of restrictive cardiomyopathy. Any cause of acute pericarditis may progress to constrictive pericarditis through fibrotic organisation of the acute inflammation, but tuberculosis is historically the most common cause. Most episodes of acute pericarditis do not reach this end-point.

Tamponade

Tamponade is an extreme form of a pericardial effusion in which the volume of fluid that has accumulated is sufficient to compress the atria and their inflow veins and prevent filling of the heart. This produces severe cardiac failure or cardiac arrest with pulseless electrical activity. The cause is usually myocardial rupture, aortic dissection, trauma or severe acute pericarditis.

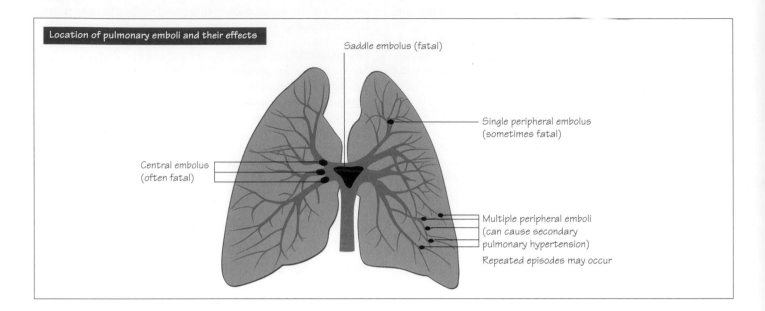

Location of pulmonary emboli and their effects

Saddle embolus (fatal)

Single peripheral embolus (sometimes fatal)

Central embolus (often fatal)

Multiple peripheral emboli (can cause secondary pulmonary hypertension)

Repeated episodes may occur

Pulmonary embolism

Pulmonary embolism (PE) is a condition in which an embolism impacts within the pulmonary vasculature. The risk factors for PE are largely the same as those for deep vein thrombosis due to the fact that most pulmonary emboli arise from the deep veins of the lower limb and pelvis. The right side of the heart is a much rarer source of pulmonary emboli.

Although most pulmonary emboli are thromboemboli, other rare sorts occur:
- Bone marrow/mature adipose tissue – seen after fractures.
- Amniotic fluid.
- Tumour cells.
- Air.

A thromboembolus will have the shape of the vessel in which it developed, not that of the vessel in which it impacts, though it may become coiled *en route*. It possesses a structure and lines of Zahn. Fibrous adhesions to the vessel wall may be seen in established cases. This is in contrast to clot that develops in the pulmonary arteries postmortem, which is softer, ramifies along the branches of the pulmonary vascular tree and lacks a structure. Separation of the serum and cellular components of a postmortem clot is referred to by the less than pleasant term of 'chicken fat and redcurrant jelly'.

The clinical presentation depends upon the size of the PE but the basic pathophysiological changes are common.
- A PE will result in a region of lung that is ventilated but suddenly no longer perfused. If this region is sufficiently large, the volume of lung tissue lost for gas exchange will be sufficient to produce hypoxia. Loss of blood flow results in a decrease in surfactant production within a few hours, with consequent atelectasis in 12–15 hours.
- A PE reduces the cross-sectional area of the pulmonary vasculature. As flow remains the same, the resistance increases. However, approximately 50% of the pulmonary bed must be lost before this causes pulmonary hypertension.

Assuming the patient survives the PE, fibrinolytic processes can remove the embolus within 2 weeks.

In some individuals there are multiple small pulmonary emboli, which affect the periphery of the lungs. This process causes a gradual occlusion of the pulmonary vasculature and may reflect defective mechanisms for removing emboli rather than excessive generation.

Pulmonary infarction

Pulmonary infarction is necrosis of part of the lung due to a disruption of its blood supply. As the lung has a dual blood supply from the bronchial and pulmonary arteries, infarction is rare, even in pulmonary embolism. Those situations in which it does occur tend to be those in which there is impaired bronchial arterial flow and raised pulmonary venous pressure, such as in mitral stenosis.

The infarct is a wedge-shaped, well-demarcated region of necrosis, the apex of which is directed towards the hilum of the lung and the base towards the pleural surface.

Pulmonary hypertension

Pulmonary hypertension is an arterial pressure within the pulmonary circulation of more than 30 mmHg. Primary pulmonary hypertension is rare but numerous secondary causes exist:
- Congenital heart disease with shunts.
- Increased left atrial pressure.
- Pulmonary embolism.
- Chronic obstructive pulmonary disease (COPD).
- Interstitial lung disease.
- Granulomatous lung disease (sarcoidosis).
- Scleroderma.
- Systemic lupus erythematosus (SLE).
- Rheumatoid arthritis.
- Parasitic lung disease.
- Sickle cell disease.
- Chronic liver disease.

As a general rule, any chronic condition of the lungs that disrupts ventilation can theoretically cause secondary pulmonary hypertension.

Systems pathology

Primary pulmonary hypertension

Primary pulmonary hypertension is a rare condition of unknown aetiology that spans a wide age range, but tends to present in children under 10 years or in the third and fourth decades. The male : female ratio is 10 : 17.

The basic pathological lesion is plexogenic pulmonary arteriopathy. Initially, there is hypertrophy of the media of the small pulmonary arteries, making them resemble systemic arterioles. Smooth muscle cells then migrate into the tunica media where they proliferate and produce extracellular matrix proteins, causing fibroelastic thickening of the intima. This results in occlusion of the arteriole, which is followed by dilatation elsewhere in the circulation.

Localised dilatation is seen as clusters of thin-walled vessels that are proximal to the sites of occlusion. These are called angiomatoid lesions. Proliferation of myofibroblasts within the lesions gives the plexiform pattern.

In 10% of cases of primary pulmonary hypertension, the pathology is centred on the veins rather than the arterioles. This is pulmonary veno-occlusive disease and shows widespread proliferation and fibrosis in the intima of the veins. The process may extend to the arterioles.

Pulmonary venous hypertension

This reflects left heart failure, with back transmission of the increased filling pressures in the left atrium to the pulmonary circulation. The increased pressure can lead to oedema and extravasation of erythrocytes, the latter causing haemosiderin deposition. The iron can induce a fibrotic response, along with a brown discolouration. The iron may also act as a focus for calcium deposition and the formation of small mineralised bodies, or microlithiasis. Rarely, there can be osseous metaplasia.

Clinical correlations

Whereas the left ventricle is capable of generating pressures of up to 300 mmHg in the face of a sudden challenge, without the need to adapt, the right ventricle is a much lower pressure system and is considerably less tolerant of sudden increases in afterload. Hence a massive PE, which will place a sudden strain on the right ventricle, can precipitate acute right heart failure.

Hypoalbuminaemia is an important cause of peripheral oedema but it seldom induces pulmonary oedema. This is due to the much lower pressure in the pulmonary circulation. As a rough guide, pulmonary oedema will not arise due to hypoalbuminaemia unless the albumin is less than 0.57 of the pulmonary arterial pressure.

Systems pathology

Systems pathology

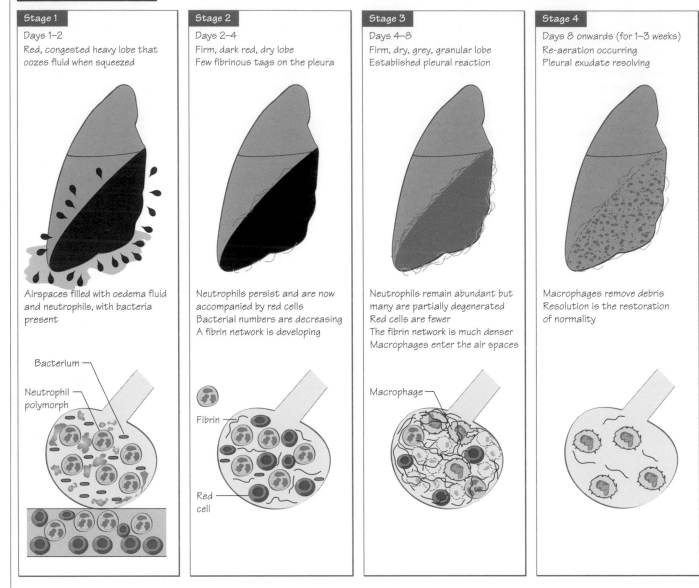

Features of lobar pneumonia

Stage 1

Days 1–2
Red, congested heavy lobe that
oozes fluid when squeezed

Airspaces filled with oedema fluid
and neutrophils, with bacteria
present

Bacterium

Neutrophil
polymorph

Stage 2

Days 2–4
Firm, dark red, dry lobe
Few fibrinous tags on the pleura

Neutrophils persist and are now
accompanied by red cells
Bacterial numbers are decreasing
A fibrin network is developing

Fibrin

Red
cell

Stage 3

Days 4–8
Firm, dry, grey, granular lobe
Established pleural reaction

Neutrophils remain abundant but
many are partially degenerated
Red cells are fewer
The fibrin network is much denser
Macrophages enter the air spaces

Macrophage

Stage 4

Days 8 onwards (for 1–3 weeks)
Re-aeration occurring
Pleural exudate resolving

Macrophages remove debris
Resolution is the restoration
of normality

Definition

Pneumonia is an acute infection of the lower respiratory tract in which there is filling of the alveolar spaces by exudate.

Epidemiology

Pneumonia is a common illness, with an incidence of 100–300 per 100 000 per year. The disease tends to present in the very young and the elderly, although no age group is exempt. The overall male to female ratio is equal, although some variations occur within the subtypes, specifically *Klebsiella*, which is more common in males.

Microbiology

Streptococcus pneumoniae accounts for the majority of cases; it is worth emphasising that ciprofloxacin, an otherwise popular broad spectrum antibiotic, is not effective against *S. pneumoniae*. The second commonest causative organism is *Mycoplasma pneumoniae*. This typically affects previously healthy adults and is community acquired.

Other important organisms are *Haemophilus influenzae* (patients with chronic obstructive pulmonary disease), *Legionella pneumophilia* (Legionnaire's disease), *Klebsiella pneumoniae* (diabetic males, especially alcoholics), *Pseudomonas aeruginosa* (patients with bronchiectasis and the immunosuppressed), *Staphylococcus aureus* (post influenza, can be a serious, destructive infection) and *Pneumocystis carinii* (a fungal pneumonia encountered in immunosuppressed patients, particularly AIDS).

The spread of the infection is by droplets and the inhalation route. Other than the extremes of age and immunocompromisation, predisposing factors encompass conditions in which there is impaired clearance of secretions from the distal airways, such as ciliary dysfunction (smokers), bronchiectasis and obstruction by a tumour.

Pathology

The traditional division is into lobar pneumonia and bronchopneumonia. Both of these share the process of consolidation, in which the distal airspaces are filled with an acute inflammatory exudate. Lobar pneumonia tends to affect healthy adults; bronchopneumonia is encountered in the elderly and the debilitated.

Other classifications reflect the pattern of acquisition and show a division into community acquired, hospital acquired, pneumonia in the immunocompromised and aspiration pneumonia. This division has the advantage of indicating the likely agents and therefore can guide treatment.

Lobar pneumonia

The four stages of lobar pneumonia are a staple feature of pathology textbooks. However, perhaps the most crucial feature to remember is that lobar pneumonia occurs in previously fit and healthy people and therefore has an excellent prognosis. As the name implies, lobar pneumonia affects one lobe and is clearly confined to that lobe.

Stage 1 The first stage is **acute congestion** and lasts 1–2 days. Faced with the initial infectious challenge, there is an acute inflammatory response. Hence, there is oedema and an exudate into the airspaces that is rich in neutrophils and organisms. The capillaries are congested. Macroscopically, this produces an affected lobe that is heavy, dark and red and yields abundant fluid when squeezed.

Stage 2 The second to fourth day is the stage of **red hepatisation**, so-called due to the resemblance of the involved lobe to liver. The neutrophils persist in the exudate and are accompanied by erythrocytes, but a network of fibrin has developed. The affected lobe is still heavy and dark but is now firm and dry. Pleural involvement is also now seen as grey-white friable tags of fibrin.

Stage 3 Days four to eight are **grey hepatisation**. The network of fibrin has become denser. The erythrocytes are now sparse, explaining the loss of the red colour. Neutrophils remain present, but many are now degenerating. The lobe is still firm and dry but is now granular and grey. The pleural reaction is more established.

Stage 4 From day eight onwards is **resolution**. Macrophages enter the fray to clear up the exudate and debris in the airspaces, assisted by fibrinolytic enzymes. Resolution also occurs on the pleura, but the process here can incorporate fibrosis, leading to adhesions between the visceral and parietal pleura. Full resolution and re-aeration of the airspaces requires 1–3 weeks.

Bronchopneumonia

By contrast with lobar pneumonia, bronchopneumonia is centred on the bronchioles and alveoli and is not lobe specific. Consolidation develops in a manner similar to the stages of lobar pneumonia but macroscopically is more widespread and scattered, rather than being demarcated to one lobe. Squeezing the cut surface of an affected lung will cause beads of pus to be produced from the involved airways.

Resolution of bronchopneumonia is not as complete as in lobar pneumonia. The extension of the process into the bronchioles leads to damage and fibrosis there. In extreme cases, this generates bronchiectasis.

At postmortem, lobar pneumonia is a rare finding because it is very seldom fatal. Consolidation in general yields lung tissue which has a more solid, but also rotten, feel to it; normal lung behaves like a sponge when pressed with a thumb whereas consolidated lung gives way like soft cheese.

Clinical correlations

The presence of a productive cough is evident from the process of consolidation described above. The lower lobes are most prone to bronchopneumonia in debilitated individuals as these lobes suffer from the gravitational accumulation of secretions, which can be exacerbated by muscular weakness that impairs the ability to expectorate the secretions.

Extension of the infection to the pleural surface yields pleurisy. This is an important phenomenon as the pleuritic pain that results from deep breathing or coughing conflicts with the need to do so to clear the inflammatory exudate.

Staphylococcus aureus pneumonia is often a secondary phenomenon that occurs in people who are already suffering from acute airway damage, such as in whooping cough or influenza. It is rapidly progressive, haemorrhagic and destructive, with a tendency to form abscesses or may cause rapid deterioration and death.

Systems pathology

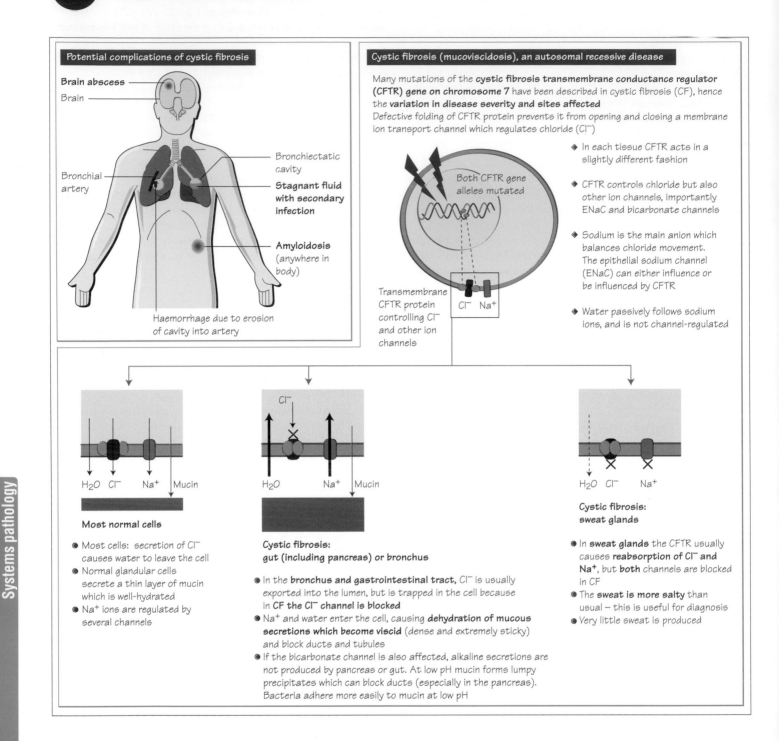

Potential complications of cystic fibrosis

Brain abscess

Brain

Bronchial artery

Bronchiectatic cavity

Stagnant fluid with secondary infection

Amyloidosis (anywhere in body)

Haemorrhage due to erosion of cavity into artery

Cystic fibrosis (mucoviscidosis), an autosomal recessive disease

Many mutations of the **cystic fibrosis transmembrane conductance regulator (CFTR) gene on chromosome 7** have been described in cystic fibrosis (CF), hence the **variation in disease severity and sites affected**

Defective folding of CFTR protein prevents it from opening and closing a membrane ion transport channel which regulates chloride (Cl^-)

Both CFTR gene alleles mutated

Transmembrane CFTR protein controlling Cl^- and other ion channels

Cl^- Na^+

◆ In each tissue CFTR acts in a slightly different fashion

◆ CFTR controls chloride but also other ion channels, importantly ENaC and bicarbonate channels

◆ Sodium is the main anion which balances chloride movement. The epithelial sodium channel (ENaC) can either influence or be influenced by CFTR

◆ Water passively follows sodium ions, and is not channel-regulated

H_2O Cl^- Na^+ | Mucin

Most normal cells

● Most cells: secretion of Cl^- causes water to leave the cell
● Normal glandular cells secrete a thin layer of mucin which is well-hydrated
● Na^+ ions are regulated by several channels

Cl^-

H_2O Na^+ | Mucin

Cystic fibrosis: gut (including pancreas) or bronchus

● In the **bronchus and gastrointestinal tract**, Cl^- is usually exported into the lumen, but is trapped in the cell because in **CF the Cl^- channel is blocked**
● Na^+ and water enter the cell, causing **dehydration of mucous secretions which become viscid** (dense and extremely sticky) and block ducts and tubules
● If the bicarbonate channel is also affected, alkaline secretions are not produced by pancreas or gut. At low pH mucin forms lumpy precipitates which can block ducts (especially in the pancreas). Bacteria adhere more easily to mucin at low pH

H_2O Cl^- Na^+

Cystic fibrosis: sweat glands

● In **sweat glands** the CFTR usually causes **reabsorption of Cl^- and Na^+**, but **both** channels are blocked in CF
● The **sweat is more salty** than usual – this is useful for diagnosis
● Very little sweat is produced

Definition

Bronchiectasis is an abnormal and irreversible dilatation of the bronchi.

Causes

The underlying mechanism is frequently a chronic necrotising infection of the bronchi and bronchioles. This makes many of the causes relatively predictable:

- Cystic fibrosis.
- Severe childhood lung infection.
- Pneumonia, specifically severe forms, such as due to *Staphylococcus aureus* or *Klebsiella*.
- Tuberculosis.
- Allergic aspergillosis.
- Hypogammaglobulinaemia.
- Kartagener's syndrome.
  Other causes exist but are rare.

Epidemiology

Bronchiectasis can be regarded more as a complication of other conditions, rather than a disease in itself. Having a diverse set of underlying aetiologies, its epidemiology is varied and follows that of the associated causes.

Pathology

As with emphysema, the definition summarises the fundamental aspects of the pathology. Three main patterns of bronchial dilatation are described. In the cylindrical form, the bronchi are uniformly dilated tubes. The varicose variant has irregular beaded dilatation. The saccular type features bronchi with a ballooned, blind-ending sac at their periphery.

All three patterns have the same underlying process, which is one of chronic, destructive inflammation affecting the walls of medium-sized airways. This destruction is followed by fibrosis. The fibrosis is a functionally inadequate attempt at repair. The smaller airways can be obliterated by the combination of destructive inflammation and the subsequent fibrosis.

The inflammatory process induces an increase in the vascularity of the bronchial wall, which can culminate in anastamoses between the bronchial and pulmonary circulations. The dilated airways and the cavities that develop in bronchiectasis are initially lined by respiratory ciliated columnar epithelium but, as with chronic irritation in chronic bronchitis, squamous metaplasia may supervene.

Clinical correlations

In common with cavities elsewhere in the body, those of bronchiectasis are susceptible to the accumulation of secretions. Stagnant secretions permit colonisation by organisms and infection. This can lead to pneumonia or a lung abscess. In addition, because of the increased vascularity that may be associated with bronchiectasis, the infection can involve the walls of blood vessels, from which septic emboli and distant abscesses arise. The brain is particularly affected by abscesses of bronchiectatic origin.

The abnormally dense and anastamosing network of vessels in bronchiectasis is susceptible to haemorrhage if further damage or inflammation occurs. Hence, bronchiectasis can be complicated by massive haemoptysis.

Bronchiectasis is a chronic inflammatory condition, so may therefore be complicated by amyloidosis.

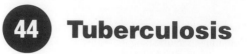

Systems pathology

Tuberculosis and its complications

Primary complex (Ghon complex): Granulomatous inflammation with caseation is seen here and in enlarged hilar lymph nodes

Hilar lymph nodes

Ghon focus

The Ziehl-Neelsen stain demonstrates MTB within a Langhan's giant cell: the red stain cannot be washed out of the waxy bacterial coat by either acid or alcohol, hence the term 'alcohol-acid fast bacilli', or AAFB

Caseous necrosis replaces renal parenchyma

Extrapulmonary tuberculosis, e.g. kidney
Any part of the body may be involved by tuberculosis. It is thought that organisms reach these sites via the blood stream However **intestinal tuberculosis** may occur due to infection from swallowed sputum containing Mycobacterium tuberculosis hominis or from drinking non-pasteurised milk from cattle infected with Mycobacterium tuberculosis bovis

Possible sequelae of primary tuberculosis

Secondary/reactivation TB with cavitation – the cavity may later become colonised by fungus

Miliary tubercles in lung parenchyma. Similar nodules may be scattered throughout the body (May occur with either primary or secondary TB)

TB bronchopneumonia: cavitating TB breaks into a bronchus and spreads along the bronchial tree to cause consolidation in the lung parenchyma

TB empyema
The tuberculous cavity breaks through the visceral pleura and caseous material spreads into the pleural space

Granulomatous inflammation in tuberculosis

Simultaneous attempt to engulf the same AAFB

Multinucleate giant cell

PMN

AAFB

Macrophage

AAFB encountered: the innate immune system is activated, but cannot kill it

Activated macrophage phagocytoses AAFB

Epithelioid giant cell

Epithelioid giant cell granuloma, under T cell regulation

Caseous necrosis

Caseous necrosis is typical of TB but not of other granulomatous conditions

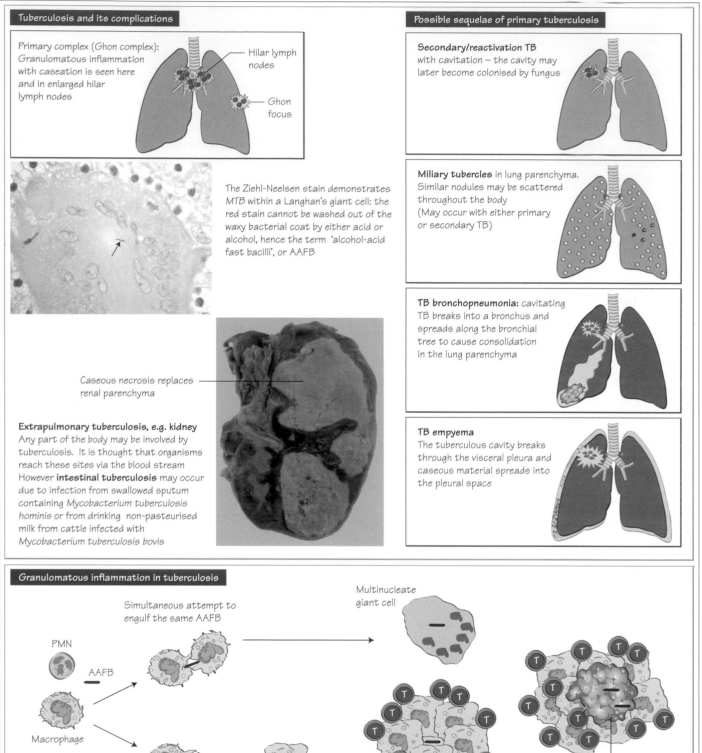

Tuberculosis (TB) is a major problem in developing countries, especially in those people with impaired immune function.
- About one-third of the world's population is subclinically infected with latent *Mycobacterium tuberculosis*, which can reactivate years later – infecting future generations.
- Ninety-five per cent of people exposed to the TB bacillus develop latent TB; only 5% initially develop active disease.
- Reactivation and new infections account for approximately 8 million new cases of TB worldwide.
- About 3 million people per year die of TB.
- Chronic alcoholism, diabetes mellitus and immunosuppression (e.g. HIV/AIDS or steroid treatment) increase the risk of acquiring new infection or of reactivating latent infection.

Primary TB: This is usually pulmonary, after inhalation of aerosolised *M. tuberculosis*, which can survive outside the body for hours or days.
- Inhaled *M. tuberculosis*, phagocytosed by alveolar macrophages, evades killing by inhibiting phagolysosome formation.
- The bacillus has a waxy, lipid-rich cell wall that influences its antigenicity and virulence.
- Activated epithelioid histiocytes (macrophages) wall off the infection site by forming granulomas. Giant cells form when macrophages fuse. The response to TB infection is an example of type IV hypersensitivity.
- The granulomas undergo central caseous necrosis – this resembles white, crumbly cheese. The granulomas coalesce and break down, releasing infected material into the lungs and causing a cough, often with bloodstained sputum.
- The initial infection site, about 2–3 mm across, in peripheral lung tissue is the 'Ghon focus'. The draining hilar lymph nodes become infected and develop granulomas. The Ghon focus plus enlarged hilar lymph nodes is the 'Ghon complex'.

Secondary TB: This may be due to reactivation of the primary infection or to re-infection, usually in the apex of the lung, where cavitation (several centimetres across) is often seen. During the initial infection, TB bacilli are carried via lung lymphatics to the nodes and to other parts of the lung via lymphatics and capillaries.

Miliary TB: Blood-borne mycobacteria may disseminate to any part of the body, where tubercles resembling scattered millet seeds set up new foci of infection. This can occur in either primary or secondary TB if the infection erodes a major blood vessel. The damage seen in the affected tissues is the result of a type IV hypersensitivity reaction.

The survival of *M. tuberculosis* within macrophages and giant cells relies on its ability to:
- Prevent lysosomal fusion with the phagocytosed mycobacterium, which would normally cause bacterial killing.
- Prevent the pH of the endosome from dropping below pH 6.2.
- Prevent the release of highly potent killing oxidative radicals.
- Block apoptosis, procuring an immunological 'safe haven' in which to grow.

Sequelae following TB infection
- **Miliary TB**: see above.
- **Latent disease**: bacilli can survive in walled-off granulomas for decades.
- **Reactivation of latent disease**: this typically occurs in apical lung and may follow immune suppression, e.g. steroid therapy. The oxygen tension is highest in the lung apex, and is preferred by TB bacilli. Macrophages

function better in low oxygen tensions, as in the inflammatory milieu.
- **Tuberculous bronchopneumonia**: bronchial erosion permits the infection to spread via the bronchial tree.
- **Pneumothorax secondary to TB**: the inflammatory process erodes the bronchus and pleural membranes, allowing air into the pleural space and causing the lung to collapse.
- **Tuberculous empyema**: the inflammatory process breaks into the pleural space and caseous, inflamed and infected debris, macrophages and lymphocytes accumulate (despite the name there are few polymorphs present) .
- **Fungal colonisation**: Colonisation of cavitating secondary TB by fungi, typically by *Aspergillus* species.
- **Extrapulmonary tuberculosis**: e.g. in kidney, Fallopian tube or elsewhere. It is usually blood-borne. However, intestinal TB may be primary (infected milk with *M. tuberculosis bovis*) or secondary (infected sputum with *M. tuberculosis hominis*).
- **TB meningitis and miliary TB**: these are seldom seen in patients who have been vaccinated with BCG.

Clinical diagnosis of TB
Symptoms and signs of TB are highly variable; often there are no symptoms if it is a primary infection. Symptoms and signs include:
- Mild chronic cough.
- Cough with bloodstained sputum.
- Fever.
- Weight loss.
- Night sweats.
- Bronchopneumonia, fever and dyspnoea.
TB can infect any part of the body, mimicking other diseases.

Mantoux test: If TB has been encountered before, circulating memory T cells generate an immune response in a few days, manifest as erythema and induration at the tuberculin protein injection site. Primary TB may take 4 weeks to induce an immune response, thus the Mantoux test may be negative in early primary infection. Surprisingly it can be negative in overwhelming infection as well.

Generating immunity
Immunity to TB can be achieved using the BCG vaccine. This live attenuated strain of *M. tuberculosis bovis* is given as an intradermal injection and elicits hypersensitivity to its antigens, generating protective T cell-mediated responses. Note that infection itself is *not* prevented, just contained, and reactivation may occur if a patient's immunity is compromised.

Since the BCG vaccine has been used, the incidence of post-primary miliary TB and of TB meningitis, more a complication in children than in adults, has plummeted. However, BCG vaccine is only partially protective against adult forms of TB.

HIV and TB
- Macrophages are a reservoir for both *M. tuberculosis* and HIV (HIV also infects CD4+ T cells).
- Immune suppression by HIV/AIDS allows reactivation of latent TB.
- TB activates T cells and macrophages, stimulating gene expression, including integrated viral genes. More HIV is thus produced, which can infect further macrophages and CD4+ lymphocytes.
- HIV affects approximately 40 million people worldwide. TB is the major cause of death in 35% of HIV-positive patients, with the exception of those treated with HAART.

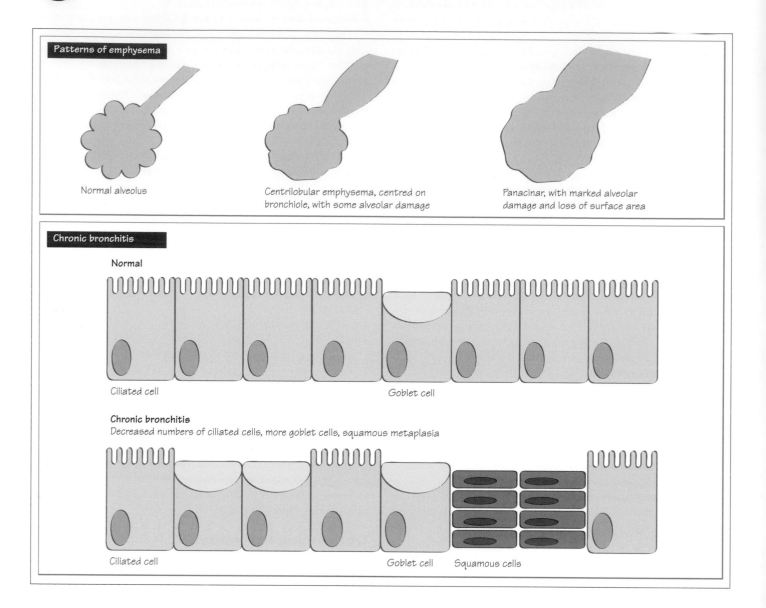

Patterns of emphysema

Normal alveolus

Centrilobular emphysema, centred on bronchiole, with some alveolar damage

Panacinar, with marked alveolar damage and loss of surface area

Chronic bronchitis

Normal

Ciliated cell

Goblet cell

Chronic bronchitis
Decreased numbers of ciliated cells, more goblet cells, squamous metaplasia

Ciliated cell

Goblet cell

Squamous cells

Definition

Chronic obstructive pulmonary disease (COPD) is a disorder in which there is an irreversible reduction of the $FEV_1 : FVC$ (forced expiratory volume in 1 second to forced vital capacity) ratio to less than 80% of that predicted in the absence of another cause.

Alternatively, COPD is the combination of chronic bronchitis and emphysema, which are defined as follows. Chronic bronchitis is a cough productive of sputum on most days of the month for 3 months of the year for two or more consecutive years, in the absence of other causes. Emphysema is dilatation of the airways distal to the terminal bronchioles with destruction of the tissues in their walls. COPD was previously referred to as chronic obstructive airways disease.

Note that chronic bronchitis is defined on clinical grounds, while emphysema has a pathological definition.

Causes

Smoking is the key aetiological factor. Environmental air pollution has a small role. Some cases of emphysema, but not chronic bronchitis, are due to α_1-antitrypsin deficiency.

Epidemiology

Presentation tends to be in middle age and onwards. As COPD is intimately related to smoking, the effects of changes in patterns of smoking on the distribution of COPD will be delayed for a few decades. Figures of 20% of the middle-aged population have been proposed as the prevalence for chronic bronchitis, but this includes subclinical cases.

Pathology

Chronic bronchitis and emphysema usually coexist, but nevertheless have different pathological features.

As chronic bronchitis is due to chronic irritation of the airways, the microscopic changes reflect this. Mucous glands are hypertrophied, and goblet cell numbers increase, while the numbers of ciliated cells decrease. The distribution of goblet cells also increases in extent, with goblet cells extending into the terminal bronchioles. Squamous metaplasia also occurs and, as with the switch to a greater degree of mucin production, is an attempt by the mucosa to defend itself against the damage induced by smoke.

The definition of emphysema given above encapsulates its pathology. The volume of the lungs increases and they may overlap the anterior borders of the heart at autopsy. However, while the lung volumes increase, the functional surface area for gas exchange decreases due to the destruction of lung tissue that is integral to emphysema. In some cases, the dilatation of the airways may lead to the formation of cystic spaces known as bullae. If these are subpleural, they may rupture, causing a pneumothorax. Much angst is needlessly expended over the distinction between centrilobular and panacinar distributions, given that the two usually coexist and the differentiation is of little to no clinical relevance in a symptomatic patient. The former type has the

changes centred on the terminal bronchioles, while the latter involves the whole of the respiratory acinus.

Clinical correlations and complications

Chronic bronchitis is associated with increased mucin production. Unfortunately, smoking impairs the function of the mucociliary escalator, which simultaneously suffers from a reduction in the number of ciliated cells. Thus, there is more mucus and an impaired ability to clear it.

As a consequence of the increased mucin production, the impaired clearance of gunge and the dilated terminal airspaces, the COPD lung is at risk of infection by bacteria of those spaces that fail to drain. Infective exacerbations of COPD are common, with *Haemophilus influenzae* being a frequent culprit. Mucopurulent material filling the airspaces of lungs that are already compromised in terms of gas transfer further exacerbates the impairment of gas exchange.

The disordered gas transfer affects pulmonary blood flow and ventilation–perfusion mismatches may develop. Further impediments to blood flow can also arise, yielding the overall result of secondary pulmonary hypertension. Chronic hypoxia leads to secondary polycythaemia.

Details of pink puffers and blue bloaters may be found in textbooks of general and respiratory medicine. These two types of patients represent extremes of disease composition, reflecting predominant emphysema and predominant chronic bronchitis, respectively. Most real patients manifest a combination of the two components of COPD. However, one of the essential differences between the two is that the pink puffer expends considerable respiratory effort (puffing) in maintaining arterial oxygen saturation (pink), whereas the blue bloater loses sensitivity to hypoxia (blue) and develops right heart failure (bloater).

Alpha-1-antitrypsin deficiency

Alpha-1-antitrypsin deficiency is an inherited defect in the enzyme α_1-antitrypsin. It presents with early onset (under 40 years) emphysema and cirrhosis. The emphysema is panacinar.

Alpha-1-antitrypsin is an antiprotease enzyme that counteracts the effects of protease enzymes which break down elastic fibres. A deficiency of α_1-antitrypsin results in an excess of protease activity, with destruction of connective tissue. Interestingly, smoking inhibits the action of α_1-antitrypsin.

The normal phenotype for the α_1-antitrypsin gene is MM. Assorted mutations exist. The disease develops in homozygous individuals; opinion is divided as to the status of heterozygotes. The most common abnormal genes are Z and S. Z has more marked effects.

• Z is carried by one in 50 European Caucasians. The mutation is glutamate 342 to lysine. The defective α_1-antitrypsin accumulates in the rough endoplasmic reticulum of the synthesising cell.

• S is carried by one in 25 European Caucasians and is due to a glutamate 264 to valine mutation. The defective enzyme has an increased susceptibility to degradation.

The development of fibrosing alveolitis

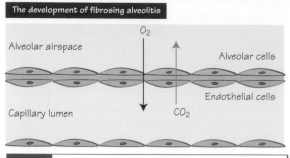

Normal

Very thin tissue layer between the endothelial cells and alveolar cells allows for quick gaseous diffusion

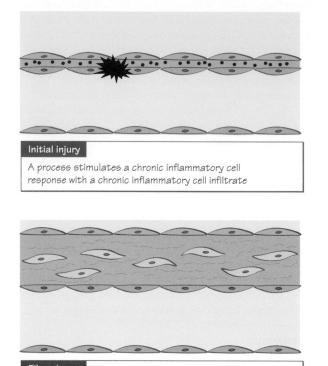

Initial injury

A process stimulates a chronic inflammatory cell response with a chronic inflammatory cell infiltrate

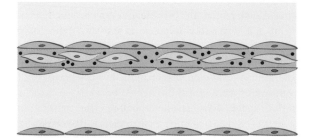

Fibroblast proliferation

In response to cytokines released by the chronic inflammatory cells, fibroblasts proliferate in the alveolar septa

Fibrosis

The fibroblasts produce extracellular matrix. This widens the alevolar septum and impairs gaseous diffusion, first for the lighter oxygen molecule, then in end-stage disease for the heavier carbon dioxide molecule

Labels in Normal diagram: Alveolar airspace, O_2, Alveolar cells, Endothelial cells, Capillary lumen, CO_2

Systems pathology

Fibrosing alveolitis

Definition

Fibrosing alveolitis encompasses a variety of conditions in which there is fibrosis of the distal airspaces.

Causes

- Cryptogenic fibrosing alveolitis.
- Extrinsic allergic alveolitis.
- Industrial lung disease, e.g. asbestos, silicosis, berylliosis, coal dust.
- Scleroderma.
- Systemic lupus erythematosus (SLE).
- Rheumatoid arthritis.
- Radiation.
- Drugs, e.g. bleomycin, amiodarone, gold.
- Renal tubular acidosis.

Epidemiology

Cryptogenic fibrosing alveolitis has an incidence of approximately two per 100 000 per year and is slightly more common in females. A wide variety of ages can be affected, but the condition tends to present around 50 years.

Pathology

The different associated conditions impart important variations to the pathological features of the disease, but there are some common themes.

The condition is a restrictive lung disorder in which fibrosis of the lung parenchyma impairs the expansibility of the lung tissue and decreases the lung volumes. The fibrosis also thickens the alveolar walls and therefore impairs gaseous diffusion between the alveoli and capillaries. As oxygen has a lower diffusing capacity than carbon dioxide, progression of the disease features the development of hypoxia before hypercapnia.

In the most advanced stages of the disease, the fibrosis distorts the macroscopic architecture of the lungs to the extent of forming a honeycomb lung, a descriptive term that encapsulates the appearance.

Pathogenesis

The precise mechanism by which the fibrosis is induced depends upon the underlying disease but the common theme is the occurrence of chronic inflammation in response to some form of stimulus or irritant. Given that fibrosis is a component of the chronic inflammatory response and repair, particularly in a prolonged process, the link between persisting activation of chronic inflammation and fibrosing alveolitis becomes evident.

In the case of industrial lung disease, the driving force is the inhaled inorganic agent, for example, coal dust. Extrinsic allergic alveolitis is discussed in more detail below but is due to an inhaled organic agent.

Scleroderma: Scleroderma is a systemic disease in which there is abnormal fibrosis in numerous organs, of which the lung is one.

Rheumatoid arthritis and SLE: These are connective tissue diseases, like scleroderma. They are associated with both circulating immune complexes (compare with extrinsic allergic alveolitis) and vasculitic processes, both of which can induce organ-based chronic inflammation and fibrosis.

Radiation: Radiation induces tissue injury and fibrosis is typically the reparative response in many organs.

Cryptogenic fibrosing alveolitis (CFA): By definition, the causative agent in CFA (also known as idiopathic pulmonary fibrosis) is not known. However, assorted other aspects of the pathology have been elucidated and one element is of important clinical relevance.

CFA is divided into two types: usual interstitial pneumonia (UIP) and desquamative interstitial pneumonia (DIP). UIP has a poorer response to steroids, shows more fibrosis and tends to progress to death within a couple of years, irrespective of steroid therapy. By contrast, DIP shows much less fibrosis, is more steroid responsive and has a much better prognosis. The term DIP reflects the presence of large numbers of mononuclear cells within the distal airspaces, which give the impression of the shedding of alveolar lining cells.

In the earliest phases of CFA, damage is induced by an unknown agent that results in leakiness of the type 1 alveolar cells and the capillary endothelial cells. Type 2 pneumocytes may proliferate. This is followed by a chronic inflammatory cell infiltrate within the interstitium. Following the chronic inflammatory cell response is fibroblastic proliferation, which ultimately progresses to severe fibrosis. In established disease, the lung will usually show an assortment of these stages distributed across different regions. However, in end stage disease, the process will have reached its fibrotic end-point and overwhelmed any of the preceding histological features.

Clinical correlations

As discussed above, there is a restrictive lung disorder, with decreased lung volumes, that is associated with hypoxia in the early stages, with hypercapnia being a late event.

Extrinsic allergic alveolitis

Definition

Extrinsic allergic alveolitis is a type III hypersensitivity disorder in which immune complexes are deposited in the walls of the distal airways in response to the inhalation of an organic agent in a sensitive individual.

Causes

The list of inhaled agents that can induce extrinsic allergic alveolitis is considerable, but among the better known or more important examples are:

- Farmer's lung: *Micropolyspora faeni* or *Thermoactinomyces vulgaris* from mouldy hay.
- Bird fancier's lung: protein from the feathers or in the droppings of birds such as pigeons, turkeys, chickens and budgerigars.
- Malt worker's lung: *Aspergillus clavutus* from mouldy barley.
- Humidifier fever: thermophilic *Actinomyces*.
- Bagassosis: *Treponema sacchari* from mouldy sugar cane.

Pathology

The inhaled agent triggers a type III hypersensitivity reaction in the distal airways. Granulomas are present in 70% of cases and can be useful in the identification of the extrinsic allergic alveolitis as the cause of fibrosing alveolitis.

The acute reaction to the agent will often cause the patient to remove themselves from the site of exposure. This resolution of the symptoms is an important diagnostic feature. However, if there is repeated re-exposure the chronic form of the disease will supervene, in which the changes of fibrosing alveolitis develop.

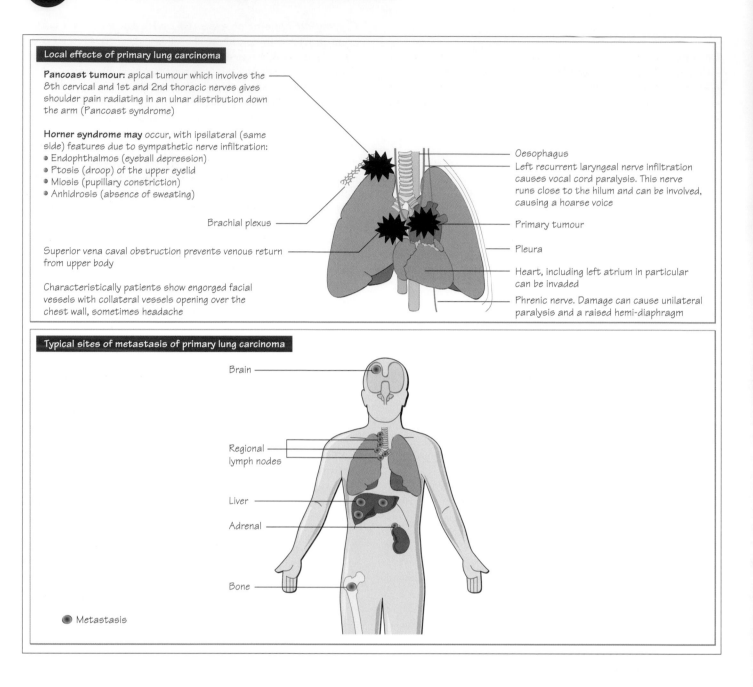

Local effects of primary lung carcinoma

Pancoast tumour: apical tumour which involves the 8th cervical and 1st and 2nd thoracic nerves gives shoulder pain radiating in an ulnar distribution down the arm (Pancoast syndrome)

Horner syndrome may occur, with ipsilateral (same side) features due to sympathetic nerve infiltration:
- Endophthalmos (eyeball depression)
- Ptosis (droop) of the upper eyelid
- Miosis (pupillary constriction)
- Anhidrosis (absence of sweating)

Brachial plexus

Superior vena caval obstruction prevents venous return from upper body

Characteristically patients show engorged facial vessels with collateral vessels opening over the chest wall, sometimes headache

Oesophagus

Left recurrent laryngeal nerve infiltration causes vocal cord paralysis. This nerve runs close to the hilum and can be involved, causing a hoarse voice

Primary tumour

Pleura

Heart, including left atrium in particular can be invaded

Phrenic nerve. Damage can cause unilateral paralysis and a raised hemi-diaphragm

Typical sites of metastasis of primary lung carcinoma

Brain

Regional lymph nodes

Liver

Adrenal

Bone

● Metastasis

110 *Pathology at a Glance.* By C.J. Finlayson and B.A.T. Newell. Published 2009 by Blackwell Publishing. ISBN: 978-1-4051-3650-1

Systems pathology

Definition

Primary lung carcinoma is a malignant tumour derived from the epithelium of the lung.

Epidemiology

Primary lung carcinoma has the infamous distinction of being the commonest malignant tumour in the United Kingdom, weighing in at approximately 40 000 new cases per year and an incidence around 65 per 100 000 per year. The male : female ratio is 3 : 2. The presentation is usually in the seventh and eighth decades.

Causes

Cigarette smoking is by far the most important causative factor, being responsible for 90% of cases of primary lung cancer. Other agents are:

- Asbestos.
- Chromium.
- Urbanisation.
- Radon gas (Cornwall and other granite-rich areas).
- Tars, soot and oil.
- Arsenic.
- Isopropyl alcohol.
- Nickel.

Histological types

The most important aspect of the pathology of primary lung carcinoma is the distinction into microscopic types of small cell and non-small cell carcinoma. Many of the general properties of these tumours have been discussed in Chapter 27.

Small cell carcinoma

Small cell carcinoma comprises 20–25% of cases of primary lung carcinoma and is derived from neuroendocrine cells within the airways and is usually found in the proximal bronchi. The term is somewhat relative to the other types of lung carcinoma, as the cells are actually two to three times the size of a lymphocyte. Partly due to its neuroendocrine derivation, small cell carcinoma is associated with a large variety of paraneoplastic syndromes, such as Cushing's syndrome, Eaton–Lambert syndrome and cerebellar degeneration.

Non-small cell carcinoma

- *Squamous cell carcinoma:* This accounts for 30–50% of primary lung carcinoma. Like small cell carcinoma, it is typically centrally located and has a tendency to cavitation. Paraneoplastic hypercalcaemia is more common with squamous cell carcinoma than the other subtypes of bronchial carcinoma.
- *Adenocarcinoma:* Adenocarcinomas contribute 20–30% of primary lung carcinomas. Unlike the other types, they are more common in women and tend to be located peripherally in the lung. As a further distinguishing feature, they have the least strong association with smoking (approximately 80%).

  One specific variant of adenocarcinoma is bronchioloalveolar carcinoma. This type grows in an unusual pattern along the surface of the airways.

  The lung is also a common site for metastasis of tumours from a variety of organs, many of which will be adenocarcinomas. Consideration of this possibility is essential in evaluating and staging an adenocarcinomatous lung tumour.
- *Large cell carcinoma:* This pragmatically named variant constitutes 10–20% of cases. Its location may be central or peripheral. The cells are large and atypical and lack evidence of differentiation that would place the carcinoma in one of the other categories.

Macroscopic features

Most lung carcinomas arise in the central bronchi where they form a mass that can ulcerate, partially obstruct or occlude the airway. Cavitation is a particular feature of squamous cell carcinoma. The more peripherally located tumours produce a mass that may distort, indurate or pucker the surface of the lung.

Spread

Organs that are susceptible to direct invasion by a primary lung carcinoma are the oesophagus, pleura, pericardium and heart. The phrenic and left recurrent laryngeal nerves may also be invaded. A Pancoast tumour is a bronchial carcinoma that is located in the apex of the lung and can therefore invade into the lower roots of the brachial plexus and the sympathetic chain.

Other than lymph nodes, distant metastases can be to a variety of sites. Primary lung carcinomas are one of the five main types of carcinoma that tend to spread to bone. There is also an unusual propensity to metastasise to the adrenal gland. The brain and liver are also susceptible.

Small cell carcinoma spreads early and is almost always disseminated by the time of presentation.

Staging

The TNM system (see Chapter 28) is employed for staging. Key features are tumour size, relationship to the carina of the trachea, invasion of adjacent organs and the presence of a pleural effusion.

Clinical correlations

- Damage to the bronchus and cavitation explain the symptom of haemoptysis.
- Obstruction of the bronchus leads to accumulation of secretions and a susceptibility to infection. Obstruction and collapse can produce dyspnoea, as may a pleural effusion.
- Invasion of the left recurrent laryngeal nerve results in a hoarse voice. Therefore, consideration of a lung primary tumour is a vital part of the investigation of a change in voice.
- Damage to the phrenic nerve can lead to paralysis of the ipsilateral hemidiaphragm. Hence, an abnormally raised hemidiaphragm found on chest X-ray should not be casually dismissed.
- Compression and invasion of the oesophagus causes dysphagia.
- Invasion of the pericardium can cause a pericardial effusion and therefore symptoms of cardiac failure. Extension to the atria may cause atrial fibrillation.

Prognosis

The prognosis for primary lung carcinoma is poor. Surgery is not appropriate for small cell carcinoma and the majority of patients with non-small cell carcinoma either present too late for surgery to be possible, or are unfit for surgery. Smoking is the key aetiological factor and is also closely related to chronic obstructive pulmonary disease (COPD). Thus, many patients with primary lung carcinoma also have COPD and cannot tolerate the loss of lung volume attendant on a lobectomy or pneumonectomy. Hence, the overall 5-year survival for primary lung cancer is 5%. Untreated small cell carcinoma has a median survival of 2–3 months; treatment may extend this to 12–18 months.

Systems pathology

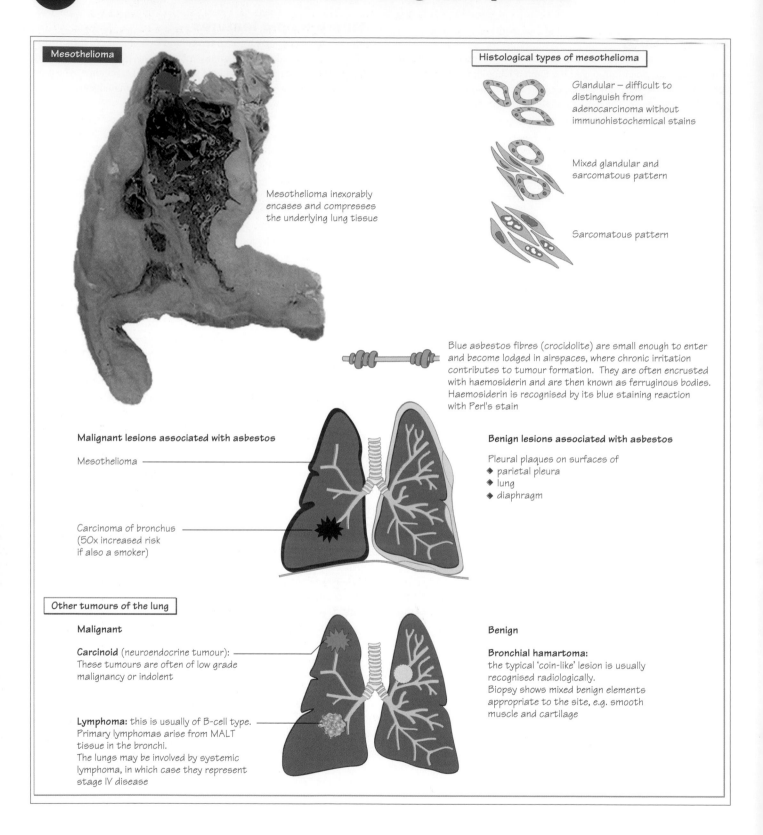

Mesothelioma

Mesothelioma inexorably encases and compresses the underlying lung tissue

Histological types of mesothelioma

Glandular – difficult to distinguish from adenocarcinoma without immunohistochemical stains

Mixed glandular and sarcomatous pattern

Sarcomatous pattern

Blue asbestos fibres (crocidolite) are small enough to enter and become lodged in airspaces, where chronic irritation contributes to tumour formation. They are often encrusted with haemosiderin and are then known as ferruginous bodies. Haemosiderin is recognised by its blue staining reaction with Perl's stain

Malignant lesions associated with asbestos

Mesothelioma

Carcinoma of bronchus (50x increased risk if also a smoker)

Benign lesions associated with asbestos

Pleural plaques on surfaces of
◆ parietal pleura
◆ lung
◆ diaphragm

Other tumours of the lung

Malignant

Carcinoid (neuroendocrine tumour): These tumours are often of low grade malignancy or indolent

Lymphoma: this is usually of B-cell type. Primary lymphomas arise from MALT tissue in the bronchi. The lungs may be involved by systemic lymphoma, in which case they represent stage IV disease

Benign

Bronchial hamartoma: the typical 'coin-like' lesion is usually recognised radiologically. Biopsy shows mixed benign elements appropriate to the site, e.g. smooth muscle and cartilage

Malignant mesothelioma

Malignant mesothelioma is a malignant tumour of the mesothelium and can affect any body cavity in which mesothelium is present (pleura, peritoneum, pericardium, scrotum) but is usually encountered in the lung. Most of the following refers to the lung.

Epidemiology

The epidemiology of mesothelioma is intimately related to exposure to asbestos, such that the vast majority of cases have a history of exposure. However, the interval between exposure and developing mesothelioma is 20–40 years and is seldom less than 15 years. Hence, the history of exposure may be forgotten by the patient unless specifically sought.

The incidence is approximately eight per 100 000 per year. Historical patterns of exposure mean that the incidence is increasing, with a peak anticipated between 2010 and 2020. The male : female ratio shows global variation, being 9 : 1 in North America, but falling closer to 1 : 1 in the UK. This is likely to reflect different patterns of exposure to asbestos. The latent interval determines the typical age of presentation.

Pathogenesis

Asbestos is the key agent and is a fibrous metamorphic mineral that is composed of hydrous magnesium silicate. Its utility in industry reflects its fire and heat resistant properties. Several different fibre types exist. The most dangerous is crocidolite, followed by amosite, with chrysotile some distance behind (the relative risk ratio is suggested to be 500 : 100 : 1). Crocidolite and amosite belong to the amphibole group. One of the features that affects toxicity is the shape of the fibres. Crocidolite is long and needle shaped, allowing it to align with the airflow and reach the distal parts of the lung.

The precise mechanism by which the fibres induce mesothelioma is unclear, but may involve induction of DNA damage and an ability of asbestos fibres to bind and concentrate other carcinogens. In this context, it should be noted that while asbestos alone doubles the risk of lung adenocarcinoma, in combination with smoking, the increased risk is substantially higher, beyond that expected from simply combining the individual risks of smoking and asbestos independently.

Pathology

Mesothelioma causes thickening of the pleura (or other mesothelial lined surface). In the early stages, this produces small nodules, mainly on the parietal pleura. As the disease progresses, the nodules increase in size and the parietal and visceral pleura thicken and fuse. The pleura can be several centimetres thick. Extension of the thickening into the pulmonary fissures is characteristic.

An effusion is usually associated with the tumour (either a pleural effusion, ascites or pericardial effusion, depending on the site of the primary).

Mesotheliomas possess a variety of histological appearances. In the simplest division, the tumours can be epithelioid (round cells), sarcomatoid (spindle cells) or both. Various patterns can be formed, including one that resembles glands. However, an invasive mode of growth is encountered throughout the variants.

Spread

Mesotheliomas grow in a relentless local fashion, extending into the underlying lung, contralateral pleura and lung, diaphragm, chest wall, pericardium and mediastinum. Mesotheliomas can metastasise to regional lymph nodes, the lung and also the liver, brain, bone and kidneys. However, presentation with disseminated disease is extremely unusual.

Prognosis

The mortality from pleural mesothelioma is effectively 100% and the median survival is 12–18 months.

Clinical correlations

Occupational exposure in one partner can also subject the other partner to asbestos if the particles are brought home on clothes. Traditionally, this happened during the preceding decades with men carrying asbestos home on their clothes which were then washed by their wives, who became exposed. However, unless a detailed history is obtained, this exposure can easily be missed.

Some forms of mesothelioma can resemble adenocarcinoma. As the pleura is a common site for metastatic adenocarcinoma, which will induce an effusion, this must be considered in the differential diagnosis. Immunohistochemical techniques can assist in resolving the issue, but the provision of complete clinical data is also very helpful.

Secondary tumours of the lung and pleura

The lungs receive the entire cardiac output every minute and this high blood flow, in conjunction with the high surface area of the vascular bed, contributes to why they are a common site for metastases. Most adenocarcinomas, including breast, can involve the lungs, as can squamous cell carcinoma. The former is more likely to be an occult primary, so caution must be employed when determining the management of a patient with adenocarcinoma in a lung biopsy in whom full staging has not yet been performed. The lung is also a frequent site for metastatic sarcomas and, in general, most self-respecting malignant tumours can find their way to the lung.

Benign lung tumours

Benign lung tumours are uncommon and are considerably rarer than malignant primary tumours. The most important is a bronchial hamartoma. This is a circumscribed mass that is composed of assorted lung mesenchymal tissues with accompanying respiratory mucosa. Cartilage is a common component. The tumour is often discovered as an incidental finding on a chest X-ray. A fine needle aspirate can make the diagnosis.

Other malignant lung tumours

While the carcinomas mentioned in Chapter 47 account for the vast majority of primary lung malignancies, other forms exist. Of these, carcinoid tumours and lymphomas are the most common. Mesenchymal malignancies are rare, as are salivary gland-type carcinomas.

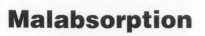

Immunological basis of coeliac disease

Gluten passively absorbed through small intestinal epithelium

Gliadin is the antigenic component of gluten

tTG in the lamina propria deamidates gluten, changing its tertiary structure

In people with HLA DQ2 or DQ8 these modified peptides closely fit the MHC II grooves and are presented to Th cells by macrophages

Activated Th cells interact with B cells and Tc cells

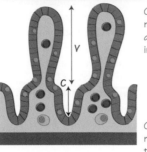

Epithelial cell destruction exceeds production and villous atrophy develops

CD8+ T cells infiltrate epithelium

Th2 predominant response generates Tc cells active against gluten, which cause apoptosis in intestinal epithelial cells if gluten is present in the diet

Antibodies from humoral response are useful diagnostically:
- Antigliadin
- Anti-tTG
- Anti-endomysial antibodies

IgA antibodies are more specific but a minority of coeliac patients lack IgA

Microscopical features of treated and untreated coeliac disease

Normal villi: villous (**V**) to crypt (**C**) ratio of 3–5:1

Normal IEL count of <25 lymphocytes/100 epithelial cells

Normal lamina propria contains no polymorphonuclear neutrophils (PMNs), moderate lymphocytes and occasional plasma cells

Gluten ingestion, microscopical damage seen in 3–5 days

Gluten free diet: return to normal takes 3–24 months

Intraepithelial lymphocytes (IEL)

Atrophy of villi may be partial or total: villous:crypt ratio <1

IEL numbers increase markedly, particularly at the villous tips

Lamina propria expansion by plasma cells, lymphocytes and occasional PMNs

Summary of causes of malabsorption and diarrhoea

Causes of malabsorption

Biliary system: obstruction to bile flow
- Gall stones

Pancreas: lack of enzyme production or obstruction to flow
- Cystic fibrosis
- Chronic pancreatitis

Small bowel
- Inflammation/Damaged absorptive surface:
  - Coeliac disease
  - Crohn's disease
  - Tropical sprue
  - Atypical mycobacteria
  - Whipple's disease
  - Lymphoma
  - Scarring interfering with absorption from small bowel
  - Ischaemia/irradiation
  - Scleroderma
- Congenitally abnormal mucosal surface:
  - Disaccharidase deficiency
  - Abetalipoproteinaemia
- Surgery:
  - Resection for stricture, fistula, etc.: short bowel
  - – decreased bile salt reabsorption → colonic irritation – secretory diarrhoea
  - Blind loop syndrome – bacterial overgrowth in redundant bowel

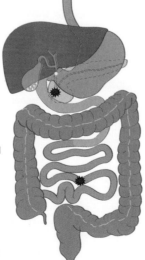

Causes of diarrhoea

Pancreas and gall bladder
- Loss of bile salts or pancreatic enzymes, e.g. chronic pancreatitis (steatorrhoea – pale, floating, offensive stools due to fat malabsorption – may be prominent)

Small bowel
- Malabsorption:
  - Coeliac disease
  - Others
- Infective enteritis:
  - Enterovirus
  - Bacteria, e.g. Salmonella, Bacillus cereus, Staphylococcus aureus
  - Protozoa, e.g. giardiasis

Small or large bowel
- Crohn's disease
- Tuberculosis
- Yersiniosis
- Neuroendocrine tumour

Large bowel
- Ulcerative colitis
- Infective colitis
  - Bacteria: Shigella, Salmonella, Campylobacter
  - Colitis due to Clostridium difficile toxin
  - (pseudomembranous colitis) Protozoa: amoebiasis
- Other colitides:
  - Collagenous/lymphocytic colitis
  - Ischaemic colitis
- Neoplasms
  - Large villous adenoma
  - Adenocarcinoma (especially rectal)

Malabsorption

This can occur at any stage of the absorptive pathway.

Loss of enzymes:

- Brush border enzymes, which digest lactose/milk fat: congenital disaccharidase deficiency.
- Pancreatic enzymes, which digest carbohydrate, fat or protein: e.g. destruction of parenchyma in chronic pancreatitis, or stricture of pancreatic duct due to cystic fibrosis.

Lack of bile salts for fat emulsification:

- Common bile duct obstruction by gallstones.
- Carcinoma of the head of the pancreas.

Lost or damaged absorptive surface:

- Gluten-sensitive enteropathy (see below).
- Tropical sprue (rare chronic bacterial infection).
- Crohn's disease.
- Blockage in absorptive pathway:
  - Whipple's disease: rare chronic bacterial infection.
  - Malignant lymphoma in the small bowel: rare, either MALT lymphoma (Chapter 95) or gluten enteropathy-associated T cell lymphoma (EATCL), which is rapidly fatal.
  - Scarring from irradiation.
  - Fibrosis associated with scleroderma.
  - Congenital deficiency in transport protein: e.g. abetalipoproteinaemia, where fat globules accumulate in the intestinal epithelium.

Loss of bowel, usually by surgery:

- Resection for stricture (e.g. Crohn's disease): shorter bowel, so less reabsorption of bile salts; causes secretory diarrhoea by irritation of the colonic mucosa. If less than 60–100 cm of small bowel remains, there may be malabsorption of nutrients.
- Blind loop syndrome: antral gastrectomy with the formation of a blind loop may allow bacterial overgrowth in the redundant small bowel. The bacteria metabolise and utilise nutrients and interfere with absorption.

Gluten-sensitive enteropathy or coeliac disease (idiopathic or non-tropical sprue)

Coeliac disease is an aberrant autoimmune reaction to gluten, the protein found in wheat, rye and barley, in people susceptible for an unknown reason. It is strongly associated with human leucocyte antigen (HLA) -DQ2 (c. 95% of cases) and -DQ8 (c.5%). The incidence is increased in patients with type I diabetes mellitus and autoimmune thyroid disease. It is a common, often subclinical, cause of malabsorption, with the highest prevalence in Ireland (one in 100). In the rest of northern Europe the prevalence is one in 300. HLA-DQ2 is rare in the Chinese and Japanese, who seldom develop coeliac disease. Monozygotic twins show strong concordance for the disease (75%); 11–13% of dizygotic twins or other siblings are affected.

While HLA-DQ2 is widely present throughout the world, only a small proportion of these people develop coeliac disease. Although many patients present in childhood, some are not diagnosed until several decades later. It may be that an enteric infection either renders the small bowel permeable to incompletely digested, larger protein molecules or an infective agent shows sequence homology with the protein and an immune response cross-reacts with small bowel epithelium.

Villous destruction by Tc cells impairs small bowel absorption. Symptomatology is proportional to the length of bowel involved. Note that vitamin B12 is absorbed in the terminal ileum and is usually spared.

Presenting symptoms can be dramatic – e.g. profuse diarrhoea – but are more usually subtle, e.g. anaemia (iron deficient, folate deficient or a mixed picture), bloating, weight loss or general malaise. Long-term risks include osteoporosis and malignancies such as EATCL, non-Hodgkin B cell lymphoma, adenocarcinoma of the small bowel and oesophageal carcinoma.

Diagnostically useful antibodies are formed against:
- Gliadin.
- tTG – the most sensitive.
- Endomysium (the membrane surrounding muscle fibres) – the most specific.

Since the antibodies are mainly produced in the mucosa-associated lymphoid tissue, they are largely of IgA type, though some coeliac patients lack the ability to make IgA and produce IgG instead.

The figure illustrates the mechanisms, which explain the microscopical features seen in coeliac disease:
- Lamina propria inflammation.
- Increased lymphocytes within the surface epithelium.
- Villous atrophy caused by loss of epithelial cells and crypt hyperplasia as the stem cells in the crypts proliferate in an attempt to replace destroyed enterocytes.

Treatment is a gluten-free diet. In most coeliac patients, oat-based food is permissible, since it's major protein is avenin. It can take 3 months to 2 years for the intestinal mucosa to return to normal, but 3–5 days for all the clinical and microscopical features to re-establish if the gluten free diet is breached just once.

Diarrhoea

One of the main presenting complaints of malabsorptive conditions is diarrhoea, defined clinically as the excretion of >300 g of faeces per day, rather than the number of times the bowels are opened per day. Causes of diarrhoea include:
- Coeliac disease.
- Laxatives.
- Failure to reabsorb bile salts if the small bowel is shortened or damaged – normally 95% of salts are reabsorbed and recycled. They irritate the colonic epithelium.
- Neuroendocrine tumours ('carcinoid tumours') may cause diarrhoea by the secretion of gut-associated hormones.
- Some drugs interfere with water absorption (e.g. NSAIDs, some laxatives).
- Infection is the commonest cause of diarrhoea, often of secretory type, which may be due to direct invasion by the bacterium or to a toxin.
- Toxins:
  - Cholera toxin acts on cAMP in the colonic mucosa to cause the excretion of chloride ions and water, and prevent water absorption, producing a rapidly dehydrating form of diarrhoea, recognised clinically as the 'rice water stool'.
  - The toxin of *Clostridium difficile* also causes profuse secretory diarrhoea. It is a serious complication of antibiotic therapy, which destroys the normal gut flora and allows *C. difficile* to overgrow.

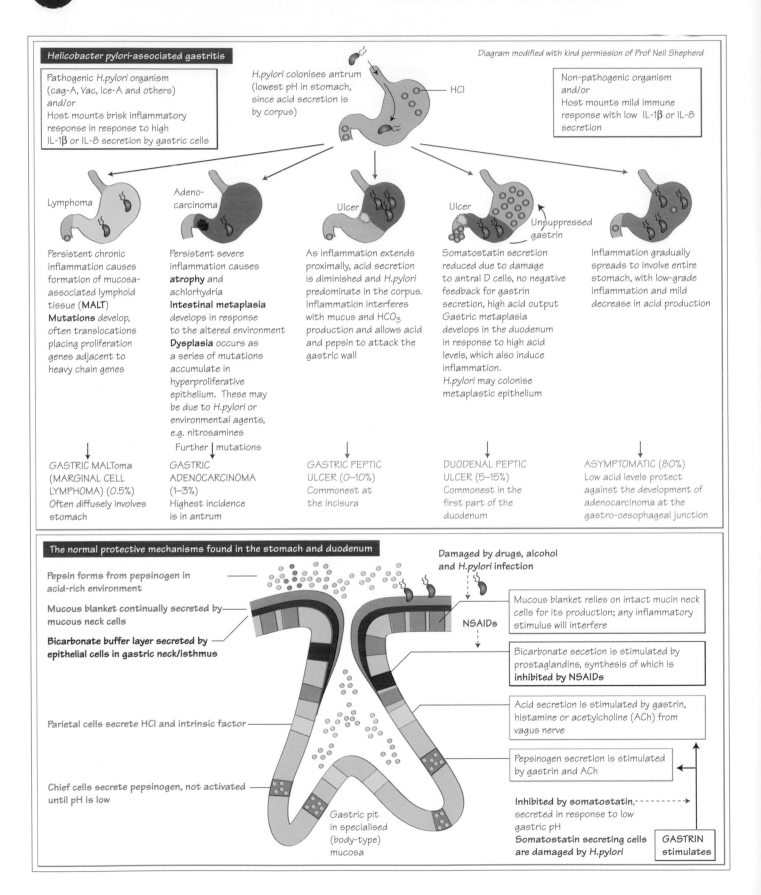

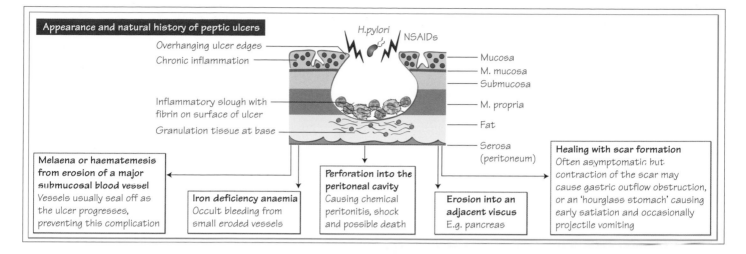

Appearance and natural history of peptic ulcers

- Overhanging ulcer edges
- Chronic inflammation
- Inflammatory slough with fibrin on surface of ulcer
- Granulation tissue at base

H.pylori & NSAIDs

- Mucosa
- M. mucosa
- Submucosa
- M. propria
- Fat
- Serosa (peritoneum)

Melaena or haematemesis from erosion of a major submucosal blood vessel
Vessels usually seal off as the ulcer progresses, preventing this complication

Iron deficiency anaemia
Occult bleeding from small eroded vessels

Perforation into the peritoneal cavity
Causing chemical peritonitis, shock and possible death

Erosion into an adjacent viscus
E.g. pancreas

Healing with scar formation
Often asymptomatic but contraction of the scar may cause gastric outflow obstruction, or an 'hourglass stomach' causing early satiation and occasionally projectile vomiting

Benign peptic ulcers typically occur in the stomach and duodenum and occasionally in the lower oesophagus if there is acid reflux. Other sites include gastro-oesophageal or gastrojejunal anastomoses and rarely a Meckel's diverticulum that contains ectopic gastric mucosa.

Several different terms are employed:
- **Acute erosions**: tiny lesions with focal surface epithelial loss which occur following stress, e.g. severe burns or systemic infection.
- **Acute ulcers**: these affect the full thickness of the mucosa and do not scar – they are seen commonly in association with therapeutic drugs (e.g. aspirin) or high alcohol levels.
- **Chronic duodenal and gastric peptic ulcers**: these show penetration of deeper levels of the wall and are associated with fibrous scarring. They occur secondary to chronic gastritis, often due to infection by *H. pylori* and non-steroidal anti-inflammatory drugs (NSAIDs).

Helicobacter pylori (HP)

H. pylori is a human pathogen spread by the faecal–oral route and discovered in 1983. Infection is common worldwide and is endemic in some regions, or portions of society of low socioeconomic status, where it is usually contracted during infancy. Improvement in living conditions and hygiene, have reduced HP levels over the last two decades. Increased awareness and treatment of infection has also contributed.

H. pylori is a flagellated Gram-negative spiral coccobacillus that preferentially inhabits the acidic environment of the stomach and binds via a specific receptor on the gastric epithelium. Part of the organism's ability to survive in this location is conferred by its expression of urease, which splits urea into ammonia and carbon dioxide to liberate energy, with ammonia shielding the bacteria against gastric acid. Urease is highly immunogenic. Furthermore, contact between surface peptidoglycans and the gastric wall stimulates acute inflammation. This is usually insufficient to eradicate infection so chronic infection ensues. The organism's flagella let it burrow into the mucous barrier, which protects it from the host response and antibiotics.

Some strains of HP possess proteins that enhance the organism's pathogenicity. The cagA protein is injected into gastric epithelium and stimulates cell proliferation. The vacuolating toxin (Vac) subtype S1 induces apoptosis and punches holes in gastric epithelial cells, allowing nutrients to leak out. It also interferes with cell signalling and the T cell response. Other proteins (e.g. Ice-A) are also important.

The incidence of gastric carcinoma is high in some HP endemic regions (e.g. South America, the Far East, the West), but low in others (e.g. Africa, Asia). Therefore, while HP can contribute to the development of gastric carcinoma, pathogenicity of the organism and host susceptibility are also important.

Around 80% of people with HP gastritis never manifest clinically obvious problems; 0–10% exhibit dyspepsia without ulcer formation, and 5–15% have peptic ulcers. Only 1–3% develop gastric adenocarcinoma, while 0.5% acquire a gastric MALToma.

NSAIDs

NSAIDs inhibit cyclo-oxygenase, which catalyses prostaglandin synthesis. Prostaglandins stimulate neck and isthmic epithelial cells to secrete a buffer layer of bicarbonate, which is trapped beneath the surface mucin blanket. Blockage of this pathway renders the gastric epithelium susceptible to acid damage in areas where the mucous layer is thinned, as may happen with drug ingestion or HP infection.

Duodenal ulceration

Duodenal ulceration is strongly associated with HP infection (more than 95% association until recently, now drug-associated ulcers are increasing). Infection is most likely to have been contracted during adulthood and the antral pattern of infection predominates. *H. pylori* depresses somatostatin production by directly damaging the duodenal cells that produce it, so the normal negative feedback mechanism on antral G cells gastrin secretion is disrupted and gastric parietal cell acid output increases (these cells are spared in antral-pattern infection). The duodenum becomes inflamed and undergoes gastric metaplasia in response to elevated acid delivery from the stomach, particularly in the first part. *H. pylori* may infect the metaplastic gastric epithelium and cause further inflammation. The metaplastic epithelium may be more susceptible to the effects of NSAIDs, but gastric metaplasia may not be necessary for NSAIDs to cause duodenal ulceration.

Gastric peptic ulceration

Longer-term HP infection, which affects the corpus of the stomach, may cause peptic ulceration locally despite normal or reduced acid production. 70–80% of gastric peptic ulcers used to be HP associated, now drug-associated ulceration is increasing. Gastric peptic ulcers typically affect the incisura. The incidence of cancer associated with gastric peptic ulceration is <1%.

Pathological features of peptic ulcers

Chronic peptic ulcers have clean bases and smooth, overhanging edges. Gastric ulcers can be 1 to 10 cm in diameter. Duodenal ulcers are smaller and may be paired. Microscopical features are summarised in the diagram.

Systems pathology

Factors contributing to reflux oesophagitis and Barrett's oesophagus

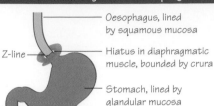

Oesophagus, lined by squamous mucosa

Z-line

Hiatus in diaphragmatic muscle, bounded by crura

Stomach, lined by glandular mucosa

Z-line

Congenitally large hiatus: part of the stomach is pulled through into the thorax

Acid reflux causes metaplasia, an alteration of lining epithelium

◆ **Normal**: there is a valve mechanism at the gastro-oesophageal junction, contributed to by pressure from the crura of the diaphragm, the angle of entry of the oesophagus and the pressures of thoracic and abdominal cavity contents

◆ **Hiatus hernia**: part of the stomach is pulled into the thorax and allows reflux of gastric contents into the oesophagus. Obesity or pregnancy increases the upward pressure on the stomach and its contents
◆ Acid damages the squamous mucosa, which may undergo Barrett's metaplasia

◆ **Barrett's oesophagus**: the sphincter permits gastric contents to reflux into the oesophagus
◆ The squamous mucosa undergoes metaplasia to develop a glandular lining which is usually a mixture of gastric and intestinal-type mucosa
◆ Secondary bile acids have carcinogenic effects

Consequences of reflux at the gastro-oesophageal junction

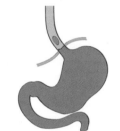

Peptic ulcer in squamous mucosa

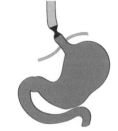

Benign peptic stricture in squamous mucosa

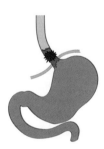

Adenocarcinoma in Barrett's metaplasia: spread of these tumours is similar to those of stomach, if present at or below the cardia.

Typical sites of spread from squamous cell carcinoma of oesophagus

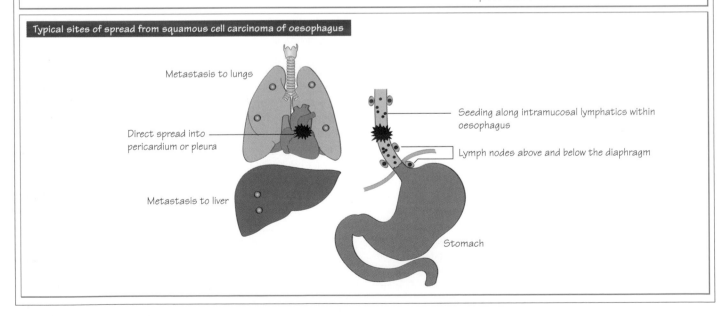

Metastasis to lungs

Direct spread into pericardium or pleura

Metastasis to liver

Seeding along intramucosal lymphatics within oesophagus

Lymph nodes above and below the diaphragm

Stomach

Gastro-oesophageal reflux disease (GORD)

GORD primarily affects the affluent Western world and is increasing in incidence – currently 20–40% of the UK population.

Aetiology and pathogenesis

Unlike the well-defined upper oesophageal striated muscled sphincter, the lower oesophageal sphincter is less clear, made of smooth muscle and its effectiveness is increased by external pressure from the surrounding diaphragmatic crura. Increased intra-abdominal pressure (from obesity, pregnancy) may cause reflux of gastric contents into the oesophagus, damaging the squamous mucosa, which has no protective mucous barrier.

In hiatus hernia, the gastro-oesophageal junction rides upwards into the chest. This removes part of the lower oesophageal sphincter control and allows reflux.

Pathology

There may be peptic-type ulceration, due to acid, which can lead to stricture formation as the oesophagus heals by fibrosis. Microscopy shows acute inflammation initially, then chronic inflammation and scarring.

About 10–15% of patients with GORD have Barrett's oesophagus (columnar lined oesophagus, CLO), in which the squamous epithelium undergoes metaplasia to gastric-type and/or intestinal-type columnar mucosa. Instead of pale pink squamous epithelium, there is velvety red mucosa similar to that of the stomach and the well-defined Z-line of the gastro-oesophageal junction is blurred and moved proximally.

CLO predisposes to the development of oesophageal adenocarcinoma and the increased incidence of CLO is one of the key reasons for the current increase in oesophageal adenocarcinoma in the West.

Treatment of CLO and GORD with acid-suppressing drugs may both improve symptoms and allow a reversal of metaplasia to normal mucosa, but the incidence of cancer in people with GORD and hiatus hernia is still 2–3 times higher than in non-dyspeptic people.

Dysplasia may arise in CLO; in 50% of people with high grade dysplasia on biopsy there is a coexisting invasive carcinoma in the oesophageal resection. If people with high grade dysplasia are observed, 80% develop invasive cancer in 2 years (the figure is 20% for low grade dysplasia). Because dysplasia and adenocarcinoma can take 15–20 years to develop, patients are often too old and infirm to survive radical surgery. New techniques, such as photodynamic therapy, show promise for the ablation of dysplasia and early cancers.

Squamous cell carcinoma

Squamous cell carcinoma (SCC) is the commonest oesophageal tumour worldwide, though in the Western world adenocarcinoma has now overtaken SCC. The geographical variation is striking, even within regions of the same country (e.g. Hoisin province in China has an incidence of 170 per 100 000 per year, Hong Kong 20 per 100 000 and the UK 3–6 per 100 000). The highest incidence occurs in Iran, Kazakhstan and China.

In the UK the incidence is falling. The male : female ratio is 3–4 : 1. There are a range of associations of different strengths.

1 Strong associations:
- Alcohol (spirits).
- Thermal damage from very hot tea.
- Smoking of tobacco or opium (especially chewing of pipe remnants).
- Link with HPV infection is 20–40% in China.

2 Less strong associations:
- Nitrosamines and fungal contamination of food.

3 Rare associations:
- Females with oesophageal webs and iron deficiency anaemia (Plummer–Vinson–Kelly (PVK) syndrome).
- Achalasia is a neuromuscular disorder in which oesophageal ganglion cells are congenitally absent or destroyed, impairing relaxation of the lower oesophageal sphincter.

Gross features

The middle third of the oesophagus is the typical site affected, especially in males, then the upper third (especially females). The tumours are usually annular and stricturing with a very poor prognosis, but occasionally SCC may present as a large polypoid mass that protrudes into the lumen with less tendency to early spread.

Microscopic features

These are as for SCC seen at other sites (Chapter 27)

Adenocarcinoma of the oesophagus

The UK incidence is 8 per 100 000 per year linked to:
- Gastro-oesophageal reflux disease and columnar metaplasia (two-fold risk): Barrett's oesophagus is very common. Estimates as to the percentage who will develop adenocarcinoma vary between 1% and 10%.
- Acidity of refluxed fluid: there is genetic variation in the gastric acidity, e.g. Scots have higher gastric acid levels than the Chinese.
- Bile in refluxed fluid increases the cancer risk.
- There is an inverse link with *H. pylori* gastritis: the decline in *H. pylori* has been linked to a rise in incidence of adenocarcinoma of oesophagus and cardia; *H. pylori*-associated adenocarcinoma of the gastric antrum is declining.

Gross features

Tumours of the gastric cardia behave like other stomach tumours, while those of the gastro-oesophageal junction and lower oesophageal tumours behave more like SCC. Adenocarcinoma is rare in the middle third of the oesophagus and only then if there is long segment columnar metaplasia.

Microscopic features

These are as for adenocarcinoma seen in the stomach (see Chapter 52).

Pattern of spread

- Direct spread along the oesophagus is typical, often utilising intramucosal and submucosal lymphatics. Direct spread through the wall into the mediastinum is common and renders complete surgical excision difficult.
- Lymphatic spread to local lymph nodes is usual at presentation, generally affecting nodes on both sides of the diaphragm and often nodes at more distant sites.
- Venous spread is also very common – though all but the very distal oesophagus drains into the systemic veins. Liver metastases are seen in almost 50% of patients, and lung metastases in about 40%.
- Transcoelomic pleural or pericardial spread is rare.

Prognosis

The 5-year survival is around 10%. Prognostic factors are the depth of mural invasion, lymph node metastases and extramural venous invasion.

Surgery is the only hope of cure. Preoperative chemoradiotherapy can downstage advanced cancers and improve outcome. Patients who have high grade dysplasia or superficial adenocarcinoma and cannot tolerate major surgery can be treated with laser ablation.

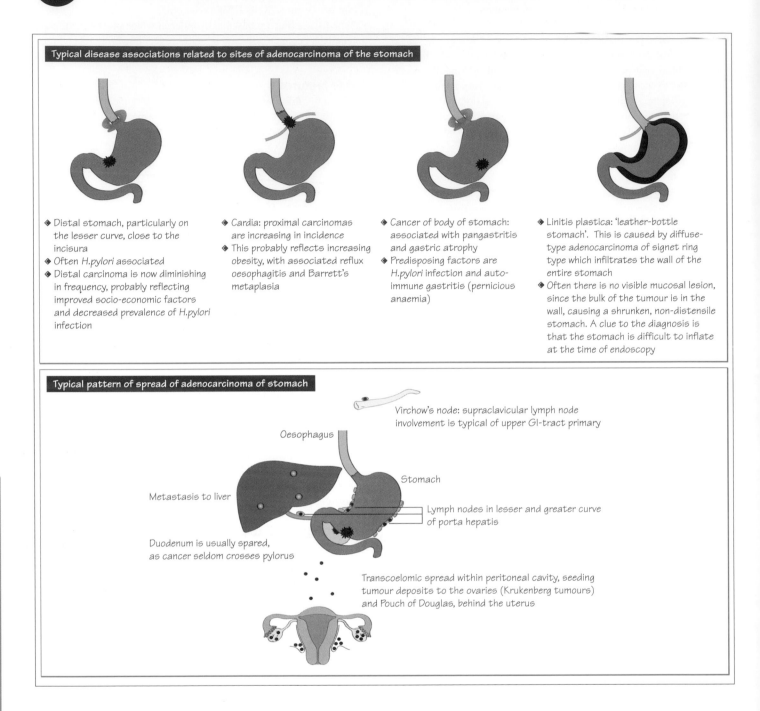

Typical disease associations related to sites of adenocarcinoma of the stomach

◆ Distal stomach, particularly on the lesser curve, close to the incisura
◆ Often *H.pylori* associated
◆ Distal carcinoma is now diminishing in frequency, probably reflecting improved socio-economic factors and decreased prevalence of *H.pylori* infection

◆ Cardia: proximal carcinomas are increasing in incidence
◆ This probably reflects increasing obesity, with associated reflux oesophagitis and Barrett's metaplasia

◆ Cancer of body of stomach: associated with pangastritis and gastric atrophy
◆ Predisposing factors are *H.pylori* infection and auto-immune gastritis (pernicious anaemia)

◆ Linitis plastica: 'leather-bottle stomach'. This is caused by diffuse-type adenocarcinoma of signet ring type which infiltrates the wall of the entire stomach
◆ Often there is no visible mucosal lesion, since the bulk of the tumour is in the wall, causing a shrunken, non-distensile stomach. A clue to the diagnosis is that the stomach is difficult to inflate at the time of endoscopy

Typical pattern of spread of adenocarcinoma of stomach

Virchow's node: supraclavicular lymph node involvement is typical of upper GI-tract primary

Oesophagus

Stomach

Metastasis to liver

Lymph nodes in lesser and greater curve of porta hepatis

Duodenum is usually spared, as cancer seldom crosses pylorus

Transcoelomic spread within peritoneal cavity, seeding tumour deposits to the ovaries (Krukenberg tumours) and Pouch of Douglas, behind the uterus

Gastric adenocarcinoma

Epidemiology

The incidence is very high in some parts of the world (highest in Japan with an incidence of 88 per 100 000, versus the UK with an incidence of 20 per 100 000). They make up 15% of GI malignancies. The male : female ratio is 2 : 1.

Risk factors

• *Helicobacter pylori* infection.
• Family history.
• Dietary nitrosamines and polycyclic hydrocarbons.
• Pernicious anaemia.
• Adenomatous polyps and polyposis syndromes.
• Blood group A.

The incidence of antral carcinomas has dropped steadily as *H. pylori* gastritis has declined. There appears to be a 'move proximally', as tumours of the cardia increase, whereas those of the corpus are unchanged.

Colonisation of the stomach by *H. pylori* is the most important factor and its effects reflect the following:

• Pathogenic strains (cagA, vac and others).

- Distribution of infection (pangastritis or corpus predominant gastritis), which may partly reflect the duration of infection, e.g. acquired in infancy or childhood.
- The host response – there is genetic variation in the genes encoding IL-1β and TNFα, both of which can suppress the level of acid production by the stomach. The rate of progression of antral to multifocal *H. pylori* gastritis is increased in patients with lower acid production.

Gross features

Gastric adenocarcinoma may be ulcerated (usual) or polypoid (rare). The ulcers differ from peptic-type ulcers by having a shaggy, necrotic base and everted, 'rolled', raised edges. However, the macroscopical distinction is not always easy and multiple biopsies from the edges of any gastric ulcer are advised.

Microscopic feature

Gastric adenocarcinoma may show an intestinal-type or diffuse pattern of glands.
- **Intestinal type**: this pattern is most associated with the pathway through intestinal metaplasia and dysplasia to cancer, as seen with *H. pylori*.
- **Diffuse type**: sheets of mucin-containing 'signet ring' cells diffusely infiltrate the gastric wall. This pattern is associated with the classic 'leather-bottle stomach'. This often shows no discernible mucosal abnormality at endoscopy, since the tumour is mainly present in the deeper layers. Suspicion is aroused in the endoscopist by the non-distensibility of the stomach, and imaging may demonstrate a thickened wall. Deep biopsies that include the submucosa may be required to make the histological diagnosis.

Pattern of spread

The figure illustrates the pattern of spread.

Prognosis

Prognostic factors are the depth of invasion, lymph node metastases and extramural venous invasion. The overall 5-year survival rate is around 12%, but is 90% for stage 1.

Surgery is the best chance of cure but most tumours present too late for curative surgery. There has been an improvement in outcome with the use of preoperative chemoradiotherapy, which can downstage advanced cancers and render them operable.

Other tumours

Lymphoma (see Chapter 95)

MALToma, more properly called 'extranodal marginal zone lymphoma of MALT type', is commonest in the stomach but can be encountered in the small or large bowel. There is no mucosa-associated lymphoid tissue (MALT) in normal stomachs – it develops in response to *H. pylori* colonisation.

MALTomas may eventually transform into high grade lymphomas, of diffuse large B cell type, which are indistinguishable in behaviour from those that arise from lymph nodes.

Neuroendocrine tumours

Neuroendocrine tumours (also known as carcinoid tumours) are rare tumours, commonest in the appendix, then ileum, then stomach and lastly colon and rectum. They occur in adults and constitute 5% of gastrointestinal tumours. Neuroendocrine tumours may also arise within the lung, where their behaviour is generally more indolent.

The tumours are often small and can secrete a variety of neuroendocrine hormones – of which 5HT (serotonin) was the first to be described. The 5HT breakdown product HIAA (hydroxyindole acetic acid) can be detected in the urine. Serotonin is inactivated in the liver so symptoms are therefore only usually seen in patients with liver metastases, whose hormones are released into the systemic blood supply.

The classic presentation is with the 'carcinoid syndrome' of episodic diarrhoea, flushing and palpitations. 5HT secretion may stimulate endocardial proliferation and cause tricuspid and/or pulmonary stenosis and/or endomyocardial fibrosis

In the stomach three patterns are recognised:
- Multiple superficial polyps: these are curable by endoscopic resection, but new lesions develop and require regular 'pruning'.
- Multiple endocrine neoplasia (MEN) associated polyps (Chapter 91) – these have a good prognosis, but require surgical removal.
- Sporadic: often have a poor prognosis, similar to adenocarcinoma.

In the small bowel, 15–35% are multiple. Appendiceal neuroendocrine tumours are often removed at appendicectomy, either as an incidental finding or as the cause of the inflammation (by obstruction of the lumen). This is usually curative.

Prognosis

This is very difficult to predict, the best indicator being the proliferation index (proportion of dividing cells). These tumours are usually more indolent than adenocarcinoma and the clinical course of metastases, resection and more metastases, may extend over several decades.

Gastrointestinal stromal tumour

These rare tumours are thought to arise from the neuronal pacemaker cells of the gut, the 'interstitial cells of Cajal'. They are commonest in the stomach and small intestine, but may occur anywhere in the GI tract and even in the mesentery or omentum. Their behaviour is difficult to predict, size and mitotic activity being the best indicators. Surgical excision is the recommended treatment, with follow-up imaging to detect those patients in whom the tumour has spread (usually to the liver).

GI stromal tumours resemble smooth muscle tumours grossly and microscopically, but immunohistochemistry shows them to be negative for smooth muscle markers and positive for CD117. This is a tyrosine kinase surface receptor molecule for which a specific receptor blocker exists (known as Glivec or imatinib, originally synthesised for the treatment of chronic myeloid leukaemia). The response to therapy in patients with metastatic GI stromal tumours has been dramatic.

Mechanical disease of the gastrointestinal tract

Systems pathology

Volvulus

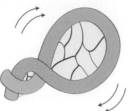

◆ Rotation of small or large bowel impedes blood supply, causing haemorrhagic infarction
◆ Infarcted bowel becomes permeable to bacteria, causing septicaemia and shock
◆ Gangrenous bowel will perforate if left; requires surgical removal of all grossly affected bowel

◆ The mesenteric arteries are thick walled and it is the thin-walled veins that succumb to the pressure exerted by torsion of the pedicle. Blood can enter the bowel but not escape, leading to haemorrhagic infarction
◆ The bowel wall appears purple due to engorgement by blood
◆ Gangrene will develop if this remains unrelieved

Intussusception

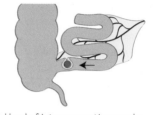
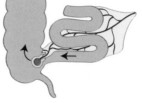
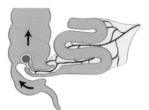

◆ Head of intussusception may be hyperplastic lymphoid tissue (young children), polyp (children/adults) or primary or secondary tumour (adults)

◆ The head of the intussusception is moved by peristalsis into adjacent bowel, carrying with it the mesentery

◆ Mesenteric vessels are compressed at the neck of the intussusception, causing haemorrhagic infarction and shock

Diverticular disease and possible consequences

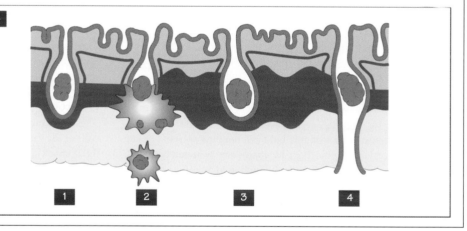

1. Diverticulum with faecolith

2. Erosion of faecolith through wall causes abscess formation, which may lead to perforation and peritonitis

3. Muscular hypertrophy, inflammation and scarring can cause stricture

4. Erosion of the tip of a diverticulum may lead to fistula formation, e.g. with bladder, vagina or Fallopian tube

Apart from strictures caused by cancer or Crohn's disease, mechanical obstruction in the GI tract is mainly due to diverticulitis, torsion (volvulus), intussusception or vascular occlusion (arterial or venous), with a smaller group of neuromuscular and other disorders.

Diverticular disease

Diverticulosis is usually asymptomatic but is common; the incidence increases with age (50% of 80-year-olds). Problems develop if inflammation or scarring supervene. The sigmoid colon is primarily affected but other regions of the colon may be involved.

The presentation varies with the severity and extent of the disease and is usually with abdominal pain, an obstructive mass or rectal bleeding. Torrential bleeding requiring blood transfusion is sometimes encountered.

Pathology

Colonic diverticula are outpouchings of the colonic mucosa and submucosa through the smooth muscle wall of the large bowel. It is believed that they arise due to prolonged high luminal pressure, which causes the mucosa to 'blow out', typically in places where the bowel wall is weaker due to penetrating blood vessels. This process is facilitated by the low fibre, high carbohydrate Western diet that requires more peristaltic effort to propel faeces through the colon. Hence, the smooth muscle hypertrophies, making the wall thick and stiff and therefore vulnerable to blow out through zones of relative weakness.

Faeces within a diverticulum may erode and ulcerate the wall, causing inflammation and sometimes perforation. This is diverticulitis. Consequences include stricture, abscess, fistula formation or peritonitis.

Treatment

A high fibre diet improves faecal transit and reduces the risk of complications in diverticulosis. Surgical resection is often required for those with a stricture, fistula or inflammatory mass.

Volvulus

Volvulus is the rotation of a portion of bowel on its pedicle. The principal site is the sigmoid colon, classically a long, faecally loaded sigmoid colon with a pendulous mesentery. Caecal and small bowel volvulus are rarer. Twisting of the pedicle of the bowel compresses the thin-walled mesenteric veins but arterial flow is protected by the thicker, muscular arterial walls. Blood enters the bowel but cannot escape. Thus, the bowel becomes engorged with stagnant blood, causing venous infarction.

Gross and microscopic pathology

The affected segment is haemorrhagic or purple/black. Microscopically, the bowel wall structures are effaced by haemorrhage and appear as ghosted outlines.

Treatment

If surgical intervention is sufficiently early it may be possible to untwist the rotated bowel and secure it to the abdominal wall to prevent recurrence. Steps must then be taken to avoid the precipitating cause.

Often infarction has already occurred and the necrotic bowel must be excised. If surgery is delayed, gangrene will occur and bacteria from the faeces will seep into any functional veins, causing septicaemia, or perforation and faecal peritonitis will supervene.

Intussusception

Intussusception is a disorder in which part of the bowel is drawn into and basically swallowed by another due to peristalsis. The affected piece of bowel must have a long enough mesentery to be mobile, thus the small bowel, notably the terminal ileum is the usual site.

Intussusception usually occurs in young children secondary to small intestinal lymphoid hyperplasia due to viral infection (e.g. Peyer's patches in the terminal ileum). This bulky lymphoid hyperplasia acts like a food bolus and is pushed by peristalsis along the bowel. However, the 'bolus' is connected to the bowel wall. Hence, this mural attachment is pulled in and 'sleeved' by adjacent bowel, together with the mesentery and blood vessels. Haemorrhagic infarction ensues because the thin-walled mesenteric veins are compressed but the thick-walled arteries remain patent.

Peutz–Jeghers polyps are rare hamartomatous polyps which may head an intussusception. Affected children have a syndrome with pigmentation of the lips and buccal mucosa and an increased risk in adulthood of gastrointestinal tract disease and malignancies (e.g. breast).

The nidus in older children and adults who develop intussusception may be a pedunculated tumour, often a benign polyp but occasionally a malignant polypoid tumour. The presentation is with obstruction and abdominal pain. Sometimes a mass is palpable. It is important to remember that other than young children, intussusception is usually due to a neoplasm.

Gross and microscopic pathology

As in volvulus, there is haemorrhagic necrosis of the affected segment. Microscopically there is haemorrhagic necrosis.

Treatment

If reversed before infarction has occurred, the bowel may be saved. In neonates, a barium enema may achieve this without the need for surgery. Infarcted tissue must be excised.

Other causes of bowel infarction
Arterial thromboembolic disease

This is usually the result of atheroma affecting the aorta and superior/inferior mesenteric arteries. Fragments of thromboembolus, often containing cholesterol-rich atheromatous debris, shower into the vascular arcades supplying the bowel, which are extensively cross-linked so this seldom causes large segments of bowel to infarct. Presentation is with fleeting episodes of colicky abdominal pain, subacute obstruction or (typically) GI bleeding. Often there is little to see at colonoscopy.

Patients with atheromatous stenosis of the mesenteric artery origins may develop 'mesenteric angina' – severe abdominal pain after eating, as the increased demand for blood flow to the gut cannot be met. Arterial stents, inserted via a catheter in the femoral artery can produce a dramatic improvement.

Vasculitis

Arterial or venous inflammation may lead to infarction at unpredictable locations. Henoch–Schönlein purpura typically affects children and has a good prognosis, but other forms of vasculitis, such as microscopic polyarteritis, can have a poor outcome.

Spontaneous venous thrombosis

This is rare and sometimes follows sepsis or occasionally occurs in prothrombotic syndromes.

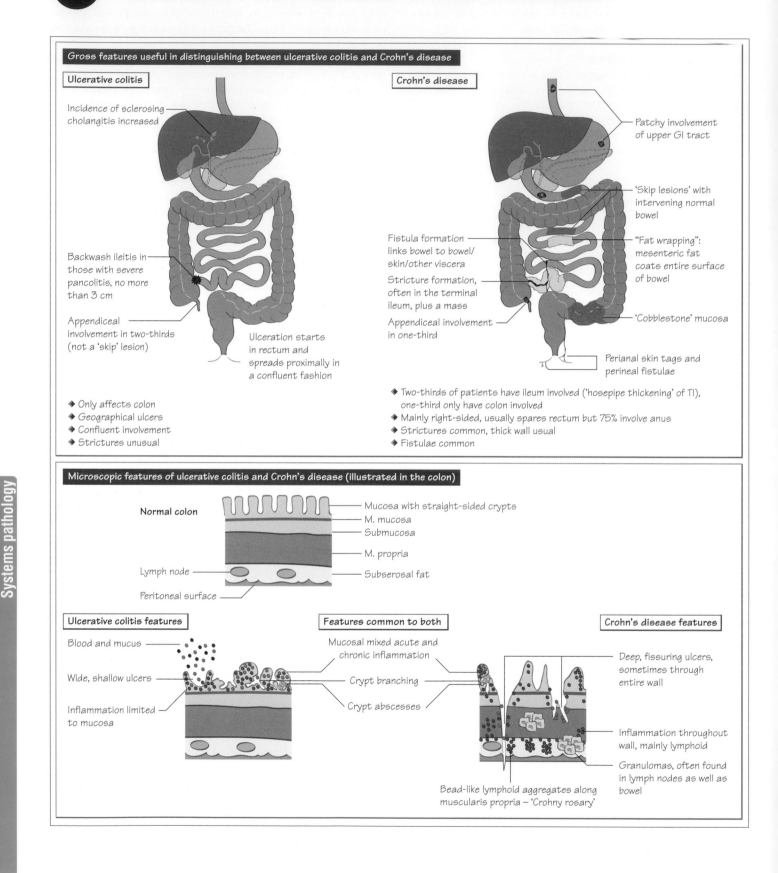

Gross features useful in distinguishing between ulcerative colitis and Crohn's disease

Ulcerative colitis

Incidence of sclerosing cholangitis increased

Backwash ileitis in those with severe pancolitis, no more than 3 cm

Appendiceal involvement in two-thirds (not a 'skip' lesion)

Ulceration starts in rectum and spreads proximally in a confluent fashion

◆ Only affects colon
◆ Geographical ulcers
◆ Confluent involvement
◆ Strictures unusual

Crohn's disease

Patchy involvement of upper GI tract

'Skip lesions' with intervening normal bowel

Fistula formation links bowel to bowel/ skin/other viscera

"Fat wrapping": mesenteric fat coats entire surface of bowel

Stricture formation, often in the terminal ileum, plus a mass

'Cobblestone' mucosa

Appendiceal involvement in one-third

Perianal skin tags and perineal fistulae

◆ Two-thirds of patients have ileum involved ('hosepipe thickening' of TI), one-third only have colon involved
◆ Mainly right-sided, usually spares rectum but 75% involve anus
◆ Strictures common, thick wall usual
◆ Fistulae common

Microscopic features of ulcerative colitis and Crohn's disease (illustrated in the colon)

Normal colon

Mucosa with straight-sided crypts
M. mucosa
Submucosa
M. propria
Subserosal fat

Lymph node
Peritoneal surface

Ulcerative colitis features

Blood and mucus

Wide, shallow ulcers

Inflammation limited to mucosa

Features common to both

Mucosal mixed acute and chronic inflammation

Crypt branching

Crypt abscesses

Bead-like lymphoid aggregates along muscularis propria – 'Crohny rosary'

Crohn's disease features

Deep, fissuring ulcers, sometimes through entire wall

Inflammation throughout wall, mainly lymphoid

Granulomas, often found in lymph nodes as well as bowel

Definition

- Ulcerative colitis is a chronic inflammatory disorder of uncertain aetiology that involves only the large bowel of the gastrointestinal tract but can also have extra-GI manifestations.
- Crohn's disease is a chronic inflammatory condition of unknown aetiology that can affect the entire gastrointestinal tract and may have extragastrointestinal manifestations.

The two conditions are collectively known as inflammatory bowel disease (IBD).

Epidemiology

The UK prevalance of ulcerative colitis is 80–160 per 100 000, while Crohn's disease is 40–80 per 100 000. The annual incidences are 14 and 7 per 100 000, respectively.

Crohn's has a peak onset at 20–30 years and a second smaller peak from 60 to 70 years. Ulcerative colitis has a less defined and broader age range, though patients are often children or young adults.

Aetiology and pathogenesis

The two diseases possess considerable clinical and pathological overlap. Families with a high incidence of IBD may include patients with either condition. Both can affect the colon, but only Crohn's involves the small bowel and rarely the stomach, oesophagus and pharynx. Both relapse and remit.

Curiously, smoking increases the incidence and severity of Crohn's attacks and is said to double the risk of disease onset, but diminishes the severity and likelihood of relapse in ulcerative colitis.

Genetic factors appear to be important in modulating the patient's response to a gut mucosal-damaging stimulus, which may be infective or environmental. Some Crohn's families have an abnormal NOD2 gene. The gene product helps modulate gut mucosal inflammation. The immune response is directed along the Th1 pathway rather than the Th2. The abnormal inflammatory response may involve failure to downregulate cytokine release and recruitment and activation of inflammatory cells following stimulation by gut bacteria.

The presence of p-ANCA in 70% of IBD patients also implicates disordered immune function.

Mycobacteria have been postulated as causative organisms in Crohn's disease but this is disputed.

Due to the different clinical behaviour of the two diseases, notably the propensity of Crohn's to recur after surgery and the unsuitability of Crohn's to the creation of a neorectum after colectomy, distinction between the two is vital and is largely based upon pathological factors.

Gross features

Ulcerative colitis commences at the rectum and spreads proximally in a *continuous* manner but affects only the colon (with backwash ileitis being permissible in severe disease). By contrast, Crohn's disease can involve any part of the GI tract, has a *discontinuous* distribution and most commonly affects the terminal ileum; colonic Crohn's disease often spares the rectum.

Ulcerative colitis features geographical, confluent ulcers; Crohn's has tiny aphthous ulcers or a cobblestone mucosa. Fat-wrapping is found in Crohn's but not ulcerative colitis; fistulae and strictures are a feature of Crohn's but not ulcerative colitis.

Microscopic features

Both diseases demonstrate mixed acute and chronic inflammatory cell infiltrates within the bowel mucosa. The inflammation is associated with mucosal damage, which manifests as distortion of the architecture of the glandular crypts and crypt atrophy. The inflammation includes inflammation of the crypts themselves (cryptitis) and small abscesses within the crypts.

The inflammation in ulcerative colitis is confined to the mucosa (with some deeper extension permissible in fulminant disease), whereas it is transmural in Crohn's. This transmural ulceration in Crohn's often features 'knife-like' fissuring ulcers and bead-like lymphoid aggregates along the serosa.

Non-caseating granulomas are common in Crohn's, including in regional lymph nodes. Care must be taken in interpreting the diagnostic significance of small granulomas that are associated with damage to mucosal crypts as these can be found in either condition, but submucosal granulomas are a very powerful distinguishing feature.

The transmural inflammation in Crohn's disease explains the association with fistulae, strictures and fat wrapping.

Clinical features

Ulcerative colitis

The typical presentation is with diarrhoea, which is often severe and is accompanied by rectal bleeding and copious mucus. Contact bleeding is found at endoscopy. Toxic megacolon is an emergency complication characterised by acute colonic dilatation associated with a high risk of perforation. It occurs in 5–10% of patients, often as the first attack.

Crohn's disease

The presentation of Crohn's is more variable than ulcerative colitis due to the various parts of the GI tract that can be affected. Diarrhoea develops in 80% although rectal bleeding is rare. Constipation may be encountered and rarely bowel obstruction. Abdominal pain occurs in 50%. Ileocaecal disease can cause a right iliac fossa mass.

An anal skin tag is present in 75% of patients with colonic disease and 33% of these feature a granuloma. By contrast the tag is found in only 25% of those with ileal-based Crohn's disease.

Weight loss is common (70%), while outright malabsorption suggests terminal ileal disease.

Perineal fistula formation ('watering can perineum') is rare but highly suggestive of Crohn's, whereas anal fissures are common but also occur in other diseases.

Extraintestinal disease

Both conditions can show fever, anaemia and uveitis. Skin manifestations include erythrema nodosum and pyoderma gangrenosum. Ulcerative colitis may feature sacroileitis or primary sclerosing cholangitis.

Prognosis

Colectomy is curative in ulcerative colitis, whereas it only addresses local disease in Crohn's. Approximately 50% of patients with Crohn's will require an operation and of those, half again will need one or more subsequent procedures.

The risk of colorectal carcinoma is elevated in ulcerative colitis. The risk increases with the extent of the disease and the duration of active episodes. Overall, the risk is around 16.5% after 30 years.

The risk of colorectal carcinoma in longstanding Crohn's is equally elevated and there is a slightly increased incidence of lymphoma.

Systems pathology

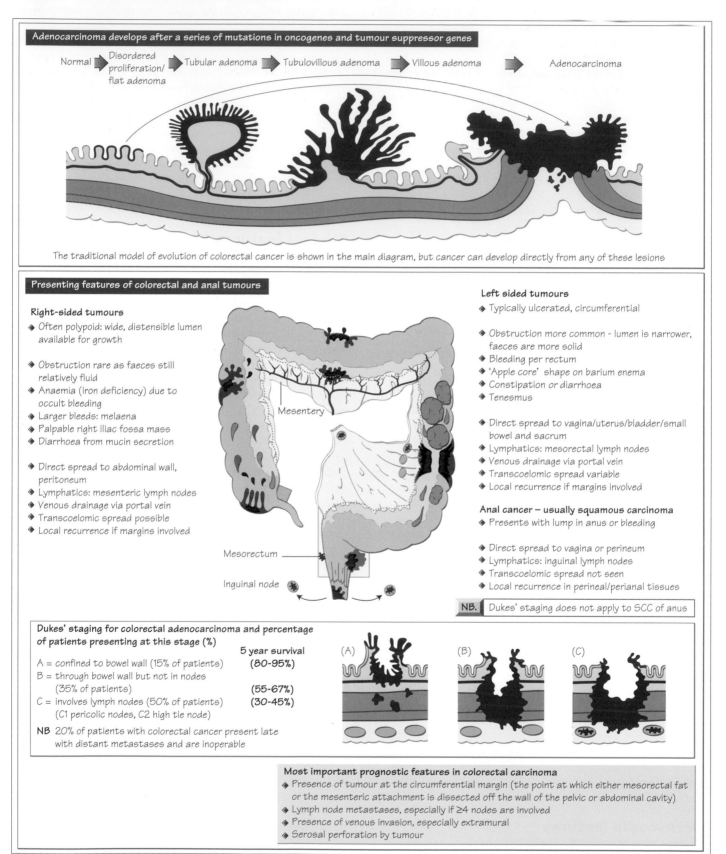

Adenocarcinoma develops after a series of mutations in oncogenes and tumour suppressor genes

Normal → Disordered proliferation/ flat adenoma → Tubular adenoma → Tubulovillous adenoma → Villous adenoma → Adenocarcinoma

The traditional model of evolution of colorectal cancer is shown in the main diagram, but cancer can develop directly from any of these lesions

Presenting features of colorectal and anal tumours

Right-sided tumours

- Often polypoid: wide, distensible lumen available for growth

- Obstruction rare as faeces still relatively fluid
- Anaemia (iron deficiency) due to occult bleeding
- Larger bleeds: melaena
- Palpable right iliac fossa mass
- Diarrhoea from mucin secretion

- Direct spread to abdominal wall, peritoneum
- Lymphatics: mesenteric lymph nodes
- Venous drainage via portal vein
- Transcoelomic spread possible
- Local recurrence if margins involved

Mesentery

Mesorectum

Inguinal node

Left sided tumours

- Typically ulcerated, circumferential

- Obstruction more common - lumen is narrower, faeces are more solid
- Bleeding per rectum
- 'Apple core' shape on barium enema
- Constipation or diarrhoea
- Tenesmus

- Direct spread to vagina/uterus/bladder/small bowel and sacrum
- Lymphatics: mesorectal lymph nodes
- Venous drainage via portal vein
- Transcoelomic spread variable
- Local recurrence if margins involved

Anal cancer – usually squamous carcinoma
- Presents with lump in anus or bleeding

- Direct spread to vagina or perineum
- Lymphatics: inguinal lymph nodes
- Transcoelomic spread not seen
- Local recurrence in perineal/perianal tissues

NB. Dukes' staging does not apply to SCC of anus

Dukes' staging for colorectal adenocarcinoma and percentage of patients presenting at this stage (%)

	5 year survival
A = confined to bowel wall (15% of patients)	(80-95%)
B = through bowel wall but not in nodes (35% of patients)	(55-67%)
C = involves lymph nodes (50% of patients) (C1 pericolic nodes, C2 high tie node)	(30-45%)

NB 20% of patients with colorectal cancer present late with distant metastases and are inoperable

(A) (B) (C)

Most important prognostic features in colorectal carcinoma
- Presence of tumour at the circumferential margin (the point at which either mesorectal fat or the mesenteric attachment is dissected off the wall of the pelvic or abdominal cavity)
- Lymph node metastases, especially if ≥4 nodes are involved
- Presence of venous invasion, especially extramural
- Serosal perforation by tumour

Adenomatous polyps

Adenomas are the most clinically important polyp type in the gastrointestinal tract, since they are dysplastic and thus predisposed to develop cancer. The main other type of GI polyp is the hyperplastic polyp. Interest is growing in 'serrated adenomas', which combine adenomatous and hyperplastic features.

'Pedunculated' polyps have stalks, those without are 'sessile'. They may have a tubular, tubulovillous or villous morphology. The risk of cancer development increases with adenoma size (>10 mm), severity of dysplasia and extent of villous architecture. Recently, non-polypoidal 'flat' adenomas have been described and appear to carry a high cancer-risk.

In the 1980s, Vogelstein et al. characterised many of the mutations present in the polyp–carcinoma sequence. Progressive accumulation of mutations occurs in adenomas prior to the development of colonic adenocarcinoma. Colorectal cancer became the exemplar of the 'multi-hit hypothesis' of carcinogenesis. A person with one adenoma will usually develop others. Regular colonoscopy is important, to identify and remove these potentially cancerous lesions.

Colorectal carcinoma

Adenocarcinoma comprises 98% of colon cancers. Rarely other tumours such as lymphoma, neuroendocrine tumour (carcinoid) or sarcomas are seen, but will not be discussed further.

Epidemiology

Colorectal carcinoma (CRC) is the third commonest cancer in the UK, causing 16 000 deaths in 2006. The UK incidence of 37 per 100 000 population compares poorly with 2.5 per 100 000 in Nigeria.

Men are affected slightly more than females; 80% of patients are over 50 years.

Aetiology

• Carcinogens implicated in CRC include heterocyclic amines (from burned meat), higher than normal faecal bile levels (stimulated by the presence of excess fat) and reactive oxygen species due to oxidants in food and the stimulation of inflammation.
• A low dietary fibre content and lack of exercise delays stool transit, increasing exposure of the bowel wall to these agents. A high vegetable diet may protect by reducing faecal transit time, supplying antioxidants to combat free radicals, binding (by fibre) of intraluminal carcinogens and generating protective volatile fatty acids by fibre fermentation.
• Tar-related carcinogens from smoking, absorbed into the bloodstream in the lung capillaries, may exert their effects in any part of the body.
• Chronic inflammatory bowel disease carries an increased risk of CRC, which reflects the distribution of disease and the extent of large bowel affected (5–15 times increased risk in ulcerative colitis; 3 times risk in Crohn's disease).
• Genetic predisposition (5% of cases) is suspected in those patients aged 30–50 years. There is often a strong family history of CRC. Examples are:
   • Inherited adenomatous polyposis coli (APC) gene mutation (familial polyposis coli).
   • DNA mismatch repair gene mutations (hereditary non-polyposis colorectal carcinoma, HNPCC).

Pathogenesis

Two main genetic pathways have been proposed to explain the development of sporadic CRC, as well as a third one:

1 In 80–85%, the path follows the traditional adenoma–carcinoma sequence of mutations involving the *APC* gene (5q), *ras* gene (12p), loss of DCC (18q) and p53 (17p). The distribution of these tumours is mainly left sided and mirrors the incidence of adenomatous polyps.
2 In 15–20%, the path is different: mutations accumulate because of DNA mismatch repair enzyme-related deficient surveillance. Inherited HNPCC makes up around 5% of patients. The tumours are predominantly right sided and may show mucinous or signet ring change. Stage for stage, these tumours appear to have a slightly better prognosis than those in the sporadic pathway but are said to be less responsive to chemotherapy.
3 A third pathway involving serrated adenomas has recently been proposed.

Clinical features

Any persistent change of bowel habit should be investigated. Iron deficiency anaemia is assumed to be caused by GI tract bleeding unless proved otherwise (note that menstruation is the main cause of iron deficiency anaemia in premenopausal females).

Prognostic features

• Tumour stage: Dukes' staging system or TNM stage (see Chapter 28); worse if four or more nodes are involved.
• Tumour at the mesorectal or retroperitoneal surgical margin increases local recurrence rates.
• Extramural venous invasion correlates with distant spread.
• Serosal perforation by tumour increases the risk of transcoelomic spread.
• The histological grade has a lesser bearing on prognosis.

Treatment

Treatment is by surgical excision. Large invasive tumours often respond well to preoperative chemotherapy/deep X-ray therapy downstaging.

Prognosis

The UK 5-year survival approaches 50%. Distant metastases eventually develop in 70% of CRC patients, of which 30–40% involve the liver alone.

Liver metastases may be amenable to partial liver resection – 5-year survival after this procedure is 35–40%, compared with 25% in those given chemotherapy alone for metastatic disease.

Anal cancer

Anal cancer is rare. The anus is squamous lined, thus squamous cell carcinoma (SCC) is the most common type. Rarely melanoma and other tumours may develop.

SCC is strongly associated with human papilloma virus (HPV) strains similar to those associated with cervical SCC. There is often a previous history of wart virus infection, either perianal or penile warts or cervical dysplasia. Homosexuals are at greater risk. There is an increased incidence of dysplasia and carcinoma in HIV-positive patients.

Dysplasia usually precedes the development of SCC and in a high risk community anal smears are examined in much the same way as cervical screening is carried out in women.

Pattern of spread

Spread via the lymphatics to the inguinal nodes in the groin, *not* to the mesorectal nodes. The liver is *not* the usual site of blood-borne metastases since the anus is supplied by the inferior rectal artery and drainage is via the systemic veins, not the portal vein.

56 Normal liver and the effects of liver damage

Constituents of the normal liver lobule

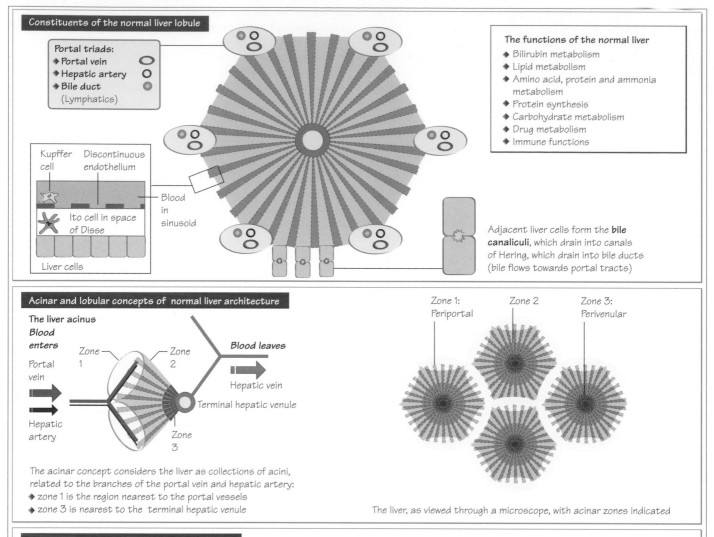

Portal triads:
◆ Portal vein
◆ Hepatic artery
◆ Bile duct
(Lymphatics)

Kupffer cell
Discontinuous endothelium
Ito cell in space of Disse
Liver cells
Blood in sinusoid

The functions of the normal liver
◆ Bilirubin metabolism
◆ Lipid metabolism
◆ Amino acid, protein and ammonia metabolism
◆ Protein synthesis
◆ Carbohydrate metabolism
◆ Drug metabolism
◆ Immune functions

Adjacent liver cells form the **bile canaliculi**, which drain into canals of Hering, which drain into bile ducts (bile flows towards portal tracts)

Acinar and lobular concepts of normal liver architecture

The liver acinus
Blood enters

Portal vein
Hepatic artery
Zone 1
Zone 2
Zone 3
Blood leaves
Hepatic vein
Terminal hepatic venule

The acinar concept considers the liver as collections of acini, related to the branches of the portal vein and hepatic artery:
◆ zone 1 is the region nearest to the portal vessels
◆ zone 3 is nearest to the terminal hepatic venule

Zone 1: Periportal
Zone 2
Zone 3: Perivenular

The liver, as viewed through a microscope, with acinar zones indicated

Effects of acute or chronic insults on the liver

Acute liver necrosis, e.g. paracetamol overdose: the acute insult causes massive hepatocyte necrosis but the liver skeleton is intact and liver regeneration can occur, providing the patient survives. The insult is not repeated and the regenerated liver is normal

Zone 1: Periportal cells survive
Zone 2: Often also affected
Zone 3: Perivenular zone necrosis, often encroaches on zone 2

Chronic liver damage: e.g. alcoholic cirrhosis
If the liver is chronically and repeatedly damaged by a stimulus, such as alcohol, which causes liver cell necrosis and inflammation, the liver structure is damaged and scarring occurs, damaging the flow of blood through the sinusoids. Scars which link zones 1 and 3 cause most disruption.
Once the liver architecture is damaged, continuing use of alcohol causes persistent inflammation. The liver forms regenerative nodules.
The combination of diffuse fibrosis disrupting the normal liver architecture and regenerative nodules is called cirrhosis

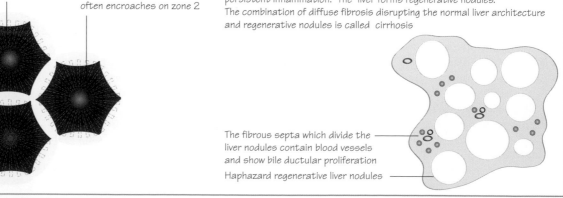

The fibrous septa which divide the liver nodules contain blood vessels and show bile ductular proliferation

Haphazard regenerative liver nodules

Normal liver

The normal liver weighs about 1500 g. Its myriad functions are summarised in the figure opposite.

The liver is composed of hepatocytes, arranged in trabeculae (walls) about 1–2 cells thick, lined by endothelial cells which are discontinuous to allow full contact between blood within the sinusoids and the hepatocytes. The space of Disse lies between the endothelium and the liver cells. Absorption and secretion of substances occurs here. Ito cells (stellate cells, which store vitamin A) lie in the space of Disse – these cells are of great importance as the source of fibrous tissue formation in chronic liver disease.

Kupffer cells, macrophages of the reticuloendothelial system, line the sinusoids and phagocytose particles and bacteria which may enter from the gut.

The blood in the sinusoids is a mixture of the portal venous supply (75%) and blood from the hepatic artery (25%), both of which run in the portal tracts, together with the bile ducts. The portal tracts ramify from the porta hepatis at the liver hilum and are supported by a sleeve of connective tissue. The periportal region is known as acinar zone 1. The blood is fed into the sinusoids and drains into the terminal hepatic venule (also known as the central vein), which then empties into the hepatic veins: the intrasinusoidal pressure equilibrates at about 3 mmHg above the inferior vena caval pressure, just enough to sustain flow.

Bile is secreted into canaliculi, formed at the junction between adjacent hepatocytes, and is massaged along from the centre of the liver lobule (perivenular region) to the portal tracts by the action of contractile cytoskeletal filaments arranged parallel to the canaliculi. The canaliculi merge with canals of Hering, lined by flattened epithelium, in the periportal region and then empty into bile ducts with cuboidal epithelium in the portal tracts, from where they drain out of the liver in the right and left hepatic ducts, which merge to form the common hepatic duct.

Acinar zone 3 is an 'at risk' region

Blood drains via several hepatic veins into the inferior vena cava, which runs for 2–3 cm and then opens into the right atrium of the heart. Increased pressure due to heart failure is easily transmitted back into the liver and readily overcomes the 3 mmHg sinusoidal pressure differential and compromises flow through the sinusoids. The liver tissue around the terminal hepatic venules (acinar zone 3) is thus easily damaged. This region of the liver has the lowest oxygen tension but curiously is the region in which the drug-metabolising enzymes are concentrated and is thus highly susceptible to toxic damage.

Cirrhotic patients have altered blood flow

The portal vein carries all the nutrients absorbed from the gut, to be metabolised and resynthesised or stored by the liver as required. The hepatic artery functions to nourish the biliary system and other liver architectural structures. If the portal supply diminishes, autoregulatory processes compensate with increased hepatic arterial flow. This is what happens in cirrhosis, as obstruction and diversion of portal blood flow leads to portal hypertension and an increased role for the hepatic arterial supply. In cirrhotic patients who bleed catastrophically from portal–systemic anastomoses, the sudden drop in systemic blood pressure and thus hepatic arterial supply leads to multifocal ischaemic necrosis of the liver.

Liver regeneration

Regeneration after acute liver cell damage

The complex metabolic functions of the liver cannot yet be reproduced by machine. In those who survive a massive acute insult, the liver's capacity to regenerate is phenomenal – it can replace between half and two-thirds of its own volume. On this basis, livers for transplantation are often split to serve two recipients.

Regeneration to replace large volume liver cell loss is performed by oval stem cells that lie adjacent to the limiting plate (the limit of the portal tracts), in the canals of Hering. They are versatile cells that can differentiate into either hepatocytes or bile ducts, and often acute regeneration is characterised by ductular proliferation as well as new hepatocyte formation.

Bone marrow stem cells can repopulate the liver, but the extent to which this mechanism is employed is not yet known. Replacement of individual damaged hepatocytes, for instance in acute hepatitis B or C virus infection, takes place by the division of adjacent hepatocytes. Liver is one of the 'permanent' type tissues in regenerative terms – it can replace damaged tissues but has little inherent mitotic activity compared with the 'labile' skin and gut epithelium.

Regeneration after chronic liver cell damage

This occurs when there is repeated or persistent inflammation, e.g. in chronic viral hepatitis, alcoholic or non-alcoholic steatohepatitis, and autoimmune or metabolic liver diseases. The skeleton of the liver is distorted by fibrosis and nodules of regeneration develop.

Hepatic failure

Liver failure is characterised by encephalopathy, bleeding and jaundice, often with hypoglycaemia, metabolic acidosis and hypoxia.

The hepatorenal or hepatopulmonary syndrome occurs in some patients – renal or pulmonary failure may develop due to reflex vasoconstriction in these organs, probably mediated by endothelin-1. The effects are to decrease glomerular flow, causing acute renal failure, and to shunt blood through the lungs, causing hypoxia.

• **Chronic hepatic failure**: this is more common than acute failure, and occurs following decompensation in a cirrhotic liver due to damage progression. It usually precedes death. In these patients the features of cirrhosis are usually also present.

• **Acute hepatic failure**: this occurs with massive liver necrosis, often secondary to a drug overdose (particularly paracetamol), infection (e.g. fulminant hepatitis A) or other toxicity (e.g. mushroom poisoning, idiosyncratic reaction to drugs such as antibiotics).

57

Jaundice, gallstones and carcinoma of the gallbladder

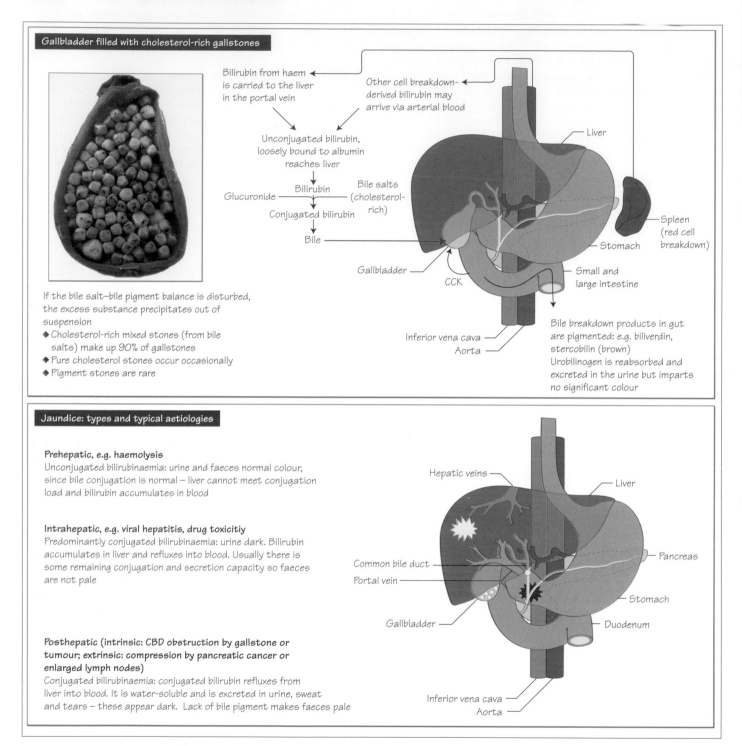

Gallbladder filled with cholesterol-rich gallstones

Bilirubin from haem is carried to the liver in the portal vein

Other cell breakdown-derived bilirubin may arrive via arterial blood

Unconjugated bilirubin, loosely bound to albumin reaches liver

Glucuronide ── Bilirubin

Bile salts (cholesterol-rich)

Conjugated bilirubin

Bile

Gallbladder

CCK

Liver

Spleen (red cell breakdown)

Stomach

Small and large intestine

Inferior vena cava

Aorta

Bile breakdown products in gut are pigmented: e.g. biliverdin, stercobilin (brown)
Urobilinogen is reabsorbed and excreted in the urine but imparts no significant colour

If the bile salt–bile pigment balance is disturbed, the excess substance precipitates out of suspension
◆ Cholesterol-rich mixed stones (from bile salts) make up 90% of gallstones
◆ Pure cholesterol stones occur occasionally
◆ Pigment stones are rare

Jaundice: types and typical aetiologies

Prehepatic, e.g. haemolysis
Unconjugated bilirubinaemia: urine and faeces normal colour, since bile conjugation is normal – liver cannot meet conjugation load and bilirubin accumulates in blood

Intrahepatic, e.g. viral hepatitis, drug toxicitiy
Predominantly conjugated bilirubinaemia: urine dark. Bilirubin accumulates in liver and refluxes into blood. Usually there is some remaining conjugation and secretion capacity so faeces are not pale

Posthepatic (intrinsic: CBD obstruction by gallstone or tumour; extrinsic: compression by pancreatic cancer or enlarged lymph nodes)
Conjugated bilirubinaemia: conjugated bilirubin refluxes from liver into blood. It is water-soluble and is excreted in urine, sweat and tears – these appear dark. Lack of bile pigment makes faeces pale

Hepatic veins

Liver

Common bile duct

Portal vein

Pancreas

Stomach

Gallbladder

Duodenum

Inferior vena cava

Aorta

Systems pathology

Causes of jaundice

Jaundice occurs when increased bilirubin is present in the blood (normal level <15 mmol/L).

Bile pigments are derived from haem, one of the major constituents of haemoglobin (Hb), also found in myoglobin and the cytochrome oxidase enzymes. Red cells are replaced every 120 days. The iron from Hb is recycled and the haem is oxidised to bilirubin, which is transported in the blood, loosely bound to albumin, to the liver. Here it is conjugated with glucuronic acid to render it water soluble for secretion into the bile.

Factors interfering with this path cause bilirubin to be retained in the body, which makes the sclera of the eye and the skin appear yellow. Bile pigments impart the colour to faecal material but do not usually affect the urine, unless bile flow is obstructed and conjugated bilirubin refluxes back into the blood and is excreted via the urine. Chronic deposition of bile pigments in the skin causes intense itching.

Causes of jaundice may be pre-, intra- or posthepatic.

Prehepatic:
• Excessive haem breakdown products in the blood overwhelm the capacity of the liver to metabolise and remove them. An example is haemolytic anaemia due to hereditary spherocytosis. The liver still conjugates bilirubin but is overwhelmed by the quantity, and jaundice is due to unconjugated bilirubinaemia.
• The urine remains a normal colour, as do the faeces.

Intrahepatic:
• Hepatitis may interfere with bile transport, conjugation or excretion. Jaundice usually reflects severe damage to the liver's synthetic or cytoskeletal mechanisms. Viral hepatitis is discussed in Chapter 60.
• Idiosyncratic drug reactions may paralyse the cytoskeletal apparatus necessary for bile movement and cause cholestasis with or without inflammation.
• Unless there is massive hepatocellular damage, the liver retains some ability to conjugate bilirubin and the stools are not usually pale, and the urine is less dark than in posthepatic jaundice.

Posthepatic:
• Bile excretion is impeded by obstruction or loss of the bile ducts.
• There is conjugated bilirubin in the blood, some of which is excreted via the urine (which appears darker than usual), whilst there is less pigment than usual in the faeces, which appear pale.
• There is impaired fat absorption which may lead to steatorrhoea (pale, offensive, bulky stools).
• Gallstones are the commonest cause, followed by carcinoma of the head of the pancreas.

Gallstones

Bile, made by the liver, is stored and concentrated in the gallbladder. It is released on demand by contraction in response to cholecystokinin (CCK) secretion by the neuroendocrine cells of the gut, the release of which is stimulated by the arrival of a fatty meal in the duodenum. Bile is a solution composed of bile salts (created by the action of 7α-hydroxylase on cholesterol, forming either chenodeoxycholate or cholate) and bile pigment (derived from the oxygenation of haem and related molecules to bilirubin). An imbalance of one of these constituents may cause precipitation out of solution and the formation of cholesterol or pigment stones, the former making up approximately 90% of stones.

Clinical features

The size, shape and number of gallstones varies considerably. Gallstones are widely prevalent in the population, particularly in middle-aged females and are often asymptomatic. They become symptomatic if they obstruct the cystic duct or common bile duct. The main symptom is usually severe pain, which may last several hours, and is often initiated by a fatty meal. It may radiate to the shoulder (reflecting the innervation of the diaphragm, which is often irritated by an inflamed gallbladder). If the common bile duct (CBD) is obstructed there is also jaundice.

Sequelae to gallstone disease
• Cholecystitis: acute or chronic (common).
• Adenocarcinoma of the gallbladder (rare).

Cholecystitis

Acute cholecystitis may follow gallstone impaction in the neck of the gallbladder or cystic duct, with erosion and ulceration and acute inflammation. Often this will settle down with conservative management, for cholecystectomy if necessary, at a later time.

However, the swelling caused by inflammation or the presence of the stone may obstruct the tiny cystic artery that supplies the gallbladder, causing infarction and gangrenous necrosis. This is a surgical emergency, as it may rupture into the peritoneal cavity, causing bile leakage and a chemical peritonitis.

Chronic cholecystitis is recognised histologically by fibrous thickening of the gallbladder wall, with chronic inflammation. Often there are out-pouchings of mucosa through the wall (similar to diverticular disease of the colon) called Rokitanky–Aschoff sinus formation. Stones may be present within these sinuses.

Adenocarcinoma of the gallbladder

Adenocarcinoma of the gallbladder comprises 95% of gallbladder carcinomas, is rare in the UK (two per 100 000) and is virtually always related to gallstone disease, though occasional cases are associated with hereditary non-polyposis colorectal carcinoma (HNPCC). Most cases arise in females aged 60–70 years. There is no association with sclerosing cholangitis or ulcerative colitis, unlike bile duct cancers.

Presentation is usually late, once spread outside the gallbladder has occurred – usually the tumour arises in the fundus of the gallbladder and thus does not cause obstructive symptoms. Occasionally a patient will have dysplasia in the gallbladder at cholecystectomy for gallstones; the operation at this, premalignant, stage is curative.

Adenocarcinoma is common in some parts of the world, e.g. South America (in Chile, Mexico and Bolivia the incidence is 21 per 100 000). This is thought to be genetic, possibly the result of the intermixing of Hispanic genes with the native American gene pool in previous centuries.

Cancer of the bile ducts (cholangiocarcinoma) is not related to gallstone disease and is discussed with liver tumours (Chapter 63).

58

Alcoholic and non-alcoholic liver disease

Effects of alcohol on the body

- Brain: Wernicke's encephalopathy, Korsakoff's psychosis
- Heart: dilated cardiomyopathy, atrial fibrillation
- Oropharynx and oesophagus: increased risk of squamous cell carcinoma
- Lower oesophagus: Mallory–Weiss tear
- Stomach: alcoholic gastritis
- Liver: fatty change, steatohepatitis, cirrhosis
- Acute and chronic pancreatitis
- Secondary effects of cirrhosis: portal hypertension, oesophageal varices, Caput Medusae, other sites of portal-systemic anastomosis include 'bare areas' of retroperitoneal wall and haemorrhoids
- Foetal alcohol syndrome may occur with ≤1 unit of alcohol/day and causes developmental abnormalities in the brain, heart, bone and genitourinary systems

- Social withdrawal, violence, traumatic injury (e.g. road traffic accidents), financial problems, psychiatric disorders

- Nervous system: Distal sensory neuropathy with typical 'glove and stocking' distribution

Metabolism of alcohol

Clinical features

Women have less alcohol dehydrogenase than men, so will achieve higher blood levels for the same dose

Genetic polymorphisms in aldehyde dehydrogenase enzymes occur, e.g. a point mutation in ~ 50% of the SE Asiatic population reduces aldehyde dehydrogenase activity, causing violent facial flushing, dizziness and nausea almost immediately after consuming alcohol

Acetaldehyde is thought to cause the foetal alcohol syndrome

Acetaldehyde causes the 'hangover' effects of excess alcohol consumption. Drugs that block acetaldehyde metabolism, causing its accumulation in the brain, are used in the treatment of alcoholism

Metabolic pathway

Alcohol

↓ Alcohol dehydrogenase in cytoplasm of liver or gastric mucosa

Acetaldehyde

↓ Aldehyde dehydrogenase in liver mitochondria

Acetic acid

Alcoholic and non-alcoholic steatosis and steatohepatitis and relationship to the metabolic syndrome (blue text)

Diabetes mellitus: lipoprotein lipase activated by hyperglycaemia mobilises FFA from fat stores

Increased dietary fat intake (obesity)

Alcohol mobilises free fatty acids (FFA) from adipocytes → FFA taken to liver ← Inherited hyperlipidaemias, e.g. abnormal apolipoprotein receptors cause decreased LDL clearance from blood

Metabolism of fatty acids and triglycerides impaired by
• competition with drugs such as alcohol
• hepatitis C virus infection (some strains)

Lipid secretion impaired by lack of protein (chronic alcoholism, protein calorie malnutrition)
Cholesterol excretion impaired by paralysis of the secretory apparatus, e.g. drugs

(Alcohol is metabolised in preference to FFA. Alcohol metabolism takes precedence over oxidisation of FFA for energy)

Fatty liver

Oxidation of fat stored in hepatocytes generates free radical formation

Fat accumulation can cause hepatocyte insulin resistance

Fat can activate angiotensin

Fat accumulation in hepatocytes may physically disrupt the normal blood flow in the hepatic sinusoids

Inflammation and fibrosis (steatohepatitis)

Type II diabetes mellitus

Systemic hypertension

Portal hypertension

The development of fatty liver disease, which may progress to steatohepatitis, fibrosis and cirrhosis is a recognised consequence of excess alcohol consumption. It has only recently been appreciated that patients who drink no alcohol may develop identical features, particularly if they suffer from the metabolic syndrome. The mechanisms are different but the gross and microscopical features are indistinguishable.

Fatty liver (steatosis): Causes include endogenous factors, such as obesity, diabetes mellitus, non-alcoholic liver disease and hyperlipidaemia, and exogenous agents such as alcohol excess, drugs (e.g. corticosteroids) or hepatitis C (some genotypes). Patients with hepatitis C virus (HCV) with fat develop fibrosis very rapidly.

Consequences of fatty liver:
- Fat is directly damaging to the hepatocytes – it can activate apoptotic mechanisms and disrupt lysosomal and mitochondrial function.
- Fatty change can trigger insulin resistance in hepatocytes.
- By physically enlarging the hepatocytes, fat can alter the microcirculation of the liver by causing sinusoidal narrowing.
- Stimulation of hepatic fibrosis through the production of fat-related cytokines (adipokines) and oxidant stress.
- Activation of angiotensin by fat, causing hypertension.

Steatohepatitis:
- The effects of fatty liver are compounded if there is also inflammation. The typical feature is acute inflammation, though some chronic inflammation is usually also present.
- Mallory's hyaline is typical of steatohepatitis – this is formed of clumps of cytoskeletal proteins.
- Fibrosis usually develops in people with extensive fatty change, both as spiky projections from the portal tracts into parenchyma and also around terminal hepatic venules.
- About 10% of chronic alcoholics develop cirrhosis.

Alcoholic liver disease
Fatty liver develops in chronic alcoholics for several reasons:
- Alcohol acts directly on peripheral fat, stimulating the break down of triglyceride and the carriage of increased free fatty acids (FFAs) to the liver, where they are taken up passively in an unregulated fashion.
- The metabolic break down of alcohol in the CYP2E1 pathway generates an excess of NADP over NADPH – a positive energy balance that the liver perceives as a stimulus to synthesise new lipid.
- The mitochondria are so busy metabolising alcohol that they have little time and space for the oxidative break down of lipid, causing accumulation of lipid in the hepatocytes.
- Acetaldehyde can bind to tubulin, impairing the transport of lipid out of the hepatocytes.
- Lipid is transported in the blood as a lipoprotein, and many alcoholics are protein deficient, thus production of lipoprotein is impaired.

The risk of liver damage in chronic alcoholics is as follows:
- **Fatty liver**: this occurs in 90% and is reversible, leaving normal liver if alcohol intake stops and there are no other factors such as obesity or diabetes which predispose to fatty liver.
- **Steatohepatitis**: this occurs in 10–35% of alcoholics. It may be acute disease, in which there is a 40–60% mortality rate for severe flare-ups, or it may be possible to see fibrosis in the background liver, indicating chronic disease. Without fibrosis, steatohepatitis is reversible. About 60% of surviving patients will eventually develop cirrhosis.
- **Perivenular fibrosis**: this usually occurs without accompanying chronic inflammation, and is seen in 40% of alcoholics but can take up to 25 years to develop.
- **Cirrhosis**: this occurs in 10–15% of alcoholics.
- **Hepatocellular carcinoma**: this supervenes in 10–15% of alcoholic cirrhotics.

Non-alcoholic fatty liver disease and non-alcoholic steatohepatitis (NAFLD/NASH)
These patients typically have type II diabetes mellitus, mainly due to insulin resistance, are often obese (though not always) and are usually aged over 45 years. About 20% of obese patients have the metabolic syndrome.

Risk factors for progression to fibrosis in non-alcoholic steatohepatitis (NASH) are: body mass index (BMI) >25 (i.e. obesity), diabetes and raised aspartate aminotransferase (AST) level. Some theories suggest that people who develop serious liver complications have a lower ability to stimulate liver progenitor cell proliferation and are 'poor healers'.

Estimates suggest that 50–70% of obese and/or diabetic people will have a fatty liver, of whom 20–30% will develop steatohepatitis with or without fibrosis and 2–5% will develop cirrhosis. The risk of hepatocellular carcinoma is not yet clear. It is thought that the changes are reversible until a late stage.

It has been postulated that bacteria, which reach the liver via the portal drainage system from the gut, may cause the production of reactive oxygen species (ROS) by Kupffer cells in the sinusoids. In a liver already compromised by the presence of large amounts of lipid, the resultant inflammation is more likely to lead to fibrosis.

Fatty liver develops in a slightly different way to that seen in alcoholic liver disease:
- Insulin resistance in type II diabetes mellitus, with resultant hyperinsulinism and an increase in blood glucose, causes activation of lipoprotein lipase in adipocytes, which release FFAs into the blood from stored triglyceride.
- Hyperglycaemia stimulates glycolysis and the release of FFAs in the liver.
- The liver passively takes up FFAs and either oxidises them in mitochondria to create energy or binds them with phospholipid and apolipoprotein to form very low density lipoproteins (VLDLs), which are secreted into the blood.

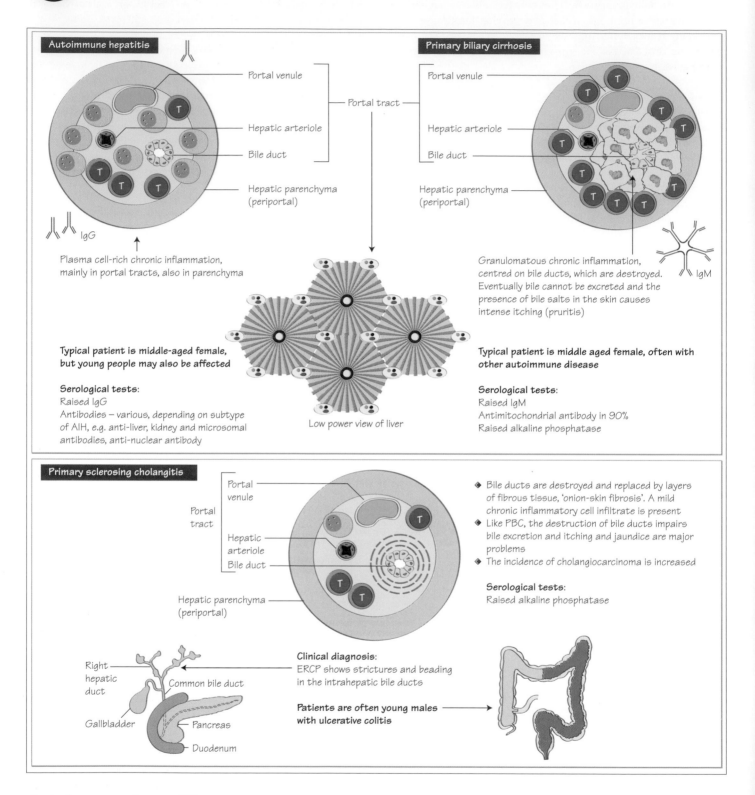

Autoimmune hepatitis

Portal venule — Portal tract
Hepatic arteriole
Bile duct
Hepatic parenchyma (periportal)

IgG

Plasma cell-rich chronic inflammation, mainly in portal tracts, also in parenchyma

Typical patient is middle-aged female, but young people may also be affected

Serological tests:
Raised IgG
Antibodies – various, depending on subtype of AIH, e.g. anti-liver, kidney and microsomal antibodies, anti-nuclear antibody

Low power view of liver

Primary biliary cirrhosis

Portal venule
Hepatic arteriole
Bile duct
Hepatic parenchyma (periportal)

Granulomatous chronic inflammation, centred on bile ducts, which are destroyed. Eventually bile cannot be excreted and the presence of bile salts in the skin causes intense itching (pruritis)

IgM

Typical patient is middle aged female, often with other autoimmune disease

Serological tests:
Raised IgM
Antimitochondrial antibody in 90%
Raised alkaline phosphatase

Primary sclerosing cholangitis

Portal venule
Portal tract
Hepatic arteriole
Bile duct
Hepatic parenchyma (periportal)

◆ Bile ducts are destroyed and replaced by layers of fibrous tissue, 'onion-skin fibrosis'. A mild chronic inflammatory cell infiltrate is present
◆ Like PBC, the destruction of bile ducts impairs bile excretion and itching and jaundice are major problems
◆ The incidence of cholangiocarcinoma is increased

Serological tests:
Raised alkaline phosphatase

Right hepatic duct
Common bile duct
Gallbladder
Pancreas
Duodenum

Clinical diagnosis:
ERCP shows strictures and beading in the intrahepatic bile ducts

Patients are often young males with ulcerative colitis

Autoimmune hepatitis
Epidemiology
Like most autoimmune diseases, autoimmune hepatitis (AIH) particularly affects middle-aged females (the female : male ratio is 8 : 1). AIH can also present in younger age groups.

Clinical features
There is no characteristic presentation; patients may be asymptomatic and have abnormal liver function tests discovered incidentally, or can present with a fulminant hepatitis or established cirrhosis.

134 *Pathology at a Glance*. By C.J. Finlayson and B.A.T. Newell. Published 2009 by Blackwell Publishing. ISBN: 978-1-4051-3650-1

Clinical diagnosis

Several types of autoimmune hepatitis exist; typical patients have abnormal liver transaminases and raised IgG levels; 80% have some/all of the following autoantibodies in their blood, but no antimitochondrial antibody:

- Antinuclear antibody.
- Anti-liver/kidney microsomal.
- Anti-smooth muscle antibodies.

Liver biopsy shows chronic inflammation with a high proportion of plasma cells. Some patients already have cirrhosis at diagnosis.

Treatment

Treatment is with steroids and other immunosuppression initially with consideration of transplantation in advanced disease.

Sequelae

As in other chronic liver disease, if untreated this can progress to fibrosis, cirrhosis and occasionally to hepatocellular carcinoma. Patients with an acute presentation with severe disease tend to progress quickly and are more likely to develop hepatocellular carcinoma.

Primary biliary cirrhosis (PBC)
Epidemiology

This disease classically affects middle-aged women (90% of patients are female), though some patients develop the disease in their twenties. PBC is an autoimmune disease of intrahepatic bile ducts. The pathogenesis is not yet fully understood.

Clinical features

There are symptoms of usually intractable itching, due to bile salt deposition in the skin, and tiredness – jaundice is a late feature.

Clinical diagnosis

There is a raised bilirubin, but the diagnostic serological tests are the presence of anti-mitochondrial antibody, specifically the PDC-E2 subtype, and raised IgM antibodies. Alkaline phosphatase (ALP) and γ-glutamyltransferase are raised, whereas transaminases are generally only slightly raised. Cholesterol is often raised.

Liver biopsy shows bile duct destruction by a CD8+ Tc lymphocytic infiltrate, associated with non-caseating granulomas either in portal tracts or parenchyma. There is much chronic inflammation and accumulation of copper and copper binding protein (copper is excreted via the bile). Curiously there is usually little bile stasis and when present this is seen in the liver lobule, not the bile ducts. There is no pus within the lumina of remaining bile ducts, unlike secondary biliary cirrhosis.

Treatment

Ursodeoxycholic acid, derived originally from the bile from bears in China, increases bile excretion and decreases the symptoms of jaundice. Transplantation is the only other effective treatment.

Sequelae

The disease inexorably progresses to a characteristic pattern of cirrhosis in which the portal tracts become linked by fibrosis 'jigsaw fibrosis',

which develops into a fine, micronodular cirrhosis over the course of about 15–20 years. The gross specimen at this stage is bright green in colour because bile is produced but cannot be exported from the liver. Death is usually due to liver failure, bleeding varices or infection.

Secondary biliary cirrhosis

This is caused by extrahepatic duct obstruction, with bile stasis and ascending infection. Causes include gallstones, obstructing carcinoma (e.g. primary cholangiocarcinoma or cancer of the head of pancreas). In children, congenital biliary atresia (a congenitally non-patent segment of common bile duct) or cystic fibrosis may cause this condition. Infection causes suppuration and abscess formation within the biliary tree, with surrounding fibrous scarring. Liver biopsy demonstrates polymorphonuclear neutrophils (PMNs) within the bile ducts and adjacent tissue, and marked fibrosis, with dilatation of bile ducts by bile. Cirrhosis supervenes later, again with a characteristic 'jigsaw' pattern.

Primary sclerosing cholangitis
Epidemiology

In the UK, primary sclerosing cholangitis (PSC) occurs in people of all ages, including young adults, and 75% of cases are associated with ulcerative colitis. The male : female ratio is 2 : 1. Interestingly, on the European continent this strong association with ulcerative colitis is not seen. Only around 4% of ulcerative colitis patients have PSC (there is a weaker relationship with Crohn's disease).

Clinical features and diagnosis

- Tiredness, itching and jaundice or a rising ALP in a patient with known ulcerative colitis is a typical presentation.
- Raised ALP levels.
- MRCP or ERCP showing bead-like dilatations and multiple strictures in the biliary tree is characteristic. Gallstone disease can cause strictures, but rarely multiple.
- Liver biopsy shows concentric periductal fibrosis ('onion skin fibrosis'), a paucity of bile ducts, copper and copper binding protein accumulation and marked fibrosis of portal tracts.
- Inflammation is variable.

Treatment

Ursodeoxycholic acid. Transplantation may be considered.

Sequelae

The disease progresses to liver failure over many years. There is a risk of cholangiocarcinoma but it is not possible to identify the at-risk group.

Bile ductular reaction

Injury to the bile ducts, as well as various other forms of liver disease, such as cirrhosis, can stimulate a proliferation of bile ductules at the limiting plate between the portal tract and the hepatocyte lobule.

Idiosyncratic drug reactions

These may present features that appear very similar to primary biliary disease or to AIH (or viral hepatitis). Drug reactions are usually divided into hepatitic or cholestatic types.

60 Viral hepatitis

Systems pathology

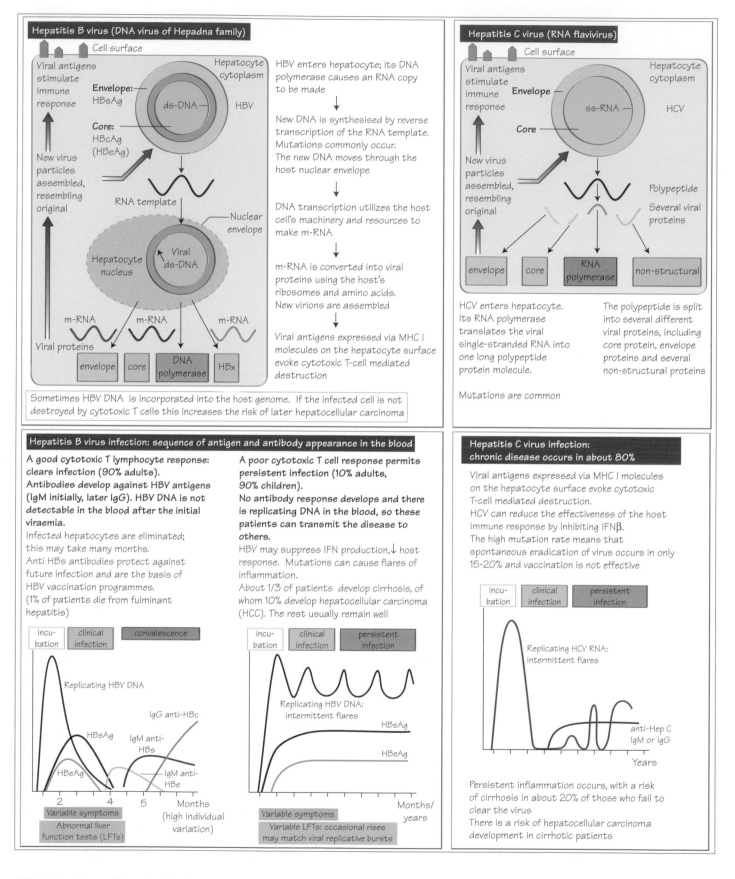

Hepatitis B virus (DNA virus of Hepadna family)

Cell surface

Viral antigens stimulate immune response

Envelope: HBsAg

Core: HBcAg (HBeAg)

ds-DNA — HBV

Hepatocyte cytoplasm

New virus particles assembled, resembling original

RNA template

Hepatocyte nucleus

Viral ds-DNA

Nuclear envelope

m-RNA   m-RNA   m-RNA

Viral proteins

envelope | core | DNA polymerase | HBx

HBV enters hepatocyte; its DNA polymerase causes an RNA copy to be made

New DNA is synthesised by reverse transcription of the RNA template. Mutations commonly occur. The new DNA moves through the host nuclear envelope

DNA transcription utilizes the host cell's machinery and resources to make m-RNA

m-RNA is converted into viral proteins using the host's ribosomes and amino acids. New virions are assembled

Viral antigens expressed via MHC I molecules on the hepatocyte surface evoke cytotoxic T-cell mediated destruction

Sometimes HBV DNA is incorporated into the host genome. If the infected cell is not destroyed by cytotoxic T cells this increases the risk of later hepatocellular carcinoma

Hepatitis C virus (RNA flavivirus)

Cell surface

Viral antigens stimulate immune response

Envelope

Core

ss-RNA — HCV

Hepatocyte cytoplasm

New virus particles assembled, resembling original

Polypeptide

Several viral proteins

envelope | core | RNA polymerase | non-structural

HCV enters hepatocyte. Its RNA polymerase translates the viral single-stranded RNA into one long polypeptide protein molecule.

The polypeptide is split into several different viral proteins, including core protein, envelope proteins and several non-structural proteins

Mutations are common

Hepatitis B virus infection: sequence of antigen and antibody appearance in the blood

A good cytotoxic T lymphocyte response: clears infection (90% adults).
Antibodies develop against HBV antigens (IgM initially, later IgG). HBV DNA is not detectable in the blood after the initial viraemia.
Infected hepatocytes are eliminated; this may take many months.
Anti HBs antibodies protect against future infection and are the basis of HBV vaccination programmes.
(1% of patients die from fulminant hepatitis)

A poor cytotoxic T cell response permits persistent infection (10% adults, 90% children).
No antibody response develops and there is replicating DNA in the blood, so these patients can transmit the disease to others.
HBV may suppress IFN production, ↓ host response. Mutations can cause flares of inflammation.
About 1/3 of patients develop cirrhosis, of whom 10% develop hepatocellular carcinoma (HCC). The rest usually remain well

incu-bation | clinical infection | convalescence

Replicating HBV DNA

IgG anti-HBc

HBsAg

IgM anti-HBs

HBeAg

IgM anti-HBe

2   4   5   Months (high individual variation)

Variable symptoms
Abnormal liver function tests (LFTs)

incu-bation | clinical infection | persistent infection

Replicating HBV DNA: intermittent flares

HBsAg

HBeAg

Months/years

Variable symptoms
Variable LFTs: occasional rises may match viral replicative bursts

Hepatitis C virus infection: chronic disease occurs in about 80%

Viral antigens expressed via MHC I molecules on the hepatocyte surface evoke cytotoxic T-cell mediated destruction.
HCV can reduce the effectiveness of the host immune response by inhibiting IFNβ.
The high mutation rate means that spontaneous eradication of virus occurs in only 15-20% and vaccination is not effective

incu-bation | clinical infection | persistent infection

Replicating HCV RNA: intermittent flares

anti-Hep C IgM or IgG

Years

Persistent inflammation occurs, with a risk of cirrhosis in about 20% of those who fail to clear the virus
There is a risk of hepatocellular carcinoma development in cirrhotic patients

 Pathology at a Glance. By C.J. Finlayson and B.A.T. Newell. Published 2009 by Blackwell Publishing. ISBN: 978-1-4051-3650-1

Viral hepatitis is inflammation of the liver due to a viral aetiology. Hepatitis viruses A to E are hepatotropic in that they specifically infect liver cells. However, other viruses such as the common Epstein–Barr virus (EBV) and cytomegalovirus (CMV) can affect the liver as part of a more systemic infection.

About 80% or more of people who contract hepatitis C will develop chronic disease, as opposed to about 10% of hepatitis B patients. It has been suggested that hepatitis C may be a worse problem than AIDS by the year 2020.

Hepatitis A

Hepatitis A virus (HAV) is a non-enveloped RNA virus of the picornavirus type that is 27 nm in diameter and has a single-stranded RNA genome 7500 nucleotides in length. Transmission is by the faecal–oral route with an incubation period of 15–45 days.

Hepatitis A is usually a self-limiting infection that is completely cleared by the liver. Recovery may take several months, but is almost always complete. Fulminant hepatitis is rare. Chronic hepatitis A does not occur.

Hepatitis B

Hepatitis B virus (HBV) is a double-stranded DNA virus 42 nm in diameter that has a genome 3200 bases long. The virus consists of a central nucleocapsid that is surrounded by an outer envelope which is derived primarily from the lipid membrane of the host cell.

HBV is a major global problem. Around 350 million people worldwide are estimated to be infective and 3000 million have been exposed. In Southeast Asia and Africa 8–10% of people have chronic HBV compared with 5% for the Indian subcontinent and the Middle East, and 1% for Western Europe and North America.

Transmission is by the parenteral route (blood, semen, vaginal secretions, saliva and even tears). The volume of infected blood that may be sufficient to transmit HBV can be as low as 1 μL. The incubation period is 30–180 days.

The most important mechanism of transmission in global terms is vertical between an infected mother and her baby at the time of birth; HBV does not cross the placenta. Children are tolerant of the infection, which becomes chronic in 90%. The tolerance persists until puberty then the immune system becomes responsive to the virus and a chronic inflammatory response develops. By contrast, chronic HBV infection occurs in only 1–10% of people who acquire the infection as an adult.

Serology

Several viral markers are important in HBV infection. The surface antigen (HBsAg) is the first marker to become raised. IgM antibodies to it are present in acute infection; IgG antibodies denote previous infection. HBsAg that persists for at least 6 months denotes chronic infection.

IgM antibodies to the core antigen (HBcAg) are the principal indicator of acute infection. The presence of the e antigen (HBeAg) implies active replication and an infective patient. If the patient has antibodies to HBeAg, they are considered not to be infective. This is important in patients with chronic HBV.

Patients with HBV DNA blood levels $>10^3$ genome copies/L are considered to be infective. This is important because some patients have mutated viruses in which HBeAg assays are unhelpful.

Clinical features

HBV typically has a flu-like prodrome that precedes the onset of jaundice. The jaundice coincides with tender hepatomegaly. Recovery from the jaundice may require several weeks and recovery from the associated fatigue can take several months.

Vaccination, available since 1982, is effective in protecting against HBV infection, even in the neonatal period.

Prognosis

- The infection is fulminant in 1%.
- Acute infection may either resolve completely or may become chronic, as indicated above. Of those patients with chronic HBV, around 0.5–2% per year spontaneously seroconvert from being HBsAg positive to negative, but the virus remains dormant and may flare up in future years.
- Those patients who remain HBeAg positive at 5 years have a 50% risk of developing cirrhosis and around 10% of these will develop hepatocellular carcinoma.
- Chronic infection acquired during the perinatal period in childhood manifests an early onset of fibrosis or cirrhosis and hepatocellular carcinoma (20–30 years).
- The use of interferon and antiretroviral agents in chronic HBV leads to about 15% of patients entering a non-replicative state in which the disease is not detectable but relapses can still occur.
- Low levels of circulating HBV DNA and high levels of transaminases (implying a robust inflammatory reaction to the virus) favour a good prognosis.

Hepatitis C

Hepatitic C virus (HCV) is a single-stranded RNA virus 30–60 nm in diameter and 9400 nucleotides long. Various genotypes exist and have different pathogenicities.

Hepatitis C is endemic in much of the world. Currently it is estimated that 170 million people are infected. Most countries report an incidence of 1.0–4.9% (in the UK it is 0.1%, and represents 25% of viral hepatitis).

Transmission is by the parenteral route, with blood being the main fluid involved; sexual transmission is less important than it is for HBV or HIV. Vertical transmission from mother to child is unusual (5–10%) and is more likely in those with high blood titres of replicating hepatitis C RNA. Transmission is mainly due to trauma at the time of birth and Caesarian section reduces the risk. Co-infection with HIV raises the risk of vertical transmission, with rates of 5.6–36% quoted in this subgroup.

HCV elicits a host CD8+ Tc cell response via type I MHC molecules on the hepatocyte surface. The risk of fibrosis is largely related to host genetic factors and the presence of fat in the liver; the liver enzymes do not accurately reflect the degree of inflammation or fibrosis and biopsy may be necessary to assess these. Patients co-infected with HIV show faster progression of fibrosis.

Replicating HCV RNA in the blood indicates current infection.

There are three common genotypes in the UK: types I, II and III. Treatment for 6 months with PEG-IFN and ribavarin can cure 80% of types II and III, whereas only 50% of type I will clear the virus. The virus can modulate its surface antigens and so far it has not been possible to create a vaccine.

Hepatitis D

Hepatitis D virus (HDV) is a defective RNA virus 36 nm in diameter that has a closed, circular genome 1679 nucleotides long. The virus requires the presence of HBV in order to replicate and is thus only ever found in people with HBV infection.

Transmission is by the parenteral route. The virus can either be contracted simultaneously with HBV or subsequently. The incubation period is 30–180 days.

HDV infection exacerbates HBV infection and the risk of fulminant hepatitis becomes 5–20%. If HDV is acquired as a co-infection, the risk of chronicity is the same as for HBV alone, but if HDV superinfects somebody with chronic HBV, chronicity is invariable. The risk of hepatocellular carcinoma is also increased.

Hepatitis E

Hepatitis E virus (HEV) is a non-enveloped RNA virus 32–34 nm in diameter and 7500 nucleotides long that has similarities with HAV.

HEV was first described in pregnant Indian women and is found in India, Asia, Africa and Central America. Transmission is by the faecal–oral route with an incubation period of 14–60 days.

Although HEV infection was previously thought to be uncommon, emerging information suggests that HEV may be far more frequent than used to be believed, in part because the presentation is often relatively non-specific or due to confusion with a drug-related hepatitis in some cases. Currently four genotypes are known, of which types III and IV are increasingly being reported in middle-aged men in the West. It has also been postulated that pigs may act as a reservoir for infection in many of these cases, although the mechanism of transmission via the faecal–oral route to humans remains in the process of being elucidated.

Fulminant hepatitis affects 1–2%, although this rises to 20% in pregnant women. Chronic HEV does not occur. Patients with chronic liver disease are at particular risk of fulminant hepatitis and death.

Hepatitis G

The hepatitis G RNA virus is a rare type of post-transfusion hepatitis.

Pathology

Acute hepatitis

Acute viral hepatitis affects the entire liver, which becomes uniformly enlarged. Many hepatocytes are swollen and vacuolated and scattered, single-cell, lytic necrosis occurs. The inflammatory cell infiltrate is composed of chronic inflammatory cells, mainly lymphocytes, as these are best adapted to dealing with a viral infection. The Kupffer cells undergo hyperplasia as part of the immune response. The changes are most pronounced in the perivenular zone.

The infection does not significantly damage the reticulin framework of the liver and this affords a scaffold on which the liver can utilise its phenomenal regenerative capacity. Once the infection is cleared, the surviving hepatocytes become hypertrophic and divide to replace their dead colleagues. Ultimately, this can lead to excellent regeneration of the liver.

If the infection is fulminant, large volumes of hepatocytes undergo necrosis. If death occurs early, the liver is normal in size but yellow due to bile staining. If death is later, the liver is shrunken, with soft haemorrhagic regions. In patients who survive, the liver's regenerative capacity can again yield good results, if the infection has been cleared.

Chronic hepatitis

This is discussed in Chapter 61.

61 Cirrhosis

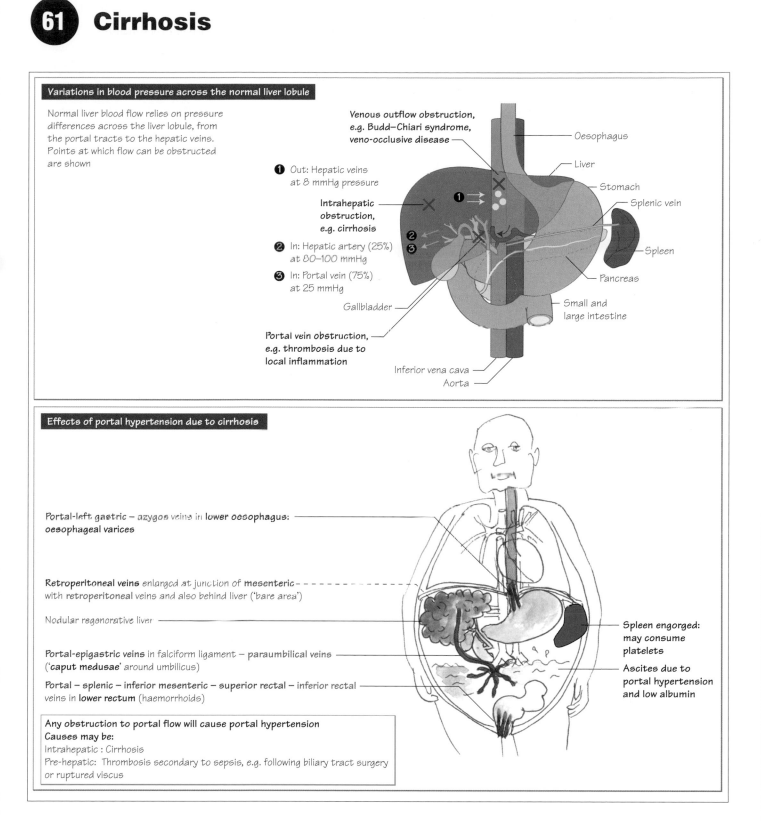

Variations in blood pressure across the normal liver lobule

Normal liver blood flow relies on pressure differences across the liver lobule, from the portal tracts to the hepatic veins. Points at which flow can be obstructed are shown

Venous outflow obstruction, e.g. Budd–Chiari syndrome, veno-occlusive disease

❶ Out: Hepatic veins at 8 mmHg pressure

Intrahepatic obstruction, e.g. cirrhosis

❷ In: Hepatic artery (25%) at 80–100 mmHg

❸ In: Portal vein (75%) at 25 mmHg

Gallbladder

Portal vein obstruction, e.g. thrombosis due to local inflammation

Oesophagus

Liver

Stomach

Splenic vein

Spleen

Pancreas

Small and large intestine

Inferior vena cava

Aorta

Effects of portal hypertension due to cirrhosis

Portal-left gastric – azygos veins in **lower oesophagus**: oesophageal varices

Retroperitoneal veins enlarged at junction of **mesenteric** with retroperitoneal veins and also behind liver ('bare area')

Nodular regenerative liver

Portal-epigastric veins in falciform ligament – paraumbilical veins (**'caput medusae'** around umbilicus)

Portal – splenic – inferior mesenteric – superior rectal – inferior rectal veins in **lower rectum** (haemorrhoids)

Spleen engorged: may consume platelets

Ascites due to portal hypertension and low albumin

Any obstruction to portal flow will cause portal hypertension
Causes may be:
Intrahepatic : Cirrhosis
Pre-hepatic: Thrombosis secondary to sepsis, e.g. following biliary tract surgery or ruptured viscus

Pathology at a Glance. By C.J. Finlayson and B.A.T. Newell. Published 2009 by Blackwell Publishing. ISBN: 978-1-4051-3650-1

Systems pathology

Definition

Cirrhosis is a chronic condition in which there is widespread, permanent disruption of the normal liver architecture by a network of anastomosing sheets and bands of fibrous tissue that divide the liver into nodules. In the UK the mortality rate due to cirrhosis has risen by 50% in the last 10 years.

Causes

In general, cirrhosis is the result of a chronic, persisting inflammatory process that damages the liver and causes hepatocyte necrosis. A list of causes is as follows:

- Post viral (hepatitis B, C and D).
- Alcohol.
- Non-alcoholic steatohepatitis.
- Autoimmune active chronic hepatitis.
- Primary biliary cirrhosis.
- Primary sclerosing cholangitis.
- Secondary biliary cirrhosis.
- Alpha-1-antitrypsin deficiency.
- Haemochromatosis.
- Wilson's disease.
- Gaucher's disease.
- Tyrosinaemia.
- Chronic right heart failure.
- Budd–Chiari syndrome.
- Veno-occlusive disease.
- Drugs and toxins – isoniazid, methotrexate, arsenic.

Hepatitis B and C (10%), alcohol (60%), biliary disease (10%) and autoimmune hepatitis (5%) are the most common in the UK, but globally HBV and HCV are the main causes. Non-alcholic steatohepatitis is also increasing in importance.

Cirrhosis is not an inevitable consequence of persisting chronic inflammation. For instance only 10–15% of chronic alcoholics develop cirrhosis.

Pathology
Chronic hepatitis

Chronic hepatitis can be caused by various conditions, including HBV, HCV, alcoholic liver disease, primary biliary cirrhosis, Wilson's disease and haemochromatosis. In all cases, there is a persisting stimulus that damages the liver and induces a chronic inflammatory response.

The inflammation in chronic hepatitis can be within the portal tract and/or the liver lobule and is composed of chronic inflammatory cells, in most cases particularly lymphocytes. Inflammation that remains confined to either of these compartments tends to be associated with only mild disease and biochemical disturbances without progression to cirrhosis. However, if interface hepatitis develops, the risk of evolution to cirrhosis becomes significant.

Interface hepatitis is also known as piecemeal necrosis and was the defining feature of the lesion that was formerly known as chronic active hepatitis. In interface hepatitis the inflammation in the portal tract disrupts the hepatocytes at the border of the portal tract and the liver lobule (the limiting plate), with hepatocyte necrosis being present.

Related to interface hepatitis is bridging necrosis. In bridging necrosis there is a zone of hepatocyte necrosis that connects two portal tracts or a portal tract and a central vein. Bridging necrosis cuts across the reticulin network and damages it.

Persisting inflammation and damage in these patterns induces fibrosis as part of the hepatic response to the injury. Initially this is seen as expansion of the portal tracts, which then extend fibrous septa. Later, these septa link portal tracts to each other, or connect portal tracts to portal veins, or both. As this bridging fibrosis progresses, the reticulin network is further damaged, thereby disrupting the scaffold for accurate regeneration. Ultimately, the fibrosis becomes so extensive that the liver is divided into multiple nodules by anastamosing bands of fibrous tissue and the derangement of the normal architecture becomes irreversible and functionally significant. During these events, the hepatocytes continue to attempt regeneration.

Cirrhosis

Like emphysema, the definition of cirrhosis encapsulates much of the key aspects of the pathology. Cirrhosis is often described as macronodular or micronodular (nodules <3 mm), but in practice most cases are of mixed type. Alcohol and primary biliary cirrhosis are two processes likely to be micronodular for some time before larger nodules develop. The nodularity is apparent on the capsular surface and cut surface of the liver. The cirrhotic liver is usually smaller than normal, but may be enlarged in early disease, or when there is marked fatty infiltration.

Microscopically, fibrous septa extend from the portal tracts to link them either to other portal tracts, or to central veins. The network of these septa produces the nodules and this change can be appreciated microscopically, particularly in micronodular cirrhosis. As well as extending septa from the portal tracts, the fibrosis also expands the size of the portal tracts.

In established cirrhosis of most causes, there is proliferation of bile ductules at the edge of the distorted portal regions. This may reflect an attempt to compensate for the compromised bile drainage that results from the cirrhotic process, or it may reflect the fact that the regeneration that attempts to oppose the cirrhosis-inducing injury occurs from pluripotential stem cells, which can form either liver cells or bile ducts.

A chronic inflammatory cell infiltrate is often present within the fibrous bands and portal regions. This usually reflects persistence of the chronic inflammatory process that produced the hepatic damage. Interface hepatitis may still be evident.

Clinical correlations

The liver has numerous functions, all of which are disrupted in cirrhosis.

- Synthetic processes are compromised due to the loss of hepatocytes. As an approximation, in a non-cirrhotic liver, the mass of the liver should be 1% of total body weight in order to provide adequate hepatic function.
- Hypoalbuminaemia is a feature of cirrhosis and can produce oedema, ascites and pleural effusions, but is not the best marker of liver synthetic function due to albumin's long half-life (6 months). Clotting factors accurately reflect the acute synthetic capacity of the liver and the international normalised ratio (INR) is most commonly used. Cirrhosis decreases the ability of the liver to produce clotting factors and so there is a coagulopathy.
- Elevated liver transaminases reflect hepatocyte damage. In advanced cirrhosis, the existing tissue loss is so great that the liver lacks the hepatocyte mass to produce an elevation in the transaminases in the face of a further insult. On the other hand, 'compensated' cirrhosis with little inflammation and delicate fibrous bands may show no abnormality in liver function tests. Therefore, a failure of transaminases to rise in cirrhosis is not necessarily a helpful feature.
- Preservation of the normal routes of hepatic blood flow is vital to permit the various detoxification processes undertaken by the liver to

occur and to allow appropriate handling of the constituents of the blood. The fibrosis in cirrhosis disrupts this normal relationship. Furthermore, as hepatocyte damage and loss underlies the cirrhosis, there is also a loss of functional liver mass.

• Detoxification of blood from the portal system before it reaches the systemic circulation is impaired. The loss of hepatocytes reduces the capacity of the liver to handle the volume of portal blood and the architectural changes permit portal blood to be shunted into the central veins without passing properly through the sinusoids. Therefore, absorbed material can enter the systemic circulation without first being processed by the liver. If these unprocessed substances reach the brain, they can induce metabolic disturbances, particularly with regard to ammonia and γ-aminobutyric acid (GABA) and are thought to be in part responsible for the complication of hepatic encephalopathy.

• Defective detoxification also has implications for drug handling. First pass metabolism is reduced and subsequent passes are also compromised, enhancing the effect of many drugs.

• Portal hypertension is a further complication that results from the distortion of the intrahepatic portal venous system. This can lead to the development of portal–systemic anastamoses. These are exaggerations of normal connections that exist between the portal and systemic venous circulations. Under normal circumstances, flow through these potential anastamoses is functionally insignificant but, in cirrhosis, it has implications for the handling of portal blood. The diagram shows the sites of these anastamoses.

• Oesophageal varices are a particular form of portal–systemic anastamosis. They arise from anastamoses between the portal veins and the left gastric/ayzgos veins in the lower oesophagus. Exposure of the systemic veins to the elevated portal pressure causes dilatation of them and they become visible as distended, tortuous vascular structures beneath the oesophageal mucosa. These distended veins are readily visible at endoscopy and are known as varices. Oesophageal varices can be vulnerable to trauma and spontaneous rupture and, if they do bleed, the haemorrhage can be rapid and massive. A variceal haemorrhage is an emergency situation and can easily be fatal. The situation is complicated by the coagulopathy that frequently coexists in cirrhosis.

• Ascites can result from hypoalbuminaemia and portal hypertension. It may be complicated by the development of spontaneous bacterial peritonitis.

• Hepatorenal syndrome is a phenomenon in which defective hepatic function induces secondary renal dysfunction (see Chapter 56).

• Hepatocellular carcinoma can complicate any cause of cirrhosis, but is most common with alcohol, hepatitis B and haemochromatosis. The frequency varies with the cause of the cirrhosis, which may reflect additional effects of the causative agent on the liver.

In summary, important complications of cirrhosis are:

• Impaired synthetic function – hypoalbuminaemia and coagulopathy.
• Impaired detoxification and drug metabolism.
• Portal hypertension – varices.
• Ascites and spontaneous bacterial peritonitis.
• Hepatic encephalopathy.
• Hepatorenal syndrome.
• Hepatocellular carcinoma.

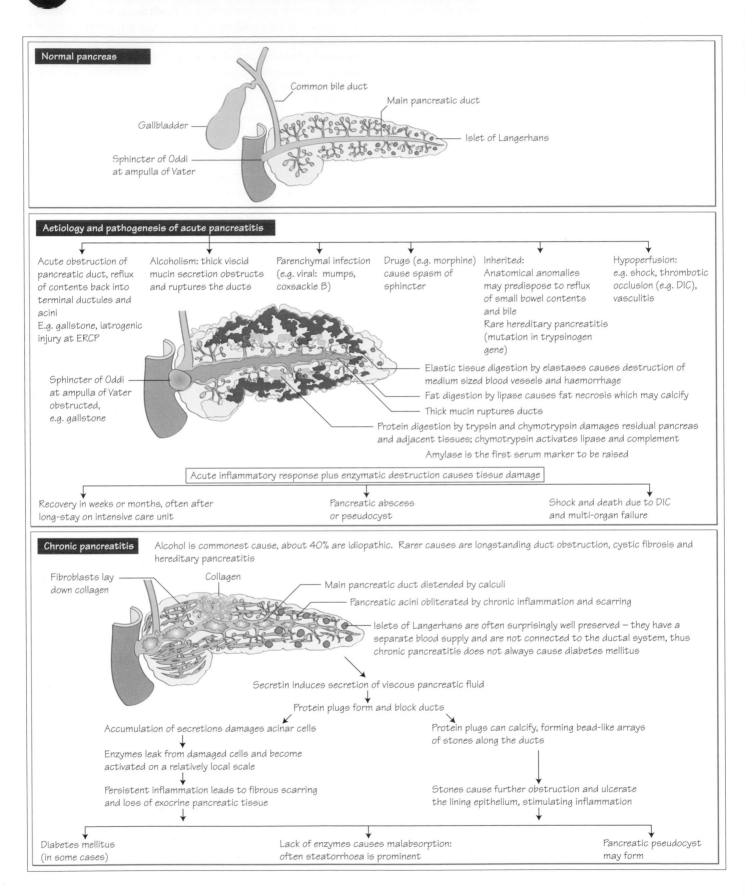

Normal pancreas

Common bile duct
Main pancreatic duct
Gallbladder
Islet of Langerhans
Sphincter of Oddi
at ampulla of Vater

Aetiology and pathogenesis of acute pancreatitis

Acute obstruction of pancreatic duct, reflux of contents back into terminal ductules and acini
E.g. gallstone, iatrogenic injury at ERCP

Alcoholism: thick viscid mucin secretion obstructs and ruptures the ducts

Parenchymal infection (e.g. viral: mumps, coxsackie B)

Drugs (e.g. morphine) cause spasm of sphincter

Inherited:
Anatomical anomalies may predispose to reflux of small bowel contents and bile
Rare hereditary pancreatitis (mutation in trypsinogen gene)

Hypoperfusion: e.g. shock, thrombotic occlusion (e.g. DIC), vasculitis

Sphincter of Oddi at ampulla of Vater obstructed, e.g. gallstone

Elastic tissue digestion by elastases causes destruction of medium sized blood vessels and haemorrhage
Fat digestion by lipase causes fat necrosis which may calcify
Thick mucin ruptures ducts
Protein digestion by trypsin and chymotrypsin damages residual pancreas and adjacent tissues; chymotrypsin activates lipase and complement
Amylase is the first serum marker to be raised

Acute inflammatory response plus enzymatic destruction causes tissue damage

Recovery in weeks or months, often after long-stay on intensive care unit

Pancreatic abscess or pseudocyst

Shock and death due to DIC and multi-organ failure

Chronic pancreatitis Alcohol is commonest cause, about 40% are idiopathic. Rarer causes are longstanding duct obstruction, cystic fibrosis and hereditary pancreatitis

Fibroblasts lay down collagen
Collagen
Main pancreatic duct distended by calculi
Pancreatic acini obliterated by chronic inflammation and scarring
Islets of Langerhans are often surprisingly well preserved – they have a separate blood supply and are not connected to the ductal system, thus chronic pancreatitis does not always cause diabetes mellitus

Secretin induces secretion of viscous pancreatic fluid

Protein plugs form and block ducts

Accumulation of secretions damages acinar cells

Protein plugs can calcify, forming bead-like arrays of stones along the ducts

Enzymes leak from damaged cells and become activated on a relatively local scale

Persistent inflammation leads to fibrous scarring and loss of exocrine pancreatic tissue

Stones cause further obstruction and ulcerate the lining epithelium, stimulating inflammation

Diabetes mellitus (in some cases)

Lack of enzymes causes malabsorption: often steatorrhoea is prominent

Pancreatic pseudocyst may form

Systems pathology

Acute haemorrhagic pancreatitis

Epidemiology and causes

The UK incidence is 20 per 100 000 per year, causing 1.6 deaths per 100 000 per year. The causes include:

- Gallstones (50%).
- Alcohol (20–25%), usually after heavy drinking.
- Idiopathic (third commonest).
- Viral (mumps, coxsackie).
- Drugs (loop diuretics, azathioprine, steroids, valproate).
- Hypertriglyceridaemia.
- Hypercalcaemia.
- Endoscopic retrograde pancreatography (ERCP).
- Trauma.
- Surgery.
- Ischaemia.
- Tumours.
- Ampullary obstruction.

Alcohol is directly toxic to pancreatic cells.

Pathogenesis

The sudden release of enzymes from the damaged pancreas into adjacent tissues causes the destruction of fat, protein and elastic tissue. Chymotrypsin activates complement and causes shock, disseminated intravascular coagulation (DIC) and haemorrhage.

Gross features

The pancreas is severely haemorrhagic and fat necrosis may cause flecks or islands of white tissue within the adjacent fat. Pseudocysts may form after the acute event – thin fluid replaces pancreatic tissue, forming a mass which may cause discomfort or become a nidus for infection – this is difficult to excise but can be drained into the stomach via an 'enterostoma'.

Microscopical features

Very little viable exocrine pancreas is identifiable within the mass of coagulative necrosis which replaces the pancreatic tissue. The islets of Langerhans are usually preserved, possibly due to their independent blood supply and lack of continuity with the ductal system.

Clinical features

There is severe acute upper abdominal pain, often radiating to the back, and vomiting. The main differential diagnosis is perforated peptic ulcer, which would cause signs of peritonitis and may lead to air under the diaphragm on plain abdominal X-ray.

The patient may develop hyopvolaemic shock due to exudation of plasma fluid into the retroperitoneal space and paralytic ileus may cause pooling of fluid in the gut. If the necrotic pancreatic tissue becomes infected by bacteria seeping from nearby, secondarily inflamed colon this is likely to trigger DIC and hyopvolaemic shock.

Clinical diagnosis

- Serum amylase levels rise quickly to very high levels. While amylase can be elevated in any abdominal inflammatory or obstructive situation, the levels in these other conditions are usually lower than those attained in fully developed acute pancreatitis.
- Pancreatic lipase is the best serological marker.
- Rosving's criteria predict a poor outcome and are: metabolic acidosis, low serum calcium, albumin, arterial oxygen, and elevated urea, glucose levels, liver transaminases, white cell count or lactate dehydrogenase.

Treatment and prognosis

Accurate diagnosis is important to avoid laparotomy, as this increases the mortality rate substantially. The episode may be acute and over in 2 days, or the patient may require prolonged supportive treatment for pain, shock, hypovolaemia, DIC and organ failure (e.g. acute renal failure and acute respiratory distress syndrome) – these patients often die but survivors can occupy intensive care beds for several weeks or months.

The mortality rate is high in patients who develop shock. Other patients may have a mild illness of short duration. The pancreas in survivors usually returns to normal.

Chronic pancreatitis

Epidemiology and causes

The UK incidence is eight per 100 000 per year; prevalence is 40–75 per 100 000. Males are affected more than females. Causes include:

- Alcohol (60–85%).
- Cystic fibrosis.
- Pancreatic neoplasm.
- Haemochromatosis.
- Obstructed pancreatic duct.
- Hyperlipidaemia.

Pathology

The underlying process in chronic pancreatitis is chronic inflammation of the pancreas, typically secondary to obstruction of the pancreatic ducts, either by abnormally thick pancreatic secretions or by a mass lesion.

The pancreas is often slightly swollen and is extremely firm, due to the fibrosis present. Dilatation of the ducts may be visible. The gross similarities with adenocarcinoma can be impossible to distinguish.

The inflammatory process destroys pancreatic acinar tissue but the islets of Langerhans are almost unscathed, set amid a sea of fibrosis. Eventually they may become damaged but this is usually late.

Clinical features and diagnosis

Abdominal pain, malaise and weight loss (seldom jaundice). The symptoms are often similar to those of pancreatic cancer. Patients may have malabsorption, particularly of fat (steatorrhoea).

Any lesion that causes long-term pancreatic duct obstruction can cause chronic pancreatitis, including a pancreatic adenocarcinoma. The diagnosis must be made by combining clinical modalities such as radiological imaging, serum enzyme and cancer marker estimations. Amylase is often slightly raised. Serum markers Ca19.9 and Ca125 may be slightly raised – high levels would increase suspicions of cancer.

Imaging may be normal or show an enlarged pancreas, similar to a tumour.

Biopsy is frowned on as many surgeons believe this may compromise curative surgery. It is difficult to know where to biopsy, since chronic pancreatitis and cancer both produce a hard, fibrotic stroma.

Bile cytology, collected at ERCP, is a non-invasive tool that can diagnose pancreatic cancer in about one-third of cases, if tumour cells are exfoliated into the bile.

Treatment and prognosis

Treatment is supportive, e.g. pain relief, abstinence from alcohol; the pancreas is scarred and recurrent episodes will worsen this – avoidance of alcohol is essential. Extensive disease depletes pancreatic enzymes, giving malabsorption that requires the use of powdered enzyme supplements. Diabetes mellitus may eventually occur, though usually late in the disease.

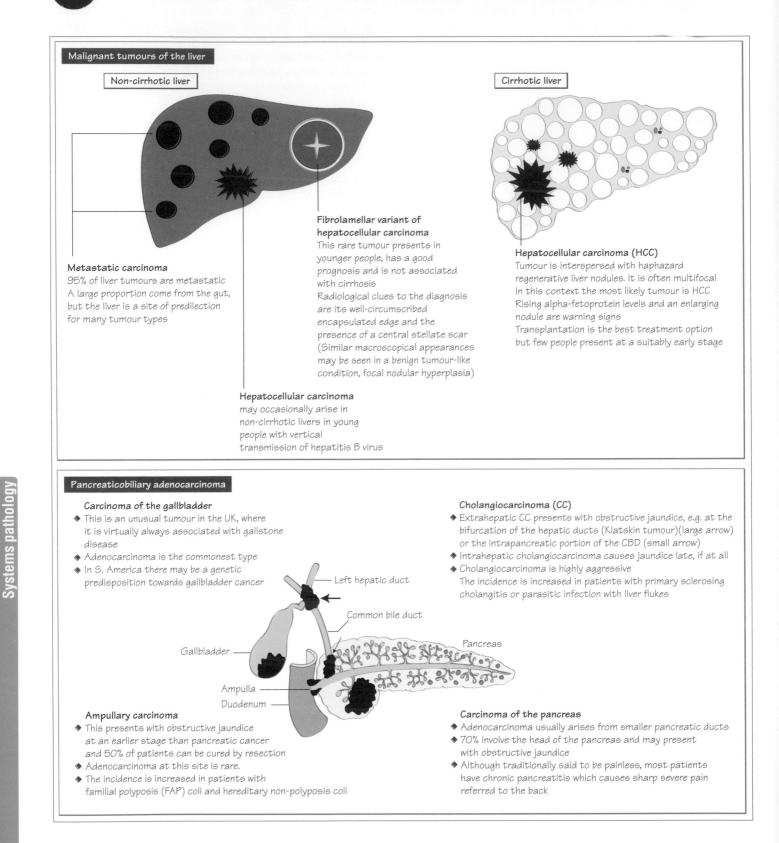

Malignant tumours of the liver

Non-cirrhotic liver

Metastatic carcinoma
95% of liver tumours are metastatic
A large proportion come from the gut, but the liver is a site of predilection for many tumour types

Fibrolamellar variant of hepatocellular carcinoma
This rare tumour presents in younger people, has a good prognosis and is not associated with cirrhosis
Radiological clues to the diagnosis are its well-circumscribed encapsulated edge and the presence of a central stellate scar
(Similar macroscopical appearances may be seen in a benign tumour-like condition, focal nodular hyperplasia)

Hepatocellular carcinoma
may occasionally arise in non-cirrhotic livers in young people with vertical transmission of hepatitis B virus

Cirrhotic liver

Hepatocellular carcinoma (HCC)
Tumour is interspersed with haphazard regenerative liver nodules. It is often multifocal
In this context the most likely tumour is HCC
Rising alpha-fetoprotein levels and an enlarging nodule are warning signs
Transplantation is the best treatment option but few people present at a suitably early stage

Pancreaticobiliary adenocarcinoma

Carcinoma of the gallbladder
◆ This is an unusual tumour in the UK, where it is virtually always associated with gallstone disease
◆ Adenocarcinoma is the commonest type
◆ In S. America there may be a genetic predisposition towards gallbladder cancer

Cholangiocarcinoma (CC)
◆ Extrahepatic CC presents with obstructive jaundice, e.g. at the bifurcation of the hepatic ducts (Klatskin tumour)(large arrow) or the intrapancreatic portion of the CBD (small arrow)
◆ Intrahepatic cholangiocarcinoma causes jaundice late, if at all
◆ Cholangiocarcinoma is highly aggressive
The incidence is increased in patients with primary sclerosing cholangitis or parasitic infection with liver flukes

Left hepatic duct
Common bile duct
Gallbladder
Pancreas
Ampulla
Duodenum

Ampullary carcinoma
◆ This presents with obstructive jaundice at an earlier stage than pancreatic cancer and 50% of patients can be cured by resection
◆ Adenocarcinoma at this site is rare.
◆ The incidence is increased in patients with familial polyposis (FAP) coli and hereditary non-polyposis coli

Carcinoma of the pancreas
◆ Adenocarcinoma usually arises from smaller pancreatic ducts
◆ 70% involve the head of the pancreas and may present with obstructive jaundice
◆ Although traditionally said to be painless, most patients have chronic pancreatitis which causes sharp severe pain referred to the back

Systems pathology

Secondary liver tumours

Ninety-five per cent of liver tumours are metastatic. The liver is the commonest site for metastatic disease, as gastrointestinal tract tumours tend to spread via the portal vein. As the liver receives over 25% of the cardiac output it is also vulnerable to metastasis of extra-intestinal tumours.

Benign primary liver tumours

Liver cell adenoma

These typically affect young female adults on the oral contraceptive pill (they may regress once this is discontinued).

Cavernous haemangioma

This is the commonest benign liver tumour, and is often found as an incidental imaging finding.

Malignant primary liver tumours

Hepatocellular carcinoma (HCC)

Hepatocellular carcinoma constitutes the majority of primary liver tumours. Globally the risk is strongly linked with hepatitis B and consuming aflatoxin-contaminated grain. Thus, HCC is very common in the Far East and Africa but rare in the UK (incidence 40 per 100 000 males in Africa and Asia, versus 1–1.6 per 100 000 in the UK, mainly in males).

In the UK, HCC is usually a complication of cirrhosis, especially cirrhosis due to haemochromatosis (develops in one-third), alcohol (arises in 10–15%), viruses, α_1-antitrypsin deficiency or Wilson's disease. The risk of HCC in a hepatitis B patient who is HBeAg-positive is 200 times that of HBeAg-negative individuals. (In the context of vertical transmission of hepatitis B, HCC may develop in young adults who do not have cirrhosis.)

Pathogenesis

DNA mutation occurs due to a variety of causes. Examples are:

- HBV can integrate into the hepatocyte genome.
- Alcohol increases the production of free radical formation.
- HCV is an RNA virus that can inhibit apoptosis.
- Iron interacts directly with DNA and generates free radicals.

Clinical detection of hepatocellular carcinoma in a cirrhotic liver

- High serum α-fetoprotein, which is usually in the thousands in HCC (normal level is <10 U/L).
- Enlarging nodule on serial ultrasound scans (but HCC is often multinodular and multifocal).
- Ascites containing tumour cells.

Gross features: The tumour may be a large single mass or multifocal, occupying much of the liver, usually with evidence of background cirrhosis.

Microscopic features: There are many patterns, most of which resemble liver cells. Demonstration of bile within the tumour is diagnostic.

Prognosis: The tumour is highly malignant and often advanced at presentation and resection or transplantation are rarely possible. Death occurs by 2 years in the majority.

(Fibrolamellar HCC is rare, affects young to middle-aged people and is not associated with cirrhosis. The prognosis is more favourable and liver resection can be curative.)

Hepatoblastoma

This is a rare childhood malignant tumour and may include mesenchymal and epithelial elements.

Angiosarcoma

These highly malignant, rapidly fatal tumours of hepatic blood vessels are rare and associated with exposure to vinyl chloride monomers, arsenic or the obsolete imaging agent Thorotrast.

Biliary tree tumours

Cholangiocarcinoma (primary bile duct adenocarcinoma)

This rare, highly malignant tumour (around one per 1 000 000 per year in the UK) is more common in males and may complicate primary sclerosing cholangitis (PSC) or parasitic disease such as the helminth *Clonorchis sinensis* (very rare in the UK). Patients with hereditary non-polyposis colorectal carcinoma (HNPCC) have an increased risk.

Obstruction to bile outflow raises serum alkaline phosphatase. Transaminases are often raised if there is associated liver damage.

Jaundice may occur before the tumour has spread outside the bile ducts. Only lower biliary tree tumours are amenable to surgery, though liver transplantation is sometimes used for higher tumours. However, distant spread is usual at presentation. Most patients die within 2 years.

Gallbladder carcinoma See Chapter 57.

Ampullary adenocarcinoma

This tumour is rare and usually presents with jaundice due to obstruction of the common bile duct. Radical surgery is required (often a modified Whipple's operation). Duodenal adenocarcinoma, often in the ampullary region, develops in 5% of FAP patients. The 5-year survival is approximately 50%.

Primary pancreatic tumours

Adenocarcinoma of the pancreatic ducts accounts for 85–90% of pancreatic carcinoma. This aggressive tumour tends to present from 60 to 80 years. The incidence is 11 per 100 000 per year in the UK. Pancreatic cancer comprised 3% of UK cancers in 2000.

There is a family history of the disease in 6%, with a five-fold risk in first degree relatives. Patients with inherited genetic mutations such as HNPCC, BRCA-1 mutations and Li–Fraumeni syndrome have an increased risk, as do those with hereditary pancreatitis.

The affected part of the pancreas is usually diffusely thickened and very firm, since most pancreatic cancers elicit a dense stromal response, but the tumour can be invisible to the naked eye.

Adenocarcinoma composed of tubules set in a desmoplastic stroma is usual, but there are several variants. Perineural infiltration is characteristic.

The only chance of cure is radical surgery (Whipple's procedure or pancreaticoduodenectomy), but few patients present before the disease has spread. The UK 5-year survival is only 2% (higher survival rates of 25–46% are quoted in the USA and Japan). The surgical mortality rate alone is around 5%.

Other pancreatic tumours

Benign tumours or tumours of the pancreatic body or tail may present as an abdominal mass or as an incidental finding during surgery for unrelated problems. Rarely, tumours may arise from the pancreatic acini (acinar tumours, of borderline or low grade malignancy) or the islet neuroendocrine cells. Even more rarely, stromal tumours may occur.

Embryonal renal development

Urachus

Cloaca makes ureter and most of the bladder

Mesonephric duct makes collecting ducts, renal pelvis, ureters and trigone of bladdder

Heart

Buds from aorta for glomeruli

Metanephros makes kidney parenchyma, tubules and Bowman's capsule

Migration path

Congenital/inherited disease of kidney

While the normal ureter implants obliquely into the bladder such that bladder contraction during micturition compresses the ureter, occluding it and preventing reflux, the duplicated ureters or those of pelvic kidneys do not implant in this oblique fashion and are therefore more susceptible to reflux and its complications

Urachal remnants may form small diverticula or separate cysts between the bladder and umbilicus

The bladder forms by folding over and fusion of the anterior abdominal wall – if this does not occur the bladder wall opens onto the abdominal surface – this is exostrophy

Hypospadias: incomplete closure of the ureteric groove can leave the ureteric opening half way down the shaft of the penis, or completely open to the surface

Renal agenesis: one kidney fails to form. Watch out for this in potential kidney donors!

Horseshoe kidney: two poles touch and fuse during migration – usually the lower poles. Often there is ureteric reduplication. Kinking of ureters over the renal arteries or inferior mesenteric artery may cause hydronephrosis

Pelvic kidney – one side fails to migrate, possibly impeded by umbilical arteries

Duplication: ureteric or even renal – there may be 3 or 4 small renal buds topping individual ureters, or ureters may be bifid and fuse later. These abnormalities are often associated with reflux and recurrent urinary tract infections

Polycystic kidney disease

Polycystic kidney disease is thought to arise because the collecting duct system (derived from the mesonephric duct) fails to unite properly with the distal convoluted tubule (derived from the metanephros). Accumulation of urine leads to ballooning of the ducts and cyst formation

Childhood PKD is recessively inherited (both paternal and maternal alleles must be mutated) and occurs in 1/5,000 births. The kidney shows fine mottling due to the presence of multiple tiny cysts which form from collecting ducts

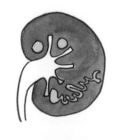

Childhood PKD

Adult PKD shows autosomal dominant inheritance (either paternal or maternal allele is mutated). It occurs in 1/500-1000 births. The disease often does not present till adulthood, when both kidneys can be massively enlarged, practically filling the abdominal cavity. Thin-walled cysts, from 1-2cm diameter, formed in any portion of the nephron, replace the kidney substance

About 15-30% of adult PKD patients have thin-walled biliary cysts in the liver and ductal cysts in the pancreas

In the embryo, the kidney develops in the pelvis, later migrating to its normal lumbar position in the posterior retroperitoneum. Its vascular supply from the aorta alters as it ascends.

The kidney is derived from three distinct elements:

1 Metanephros: this forms the renal tubules and the parenchyma.

2 Mesonephric duct: this forms the ureters, renal pelvis and collecting ducts.

3 Glomerular tufts: these are buds from the primitive aorta that invaginate into the mesonephros and stimulate tubule formation. They invaginate the end of the primitive tubules to form the Bowman's capsule.

The bladder is derived mainly from the endoderm of the cloaca, but the mesonephric duct forms the trigone of the bladder, and this is where the ureters implant into the bladder. *In utero* the bladder is continuous with the urachus in the umbilical cord – sometimes a diverticulum is left behind (urachal remnant). Rarely, a large abdominal wall defect arises and the bladder is exposed on the surface – this is exostrophy of the bladder.

The urethra forms when the urethral plate folds over to form a tube.

Renal and renal tract abnormalities are the commonest congenital and developmental abnormalities in surviving infants (around 2% of congenital malformations). There is a difference between *congenital diseases*, which are disorders of embryological development that are present at birth, and *inherited diseases*, which occur due to genetic mutations and may or may not be evident at birth.

Inherited abnormalities

Adult polycystic kidney disease (PKD) is the commonest inherited renal disease, which manifests later in life and is caused by the *PKD-1* gene.

Congenital and developmental abnormalities

Urinary tract congenital abnormalities are extremely common, for instance:

- **Kidney**:
  - Unilateral agenesis (incidence one in 500).
  - Horseshoe kidney: poles are pushed closely together during ascent; usually the lower poles fuse and cannot negotiate the inferior mesenteric branch of the aorta. Incidence is one in 600 people.
  - Pelvic kidney: failure to migrate – possibly impeded by the fork of the umbilical arteries.
- **Ureter**: e.g. duplication – early splitting of the ureteric bud into two parts.

Various degrees of ureteric duplication can occur. In some, the ureter is duplicated along its entire length, whereas in others only the upper part of the ureter is duplicated. The two components then fuse to form a common lower ureter.

Duplex ureters are associated with a duplex pelvicalyceal system within the kidney they drain. This means that the kidney is divided into two discrete units with regard to the collection and drainage of urine.

Abnormal duplication of the ureter is associated with abnormal implantation of the ureter into the bladder. Under normal circumstances, the ureter enters the bladder obliquely. This causes the ureter to be compressed when the bladder contracts and thereby provides protection against reflux of urine back into the ureter and kidney. In duplex systems, the extra ureter tends not to implant correctly and is susceptible to reflux. This can lead to dilatation of the ureter, hydronephrosis and a tendency to repeated urinary tract infections. It is usually the lower component of a duplex ureteric system that displays defective implantation.

- **Bladder**: e.g. exostrophy – failure of closure of the anterior bladder wall, with the posterior wall exposed at the abdominal surface. Bladder exostrophy is a serious condition as the bladder mucosa and, through continuity, the ureters and renal pelvicalyceal systems, are exposed directly to the external environment.
- **Urethra**: e.g. hypospadias – an incomplete fusion of the urethral groove.
- **Urachal remnant**: cyst or fistula at apex of the bladder – this is a site at which adenocarcinoma may develop.

Potter's syndrome

Potter's syndrome is an abnormality of the renal tract that is an example of a developmental abnormality known as a **sequence**. A sequence features several different components, all of which arise from one initial abnormality that then causes problems. In Potter's syndrome, this initial abnormality is bilateral renal agenesis or nonfunction. The renal agenesis means that no fetal urine is produced. This leads to oligohydramnios (reduced quantities of amniotic fluid). The oligohydramnios in turn causes the fetus to have less room inside the uterus as it is no longer floating free in amniotic fluid. The loss of space produces characteristic facial changes by mechanical effects; these include low set ears, a receding chin and a broad, flattened nose. The attitude of the lower limbs is also affected such that they are flexed at the hips and extended at the knees, giving the impression of having been 'bent up'. Also secondary to the decreased volume of amniotic fluid is pulmonary hypoplasia.

Systems pathology

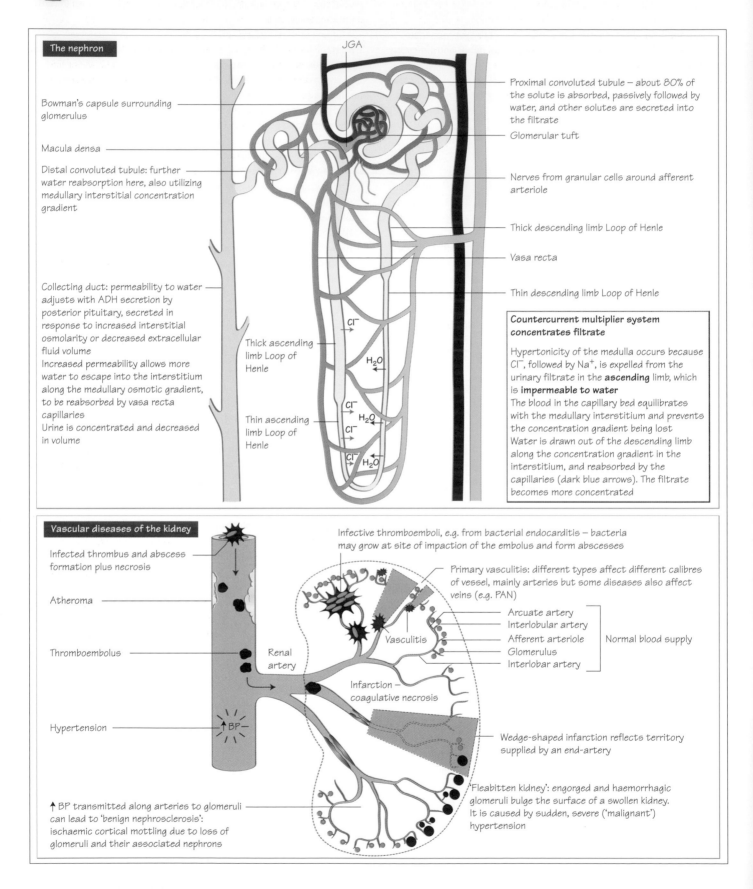

The nephron

JGA

Bowman's capsule surrounding glomerulus

Macula densa

Distal convoluted tubule: further water reabsorption here, also utilizing medullary interstitial concentration gradient

Collecting duct: permeability to water adjusts with ADH secretion by posterior pituitary, secreted in response to increased interstitial osmolarity or decreased extracellular fluid volume
Increased permeability allows more water to escape into the interstitium along the medullary osmotic gradient, to be reabsorbed by vasa recta capillaries
Urine is concentrated and decreased in volume

Proximal convoluted tubule – about 80% of the solute is absorbed, passively followed by water, and other solutes are secreted into the filtrate

Glomerular tuft

Nerves from granular cells around afferent arteriole

Thick descending limb Loop of Henle

Vasa recta

Thin descending limb Loop of Henle

Thick ascending limb Loop of Henle

Thin ascending limb Loop of Henle

Cl^- H_2O

Countercurrent multiplier system concentrates filtrate

Hypertonicity of the medulla occurs because Cl^-, followed by Na^+, is expelled from the urinary filtrate in the **ascending** limb, which is **impermeable to water**
The blood in the capillary bed equilibrates with the medullary interstitium and prevents the concentration gradient being lost
Water is drawn out of the descending limb along the concentration gradient in the interstitium, and reabsorbed by the capillaries (dark blue arrows). The filtrate becomes more concentrated

Vascular diseases of the kidney

Infected thrombus and abscess formation plus necrosis

Atheroma

Thromboembolus

Renal artery

Hypertension

↑BP

Infective thromboemboli, e.g. from bacterial endocarditis – bacteria may grow at site of impaction of the embolus and form abscesses

Primary vasculitis: different types affect different calibres of vessel, mainly arteries but some diseases also affect veins (e.g. PAN)

Vasculitis

Arcuate artery
Interlobular artery
Afferent arteriole — Normal blood supply
Glomerulus
Interlobar artery

Infarction – coagulative necrosis

Wedge-shaped infarction reflects territory supplied by an end-artery

'Fleabitten kidney': engorged and haemorrhagic glomeruli bulge the surface of a swollen kidney. It is caused by sudden, severe ('malignant') hypertension

↑ BP transmitted along arteries to glomeruli can lead to 'benign nephrosclerosis': ischaemic cortical mottling due to loss of glomeruli and their associated nephrons

The glomerulus and tubule system constitute the nephron.

Glomerulus: This is a knot-like arrangement of capillaries that invaginates the Bowman's capsule. The glomerulus is the site of filtration of the blood. The capillary endothelium is fenestrated, making it porous to all fluid and solutes, but not plasma proteins or cells. The pressure within the tuft is high, since both afferent and efferent vessels are arterioles. The hydrostatic pressure pushing the fluid out of the capillary exceeds the plasma oncotic pressure within the tuft, so filtration results.

Mesangial cells: Mesangial cells and the matrix they secrete form the supporting core of the glomerulus. Mesangial cells phagocytose particles that leak from the glomerular tuft.

Bowman's capsule: This is a cup-shaped funnel which forms in the embryo when the glomerular tuft invaginates the blind end of the developing renal tubule. The epithelial cells of the Bowman's capsule that are in contact with the capillaries of the tuft (the visceral layer) are called podocytes, because of the foot processes they extend toward the capillaries to envelope them.

A cavity separates the inner and outer (visceral and parietal) layers of epithelium; the plasma filtrate from the glomeruli is collected here and funnelled into the proximal convoluted tubule. The epithelial cells (podocytes) envelope the capillaries. Each podocyte contacts the basement membrane via further processes (pedicels), which in turn have a brush-like collection of molecules (nephrin) on their surfaces. The spaces between the pedicels are called slit pores – these permit fluid to pass into the lumen of the Bowman's capsule (Chapter 66).

Basement membrane: The basement membrane is probably the most important part of the filter system. It is made of a negatively charged collagen matrix partly formed by the epithelium (podocyte) and partly by the endothelium of the capillary. Where these layers meet, the basement membrane appears dark on electron microscopy (the lamina densa). Particles and solutes pass through, depending on their size and charge. The negative charge has a key role in preventing the filtration of low molecular weight proteins like albumin.

Blood pressure control: Blood pressure control is in part mediated by the renin–angiotensin system, which is activated by low flow rates through the glomerular tuft. Renin is secreted by cells in the macula densa, a portion of the distal convoluted tubule that lies adjacent to the juxtaglomerular complex (JGA). There are also sympathetic nerves that detect low flow in the afferent arterioles.

Vascular diseases of the kidney

If the capillaries that form the glomerular tuft are irreparably damaged, the entire nephron will usually atrophy. In order to understand renal vascular diseases, it is also important to appreciate the structure of the renal artery supply and the fact that the end branches are end-arteries and that the arterial supply to the cortex is terminal. Occlusion of an end-artery leads to infarction of the tissue in a wedge-shaped distribution distal to the obstruction. In the kidney this typically leads to coagulative necrosis.

The renal artery branches directly off the aorta at the level of T12/L1 vertebrae, just below the superior mesenteric artery origin, although one-quarter of people also have accessory renal arteries. The kidneys receive 25% of the cardiac output.

The renal arteries divide into the following sequential branches: interlobar, arcuate, interlobular, afferent arteriole, glomerulus and efferent arteriole. The efferent arteriole then either divides into capillaries which surround the collecting tubules or, if the glomerulus is close to the medulla, into the vasa recta, which extends into the medulla, beside the collecting ducts. Thus the renal vascular supply incorporates two capillary beds arranged in series – the glomerular tuft and then the capillary bed, linking the arterial and venous supplies. Draining venules form veins that mirror the distribution of the arteries and the renal vein returns blood to the inferior vena cava (IVC).

Renal artery stenosis: This is congenital or secondary to pressure, e.g. from an aberrant ureter, or atherosclerosis (usually diabetic patients). The low blood flow in the affected kidney may trigger hypertension via activation of the renin–angiotensin system – one of the rare treatable causes of hypertension.

Renal arteriole immune-mediated damage: For example polyarteritis nodosa (PAN) and Wegener's granulomatosis.

Glomerular damage: For example hypertension, immune complex diseases, disseminated intravascular coagulation and haemolytic-uraemic syndrome. Glomerulonephritis is discussed in Chapter 66.

Hypertensive damage: This may be 'benign', with hyaline thickening of afferent arterioles and interlobular and interlobar arteries, and gradual sclerosis of affected glomeruli. The loss of multiple nephrons leaves the kidney shrunken and the whole cortical surface finely puckered.

The changes of malignant hypertension occur due to rapid proliferation of smooth muscle within the affected blood vessels; ischaemia also develops due to luminal narrowing. Swelling of the kidney occurs due to oedema, secondary to excessive leakage from damaged glomerular capillaries. This is often accompanied by petechial haemorrhages, which impart a 'flea bitten' appearance to the renal cortex. Renal failure may rapidly ensue.

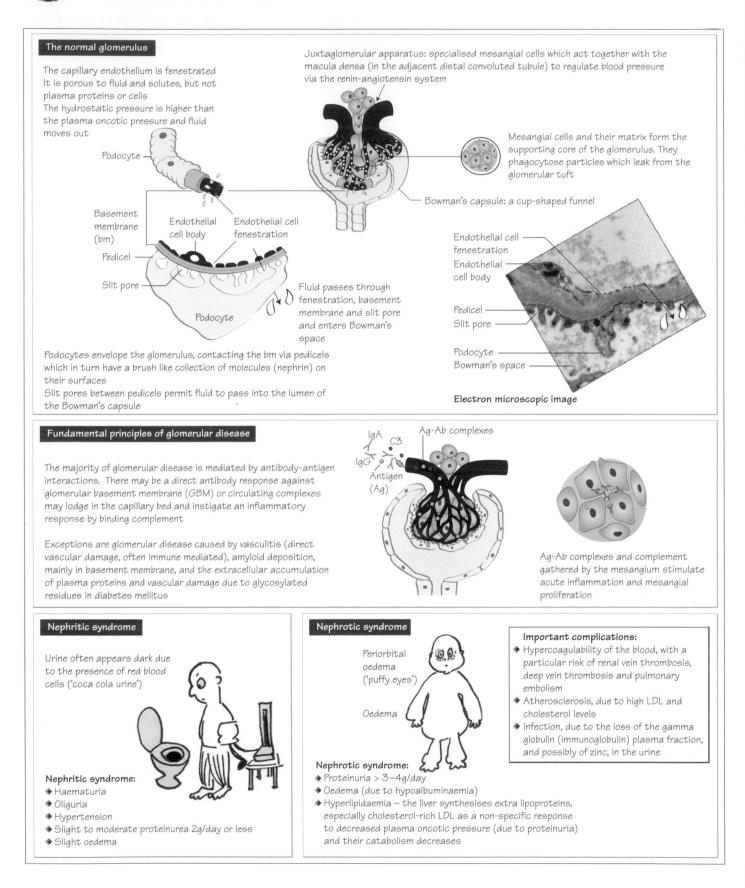

The normal glomerulus

The capillary endothelium is fenestrated
It is porous to fluid and solutes, but not plasma proteins or cells
The hydrostatic pressure is higher than the plasma oncotic pressure and fluid moves out

Podocyte

Basement membrane (bm)

Pedicel

Slit pore

Podocyte

Podocytes envelope the glomerulus, contacting the bm via pedicels which in turn have a brush like collection of molecules (nephrin) on their surfaces
Slit pores between pedicels permit fluid to pass into the lumen of the Bowman's capsule

Juxtaglomerular apparatus: specialised mesangial cells which act together with the macula densa (in the adjacent distal convoluted tubule) to regulate blood pressure via the renin-angiotensin system

Mesangial cells and their matrix form the supporting core of the glomerulus. They phagocytose particles which leak from the glomerular tuft

Bowman's capsule: a cup-shaped funnel

Endothelial cell body
Endothelial cell fenestration

Fluid passes through fenestration, basement membrane and slit pore and enters Bowman's space

Endothelial cell fenestration
Endothelial cell body

Pedicel
Slit pore

Podocyte
Bowman's space

Electron microscopic image

Fundamental principles of glomerular disease

The majority of glomerular disease is mediated by antibody-antigen interactions. There may be a direct antibody response against glomerular basement membrane (GBM) or circulating complexes may lodge in the capillary bed and instigate an inflammatory response by binding complement

Exceptions are glomerular disease caused by vasculitis (direct vascular damage, often immune mediated), amyloid deposition, mainly in basement membrane, and the extracellular accumulation of plasma proteins and vascular damage due to glycosylated residues in diabetes mellitus

IgA
IgG
C3
Antigen (Ag)
Ag-Ab complexes

Ag-Ab complexes and complement gathered by the mesangium stimulate acute inflammation and mesangial proliferation

Nephritic syndrome

Urine often appears dark due to the presence of red blood cells ('coca cola urine')

Nephritic syndrome:
◆ Haematuria
◆ Oliguria
◆ Hypertension
◆ Slight to moderate proteinurea 2g/day or less
◆ Slight oedema

Nephrotic syndrome

Periorbital oedema ('puffy eyes')

Oedema

Nephrotic syndrome:
◆ Proteinuria > 3–4g/day
◆ Oedema (due to hypoalbuminaemia)
◆ Hyperlipidaemia – the liver synthesises extra lipoproteins, especially cholesterol-rich LDL as a non-specific response to decreased plasma oncotic pressure (due to proteinuria) and their catabolism decreases

Important complications:
◆ Hypercoagulability of the blood, with a particular risk of renal vein thrombosis, deep vein thrombosis and pulmonary embolism
◆ Atherosclerosis, due to high LDL and cholesterol levels
◆ Infection, due to the loss of the gamma globulin (immunoglobulin) plasma fraction, and possibly of zinc, in the urine

Diseases of the glomeruli may be primary, in which the cause is unknown, or secondary to systemic disease. Although these are covered under the catch-all heading of glomerulonephritis, some diseases show no inflammatory component and are nowadays more commonly called nephropathy or glomerulosclerosis. If the glomerulus is destroyed by scar tissue the entire nephron (Bowman's capsule and tubular system) atrophies.

Clinical presentations vary and asymptomatic patients may be found to have haematuria, proteinuria or chronic renal failure when they have routine urine or blood tests. The most common presentations are:
• Asymptomatic haematuria – routine urine testing.
• Asymptomatic proteinuria – routine urine testing.
• Acute renal failure – presentation usually relates to an acute event that precipitates acute tubular necrosis.
• Chronic renal failure – this is often asymptomatic, but discovered on routine blood tests in a patient with heart disease, diabetes or other medical problems.
• Nephritic syndrome – described below.
• Nephrotic syndrome – described below.

Note that no test is technically 'routine'. Any time an investigation is undertaken, there should be a clear reason for performing it and an idea of how the information the investigation generates will affect the management of the patient.

Nephritic syndrome

This tends to occur in patients with proliferative glomerulonephritis – i.e. the underlying problem is caused by proliferation of the mesangium (as in immune complex diseases, like vasculitis, systemic lupus erythematosus (SLE) or IgA nephropathy), endothelium (e.g. post-infectious glomerulonephritis, the classic cause of the nephritic syndrome) or Bowman's capsule epithelium (crescentic glomerulonephritis). Mesangiocapillary glomerulonephritis can present with either nephritic or nephrotic syndrome, probably reflecting the multiplicity of underlying causes which may produce this pattern. The nephritic syndrome is also a presenting feature in malignant hypertension, which causes proliferation of smooth muscle and elastic in the arteriolar walls.

The presenting features are as follows:
• Haematuria: the urine often appears 'smoky' due to the presence of red blood cells.
• Oliguria.
• Hypertension.
• Slight to moderate proteinuria of 2 g/day or less.
• Mild oedema.

Nephrotic syndrome

This usually occurs in patients with non-proliferative glomerulonephritis. In order of likelihood these include: minimal change nephropathy, focal glomerular sclerosis, membranous nephropathy, amyloidosis, diabetes mellitus and lupus nephritis.

The presenting features are as follows:
• Proteinuria of >3–4 g/day (and consequent hypoalbuminaemia).
• Oedema (due to hypoalbuminaemia).
• Hyperlipidaemia: the liver synthesizes extra lipoproteins as a non-specific response to the decreased plasma oncotic pressure (due to proteinuria) and their catabolism decreases. There is a higher proportion of the cholesterol-rich low density lipoproteins (LDLs).

Important complications of the nephrotic syndrome are:

• Hypercoagulability of the blood, with a particular risk of renal vein thrombosis, deep vein thrombosis and pulmonary embolism. Three factors contribute to hypercoagulability:
  • Endothelial cell injury and activation (possibly partly due to increased LDL levels).
  • Increased tendency to platelet aggregation, which is normally antagonised by albumin (lost in urine).
  • An imbalance between antithrombotic proteins such as antithrombin, which are lost in the urine, and fibrinogen, whose synthesis by the liver is increased.
• Atherosclerosis, which is accelerated by the high LDLs and cholesterol levels.
• Infection, probably due to the loss of the immunoglobulins, and possibly zinc in the urine.

Secondary glomerulonephritis

Numerous causes of secondary glomerulonephritis exist. Examples include the following.

Systemic lupus erythematosus (SLE): This can produce virtually any pattern of glomerulonephritis and the subtypes of lupus nephritis are classified into five categories:
Type I: minimal change.
Type II: mesangial glomerulonephritis.
Type III: focal proliferative glomerulonephritis.
Type IV: diffuse proliferative glomerulonephritis. This is the commonest type (45–60%).
Type V: membranous nephropathy.
Types IV and V have the worse prognosis.

Systemic vasculitis: Systemic vasculitis is well placed to affect the renal arterioles, capillaries and venules and thereby induce glomerulonephritis. Fibrinoid necrosis of the vessels is typical and immunoglobulin and C3 deposition is seen.

Henoch–Schönlein purpura: Henoch–Schonlein purpura is a type III hypersensitivity disorder that is unusual in being mediated by IgA, rather than IgG. It is a form of vasculitis that tends to affect the skin, GI tract and kidney (in which there is glomerular IgA deposition and mesangial proliferation). Henoch–Schonlein purpura is more common in children and is often relatively mild and self-limiting.

Goodpasture's syndrome: This is a rare autoimmune disease in which there are circulating autoantibodies that are directed against the type IV collagen of the basement membrane of the alveoli of the lung and the renal glomeruli. The disease tends to occur in young males and most are positive for HLA-DR2.

The presentation is with haematuria and haemoptysis, possibly with other pulmonary symptoms. Prompt recognition and treatment is vital as the renal disease is rapidly progressive and usually of the crescentic glomerulonephritis type. If the renal damage reaches the stage at which oliguric renal failure develops, restoration of normal renal function is unlikely.

Others: Diabetes mellitus and amyloidosis.

The appearances of specific types of glomerulonephritis are discussed in Chapter 67.

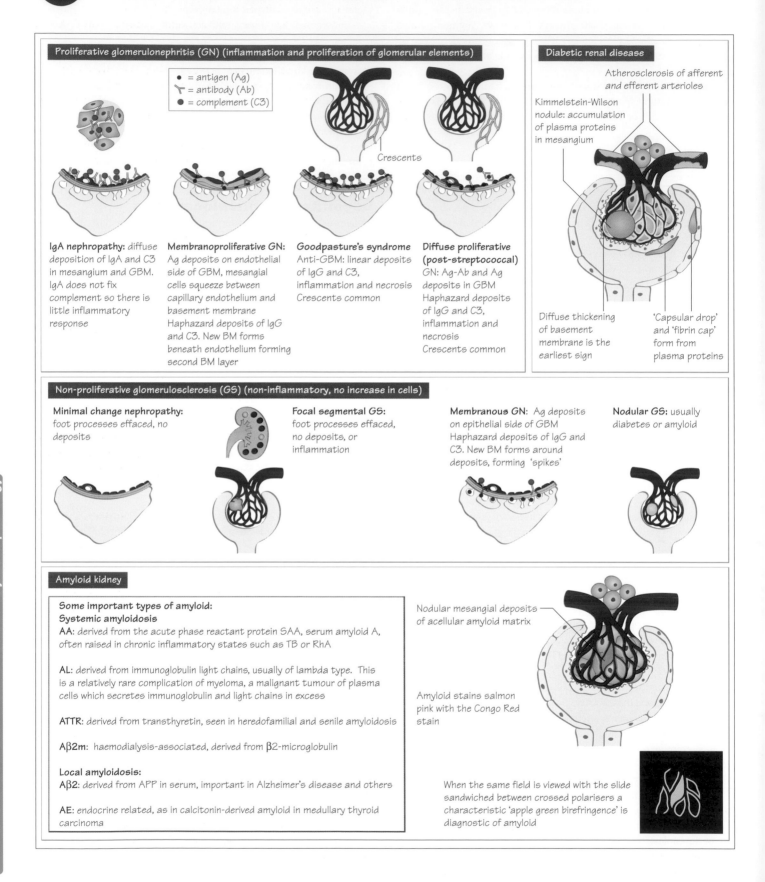

Proliferative glomerulonephritis (GN) (inflammation and proliferation of glomerular elements)

- = antigen (Ag)
- = antibody (Ab)
- = complement (C3)

Crescents

IgA nephropathy: diffuse deposition of IgA and C3 in mesangium and GBM. IgA does not fix complement so there is little inflammatory response

Membranoproliferative GN: Ag deposits on endothelial side of GBM, mesangial cells squeeze between capillary endothelium and basement membrane Haphazard deposits of IgG and C3. New BM forms beneath endothelium forming second BM layer

Goodpasture's syndrome Anti-GBM: linear deposits of IgG and C3, inflammation and necrosis Crescents common

Diffuse proliferative (post-streptococcal) GN: Ag-Ab and Ag deposits in GBM Haphazard deposits of IgG and C3, inflammation and necrosis Crescents common

Diabetic renal disease

Atherosclerosis of afferent and efferent arterioles

Kimmelstein-Wilson nodule: accumulation of plasma proteins in mesangium

Diffuse thickening of basement membrane is the earliest sign

'Capsular drop' and 'fibrin cap' form from plasma proteins

Non-proliferative glomerulosclerosis (GS) (non-inflammatory, no increase in cells)

Minimal change nephropathy: foot processes effaced, no deposits

Focal segmental GS: foot processes effaced, no deposits, or inflammation

Membranous GN: Ag deposits on epithelial side of GBM Haphazard deposits of IgG and C3. New BM forms around deposits, forming 'spikes'

Nodular GS: usually diabetes or amyloid

Amyloid kidney

Some important types of amyloid:
Systemic amyloidosis
AA: derived from the acute phase reactant protein SAA, serum amyloid A, often raised in chronic inflammatory states such as TB or RhA

AL: derived from immunoglobulin light chains, usually of lambda type. This is a relatively rare complication of myeloma, a malignant tumour of plasma cells which secretes immunoglobulin and light chains in excess

ATTR: derived from transthyretin, seen in heredofamilial and senile amyloidosis

Aβ2m: haemodialysis-associated, derived from β2-microglobulin

Local amyloidosis:
Aβ2: derived from APP in serum, important in Alzheimer's disease and others

AE: endocrine related, as in calcitonin-derived amyloid in medullary thyroid carcinoma

Nodular mesangial deposits of acellular amyloid matrix

Amyloid stains salmon pink with the Congo Red stain

When the same field is viewed with the slide sandwiched between crossed polarisers a characteristic 'apple green birefringence' is diagnostic of amyloid

Proliferative disease

Mesangial proliferation (mainly IgA nephropathy)

This is characterised by proliferation of mesangial cells – IgA and C3 are present here as clumpy deposits – but other, more variable, glomerular involvement is usually also seen. The aetiology is unknown. It is the commonest glomerulonephritis (GN) type in the Western world.

Membranoproliferative GN (mesangiocapillary GN)

Both the mesangial cells of the glomerular tuft and the basement membrane are affected. In most cases the underlying precise aetiology is unknown but the pathogenesis can be considered under three main headings:
• Thrombotic: chronic coagulative disorders, in which microthrombi form in small vessels (e.g. haemolytic-uraemic syndrome, thrombotic thrombocytopenic purpura).
• Immune disease (e.g. post-measles infection).
• Protein deposition (e.g. myeloma, amyloidosis, diabetes).

The classic lesion is the development of a double basement membrane ('tramline' pattern) due the presence of basement membrane on either side of immune complex deposits. These deposits are initially laid down on the endothelial side of the glomerular basement membrane, and are then covered by new GBM matrix secreted by endothelial cells.

A variant of mesangiocapillary GN features the nephritic factor – a circulating IgG autoantibody that is directed against the C3 convertase of the alternative pathway of the complement system. The nephritic factor/C3 convertase complex is more stable and generates excessive activated C3 (C3b).

Diffuse proliferative GN (post-streptococcal GN)

This may follow infection with a group A *Streptococcus* and develops more often after cutaneous than respiratory tract infections. It is thought that a streptococcal antigen may become trapped within the GBM, though alternative theories suggest a cross-reaction of antibodies against streptococcal antigens within the GBM. Hump-like deposits of IgG and C3 staining in the GBM are diagnostic in the correct clinical context.

Crescentic GN

Crescentic GN is a particular pattern of glomerular disease, which may be caused by many diseases. The eponymous crescents, so-called because of their shape, form when blood containing inflammatory cells leaks into the Bowman's space. Cytokines and growth factors secreted by inflammatory cells cause proliferation of the parietal epithelial cells lining the capsule and these, mixed with inflammatory cells and plasma proteins, enlarge and compress the glomerulus.

Glomerulonephritis in which at least 50% of the nephrons contain crescents is classified as crescentic GN (various percentage thresholds are given by different authorities). Clinically this is called rapidly progressive GN, and its identification is important as it indicates a swift decline in renal function unless the causative processes are counteracted.

The causes of crescentic GN can be divided into three groups:
1 Immune-pattern disease: there may be antibody/antigen complexes lodged in basement membrane (e.g. systemic lupus erythematosus (SLE), IgA nephropathy, post-streptococcal GN, membranoproliferative GN, and some drugs, such as penicillamine and bacterial endocarditis).
2 Pauci-immune disease (ANCA-associated disease): vasculitis.
3 Antiglomerular basement membrane disease (Goodpasture's syndrome).

Non-proliferative disease

Minimal change nephropathy

The podocytes are effaced, as shown on electron microscopy, and the protein loss is exclusively of albumin. No deposition of complexes, immunoglobulins or complement occurs. No changes are discernible by light microscopy. The aetiology is unknown. The prognosis is very good – about 90% recover after steroid treatment, particularly in childhood.

Focal segmental glomerulosclerosis

This tends to occur between 16 and 30 years and starts with proteinuria, soon presenting as nephrotic syndrome but also with haematuria. In many cases, hypertension is a later feature. The aetiology is unknown, though a subtype of this disease is known to occur in HIV. The prognosis is poor, renal failure is likely and the condition recurs in transplant patients.

The characteristic feature is sclerosis of the glomeruli, but in a pattern that displays only partial involvement of an affected glomerulus and involvement of only some glomeruli.

Membranous nephropathy

This accounts for one-third of adult GN. In 70% the aetiology is unknown, in others there may be circulating immune complexes to hepatitis B, syphilis, DNA (in SLE) or some drugs such as gold or penicillamine, and very occasionally to some tumours. Microscopy reveals a thickened basement membrane due to immune complex deposition and increased matrix secretion. Granular deposition of IgG and C3 along the basement membrane is typical. The prognosis is relatively poor in adults, though two-thirds of children resolve spontaneously.

Nodular glomerulosclerosis

This is the pattern typically seen in amyloidosis and diabetes mellitus. Nodular deposits are present in the mesangium and there is diffuse capillary basement membrane thickening.

Amyloidosis: Renal involvement is common in most types of amyloidosis and generally causes a nodular glomerulosclerosis. This produces progressive renal failure and death in 1–2 years. Presentation is with proteinuria or the nephrotic syndrome.

Diabetes: Thirty-five to 45% of type I and under 20% of type II diabetes mellitus patients develop renal disease. Death from renal failure occurs in 10% of diabetics. However, 50% of deaths in children with type I diabetes are due to renal failure.

While renal artery atheroma is often seen in diabetes (this site is otherwise rarely affected by atheroma), renal failure develops due to hyaline arteriolosclerosis secondary to hypertension. This causes ischaemic damage and the formation of advanced glycated end-products in the GBM and mesangium. These damage the GBM and mesangial proteins. Typical features of diabetic glomerulosclerosis are:
• GBM thickening due to deposition of advanced glycated end-products is the earliest lesion.
• Mesangial matrix expansion and later nodular change (Kimmelstein–Wilson lesion).
• The afferent and efferent arterioles typically show marked hyaline thickening, probably also due to advanced glycated end-products.
• The classic 'capsular drop' and 'fibrin cap' lesions in Bowman's capsule are thought to be due to insudation of plasma protein into epithelial cells.

Membranoproliferative GN (mesangiocapillary GN)

This occasionally presents with the nephrotic, rather than nephritic, syndrome.

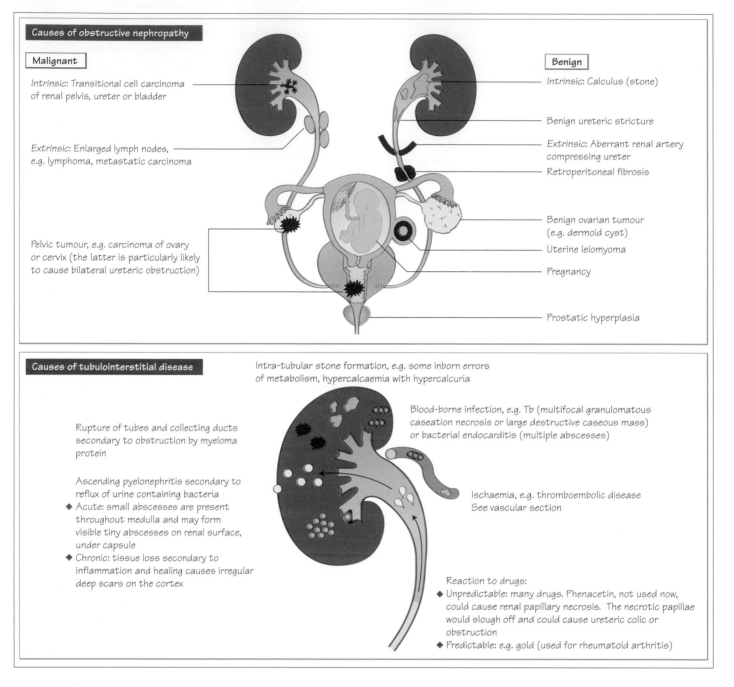

Causes of obstructive nephropathy

Malignant

Intrinsic: Transitional cell carcinoma of renal pelvis, ureter or bladder

Extrinsic: Enlarged lymph nodes, e.g. lymphoma, metastatic carcinoma

Pelvic tumour, e.g. carcinoma of ovary or cervix (the latter is particularly likely to cause bilateral ureteric obstruction)

Benign

Intrinsic: Calculus (stone)

Benign ureteric stricture

Extrinsic: Aberrant renal artery compressing ureter

Retroperitoneal fibrosis

Benign ovarian tumour (e.g. dermoid cyst)

Uterine leiomyoma

Pregnancy

Prostatic hyperplasia

Causes of tubulointerstitial disease

Intra-tubular stone formation, e.g. some inborn errors of metabolism, hypercalcaemia with hypercalcuria

Rupture of tubes and collecting ducts secondary to obstruction by myeloma protein

Ascending pyelonephritis secondary to reflux of urine containing bacteria
- Acute: small abscesses are present throughout medulla and may form visible tiny abscesses on renal surface, under capsule
- Chronic: tissue loss secondary to inflammation and healing causes irregular deep scars on the cortex

Blood-borne infection, e.g. Tb (multifocal granulomatous caseation necrosis or large destructive caseous mass) or bacterial endocarditis (multiple abscesses)

Ischaemia, e.g. thromboembolic disease See vascular section

Reaction to drugs:
- Unpredictable: many drugs. Phenacetin, not used now, could cause renal papillary necrosis. The necrotic papillae would slough off and could cause ureteric colic or obstruction
- Predictable: e.g. gold (used for rheumatoid arthritis)

There are many causes of inflammation in the tubules and interstitium (the supporting connective tissue of the kidney). The main conditions are:
- Acute tubular necrosis (ATN).
- Interstitial nephritis.
- Chronic interstitial nephritis, e.g. analgesic nephropathy.
- Metabolic disorders.
- Physical agents.
- Infection, e.g. pyelonephritis.

Acute tubular necrosis

The sudden death and sloughing off of renal tubular lining epithelium is a common sequel to shock with sustained hypoperfusion, or may be the result of direct toxic tubular damage.

Ischaemic ATN: This is commoner than toxic ATN and usually follows sudden hypovolaemia, as in severe haemorrhage, myocardial infarction or other shock, e.g. due to acute pancreatitis. It is also discussed in Chapter 17. Clinically the patient presents with oliguria or anuria and develops oedema due to failure of urine production – initially due to circulatory collapse and later because sloughed cells obstruct outflow.

Toxic ATN: Poisoning of tubular epithelium by mushrooms, drugs or suicide attempts with paraquat causes tubular necrosis, despite good glomerular blood flow. Myoglobin (which may follow severe crushing trauma) or haemoglobin (after lysis of erythrocytes, e.g. during parasite release in malaria) are also toxic to tubular epithelium.

Interstitial nephritis

Acute interstitial nephritis: This is characterised by a florid inflammatory reaction with oedema in the interstitium. Its rapid development after exposure to the causative agent means that the cause can often be identified and is usually a drug such as an NSAID or antibiotic (e.g. gentamicin, cephalosporins, cyclosporin A). However, it can also be a toxin (e.g. lead, gold, mercury) or due to an immune mechanism, either metabolic (e.g. urate), physical (e.g. obstruction) or neoplastic (e.g. myeloma). If the cause can be removed, the patient may recover completely.

Acute papillary necrosis, with sloughing of the renal papillae in both kidneys, is a severe complication seen particularly in diabetic patients with urinary tract infections (UTIs).

Chronic interstitial nephritis: The cause is often unascertainable and patients present in chronic renal failure, at a stage when the disease cannot be reversed. Chronic analgesic use is a well-recognised cause (analgesic nephropathy). This form of chronic interstitial nephritis occurs after long-term ingestion of analgesics, often combined drugs such as aspirin/phenacetin (seldom used in the UK), which synergise to cause toxic effects that lead to chronic renal papillary necrosis.

Aspirin causes papillary ischaemia and drug metabolites of phenacetin bind cellular proteins and deplete glutathione in cells. The patients have an increased risk of transitional cell carcinoma of the renal pelvis.

Metabolic disorders

Nephrocalcinosis: This occurs in patients with hypercalcaemia due to elevated urinary excretion of calcium. The urinary calcium can precipitate to form stones, usually in the renal pelvis or collecting ducts, or it may be taken up by and deposited in the renal tubules or interstitium, damaging intracellular organelles and impairing absorption.

Physical agents

Radiation: Damage presents as hypertension and renal failure.

Obstruction: For example malformation, tumour, prostatic hyperplasia and stones.

Immune-mediated disease

Vasculitis: For example polyarteritis nodosa (PAN).

Some types of glomerulonephritis: Some types of glomerulonephritis can be due to a direct immune attack on glomerular basement membrane or to circulating immune complexes lodging in the glomerular capillaries.

Infection

Urinary tract infections that involve the kidney produce pathological changes within the interstitium and/or tubules and may therefore be considered as a form of tubulointerstitial disease.

Acute pyelonephritis: Acute pyelonephritis is a bacterial infection of the kidney and is usually secondary to an infection in the lower part of the urinary tract ascending to the kidney. Thus it is seen in vesicoureteric reflux and also in obstructive uropathy. The typical causative organisms are *Escherichia coli*, *Proteus* and *Enterobacter*.

Vesicoureteric reflux is due to a congenital lack of the 'valve' effect achieved by the normal angle of entry of the ureters into the bladder, which closes the ureters during micturition. Patients with vesicoureteric reflux often also have refluxing renal papillae (which too lack the valve effect of the normal entry angle of the collecting ducts).

Tiny abscesses form in the collecting ducts and tubules in acute pyelonephritis and are visible as purulent pinpoints on the renal surface. The condition usually resolves with antibiotics, but the possible complications are renal papillary necrosis, pyonephrosis, perinephric abscess, scarring and chronic pyelonephritis.

Chronic pyelonephritis follows repeated episodes of acute pyelonephritis and displays irregular deep cortical scars on the renal surface, acute and chronic inflammation in the tubules and interstitium and deformation of the renal calyces.

Bladder infection (cystitis) is commoner in females due to their shorter urethra, to the extent that the presence of a UTI in a male should prompt a search for an underlying predisposing condition.

Other renal and urinary tract infections:
• **Bacterial**: e.g. bacterial endocarditis – which causes multiple small abscesses within the kidney.
• **Mycobacterial**: tuberculosis (miliary TB or site of secondary reactivation) may form miliary nodules (1 mm diameter) or a mass of caseous necrosis replacing the renal substance.
• **Viral**: e.g. cytomegalovirus (usually immunosuppressed patients). HIV glomerulopathy occurs before AIDS; HBV and HCV cause glomerulonephritis.
• **Fungal**: systemic candidiasis, e.g. in immunosuppression due to leukaemia.
• **Parasitic**: schistosomiasis, which is acquired via skin from water infected with *Schistosoma* larvae. *S. haematobium* homes to the bladder, causes haematuria and may ascend the urinary tract, causing scarring and granulomatous inflammation where the eggs are laid in the tissues.

Renal calculi

These affect 1–5% of the UK population (usually >30 years, with more males than females affected) and are commonest in the renal pelvis. If large, they may form a cast of the pelvis and renal calyces ('staghorn calculi'). Renal calculi form due to factors affecting the solubility of the constituents of the stone, such as the concentration of the solute and the urinary pH. The long-term presence of stones increases the risk of developing a transitional cell carcinoma.

Patients present with excruciating renal colic, aching in the loins and recurrent UTIs that fail to clear with antibiotic treatment. Ninety per cent of stones are radio-opaque and are visible on plain abdominal X-ray. The radiolucent stones are typically composed of urate, cystine or oxalic acid, without calcium.

There are different types of renal calculi:
• Calcium oxalate + calcium phosphate and uric acid (75–80%): 10% with calcium-containing stones have hyperparathyroidism or a defect in tubular reabsorption.
• 'Triple' stones (15%): magnesium ammonium phosphate (staghorn calculi) stones are radio-opaque. They may form after bacterial UTIs, e.g. with *Proteus*.
• Uric acid (6%).
• Stones in cystinuria or oxalosis (1%).

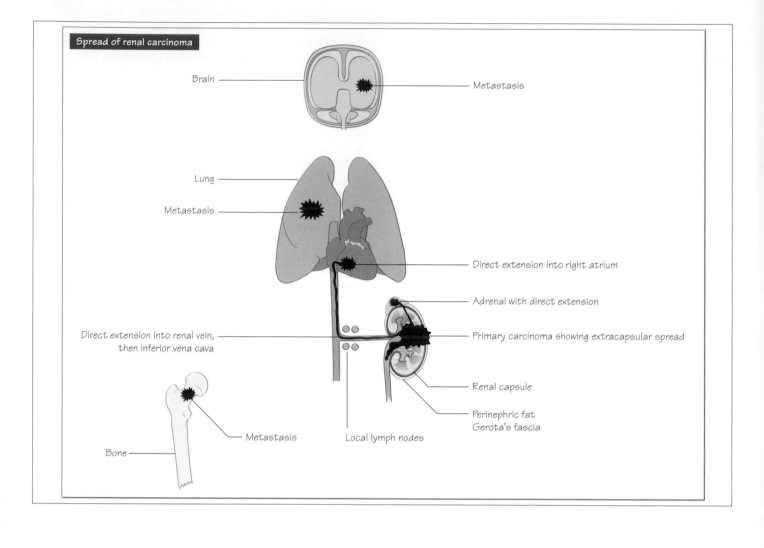

Spread of renal carcinoma

Brain — Metastasis

Lung —

Metastasis —

Direct extension into right atrium

Adrenal with direct extension

Direct extension into renal vein, then inferior vena cava

Primary carcinoma showing extracapsular spread

Renal capsule

Perinephric fat
Gerota's fascia

Metastasis

Local lymph nodes

Bone —

Systems pathology

Renal cell carcinoma

Definition
Renal cell carcinoma is a tumour that is derived from the epithelium of the proximal renal tubule.

Epidemiology
The incidence is four per 100 000 per year. The tumour is rare before 40 years and tends to present between the ages of 50 and 70 years. The male : female ratio is 2 : 1. The incidence is particularly high in Scandinavia and low in Japan.

Risk factors
- Smoking.
- Obesity.
- Cadmium.
- Coke-oven workers.
- Von Hippel–Lindau disease: 70% develop renal cell carcinoma by 60 years and the tumours are often multiple and bilateral.

Gross features
The tumour may be centred on any part of the kidney and is usually well demarcated. Compression of the adjacent renal parenchyma can give the impression of a capsule, although the tumour does not actually possess one. The cut surface is often variegated, with yellow, orange or brown regions, together with cystic change and/or haemorrhage.

Microscopic features
The majority of renal cell carcinomas are of the clear cell type and are composed of sheets of polyhedral cells that have abundant cytoplasm that is clear on staining with haematoxylin and eosin (H&E). The cells appear clear because their cytoplasm is rich in glycogen and lipid, neither of which stain with H&E. The accompanying stroma is composed of thin, fibrovascular septa.
- The papillary variant accounts for 10–15% of cases. The cells form papillary structures and have eosinophilic rather than clear cytoplasm.
- The chromophobe type occurs in 5% and features large cells with well-defined cell borders and granular cytoplasm.

Sarcomatoid change can coexist in renal cell carcinomas and is important as it indicates a worse prognosis.

Pattern of spread
Local invasion includes spread through the renal capsule into the surrounding perinephric fat and ultimately through Gerota's fascia. During this extension, the tumour may also invade the adrenal gland.

Renal cell carcinoma manifests the unusual behaviour of a tumour growing in direct extension along the major vein of the organ of origin, in this case the renal vein. The other tumour that shares this behaviour is hepatocellular carcinoma, which can grow along the hepatic vein. The direct extension of the tumour along the renal vein can be considerable, with the tumour possibly reaching the inferior vena cava and sometimes progressing into the right atrium.

The carcinoma can spread to local lymph nodes. Distant metastases are commonly to the lung and bone. The pulmonary metastases are often single and large and referred to as 'cannon-ball metastases'. The metastases of renal cell carcinoma are often highly vascular.

Staging
The TNM system is employed (see Chapter 28). The key parameters are the size of the primary, involvement of the renal vein and the degree of extension beyond the capsule.

Prognosis
The overall 5-year survival is 35–50%. Renal cell carcinoma is one of the malignancies that can characteristically recur after intervals of two decades or more.

Renal cell carcinoma idiosyncrasies
Renal cell carcinomas possess several properties that are unusual in comparison with other carcinomas:
- The grading system has four tiers rather than the usual three.
- Despite being malignant, the tumour is often well circumscribed and even appears to be encapsulated.
- The tumour can grow as macroscopically evident direct extension along major veins.
- Being disease free at 5 years does not necessarily mean cure due to the ability of the carcinoma to recur after much longer intervals.

Clinical correlations
In males, extension of a left-sided renal tumour along the left renal vein can obstruct the drainage of the left testicular vein, resulting in a left-sided varicocele. Therefore, a left-sided varicocele should warrant consideration of the state of the left renal vein.

Renal cell carcinomas can synthesise several hormones, with resultant paraneoplastic phenomena:
- Erythropoietin is normally produced by the kidney. Unregulated secretion by the tumour can cause secondary polycythaemia.
- Renin is another renally produced hormone. Tumour synthesis may result in secondary hypertension.
- Other hormones include parathyroid hormone-like substances, adrenocorticotrophic hormone, glucagon, prolactin and gonadotrophins.

Transitional cell carcinoma
Although transitional cell carcinomas are generally thought of as tumours of the bladder, they can also develop in the renal pelvis, ureter and urethra. Their presentation is typically with obstructive manifestations or haematuria.

Other tumours
Oncocytoma
This is a benign tumour that arises from the distal tubule. It tends to present around 60 years. The male : female ratio is 2 : 1.

Renal oncocytomas are circumscribed and encapsulated. Their cut surface is a homogenous brown, although larger tumours may exhibit a central stellate scar. The constituent cells possess abundant granular eosinophilic cytoplasm and can therefore resemble the cells of low grade chromophobe renal cell carcinoma.

Angioleiomyolipoma
An angioleiomyoma is a benign tumour that is composed of varying proportions of mature adipose tissue, smooth muscle and blood vessels. Approximately 75% of renal angioleiomyolipomas occur in the setting of tuberous sclerosis. The male : female ratio is 1 : 4.

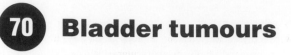

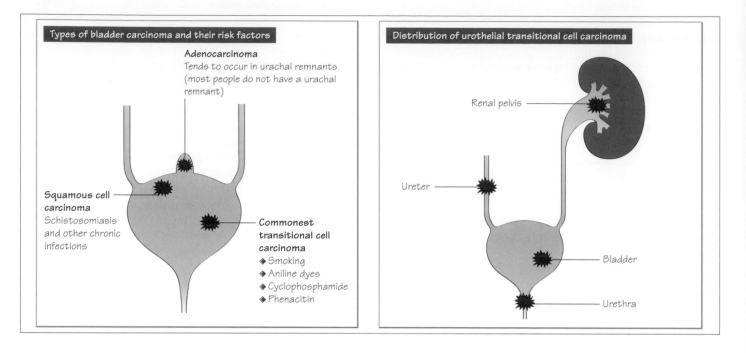

Types of bladder carcinoma and their risk factors

Adenocarcinoma
Tends to occur in urachal remnants (most people do not have a urachal remnant)

Squamous cell carcinoma
Schistosomiasis and other chronic infections

Commonest transitional cell carcinoma
◆ Smoking
◆ Aniline dyes
◆ Cyclophosphamide
◆ Phenacitin

Distribution of urothelial transitional cell carcinoma

Renal pelvis

Ureter

Bladder

Urethra

Systems pathology

Definition

Bladder cancer is a malignant tumour derived from the tissues of the urinary bladder.

Epidemiology

The incidence is 19 per 100 000 per year. The condition presents around 65 years and is rare before 50 years. The male : female ratio is 3 : 1. In general, the disease is one of industrialised countries, with the exception of regions that are endemic for *Schistosoma haematobium*.

Risk factors

• Aniline dyes that are employed in the rubber and cable industries are an important risk factor for transitional cell carcinoma of the bladder, with an increased risk of 20–60 times. Drugs such as cyclophosphamide and phenacetin have also been implicated. Smoking elevates the risk by 2–4 times.
• Urachal remnants are a risk factor for adenocarcinoma.
• Urinary schistosomiasis and other chronic bladder infections predispose to squamous cell carcinoma.

Pathology

Several subtypes are found. Transitional cell carcinoma accounts for 90%. Squamous cell carcinoma contributes 6%, adenocarcinoma 2% and the two sarcomas, rhabdomyosarcoma and leiomyosarcoma, 1% each. Small print rarities are also found.

Transitional cell carcinoma: Transitional cell carcinoma has a particular distribution within the bladder. The majority (70%) are located on the posterior and lateral walls. The trigone is affected in 20%, while the vault is relatively spared (10%).

Transitional cell carcinoma has three patterns of growth, each of which is associated with different macroscopic and cystoscopic appearances.

1 Transitional cell carcinoma in situ is confined to the epithelium. There is marked full-thickness cytological atypia, with the loss of the umbrella cells. This is seen as red patches. The cells have a tendency to be shed very easily from the mucosa, which contributes to the utility of urine cytology in diagnosis.

2 Papillary transitional cell carcinoma is present as variably sized cauliflower-like papillomatous projections from the mucosa of the bladder. The papillomas have a fibrovascular stroma and are covered by an abnormally thick layer of transitional cells that show mild to severe dysplasia. Frequently, there is no invasion of the stalk of the papillae, or only very superficial invasion, hence the good prognosis of papillary transitional cell carcinoma.

3 Fully invasive transitional cell carcinoma may have an overlying papillary component or may be an ulcer or a sessile plaque. However, regardless of the surface pattern, there is invasion of the muscularis propria of the bladder.

Adenocarcinoma: Adenocarcinoma is usually situated in a urachal remnant, although it can develop anywhere in the bladder.

Squamous cell carcinoma: This does not have a specific distribution.

Pattern of spread

The carcinoma initially invades into and through the muscularis propria of the bladder, then into the perivesical tissue from where it can enter the colon. In women, the uterus may be invaded, whereas the prostate can be infiltrated in men. The carcinoma does not cross the rectovesical pouch.

Distant metastases are to the lungs, brain, bone and liver.

Staging

The TNM system is used (see Chapter 28) and follows the model of depth of invasion through the various tissue planes of the primary organ.

Prognosis

Papillary tumours have an excellent 5-year survival. Despite being an *in situ* process, transitional carcinoma in situ has a surprisingly poor 5-year survival of only 30–40%. This reflects the fact that carcinoma in situ is a marker of generalised field change within the bladder and is a herald of a greatly increased tendency to develop a deeply invasive tumour.

The general 5-year survival is around 60%.

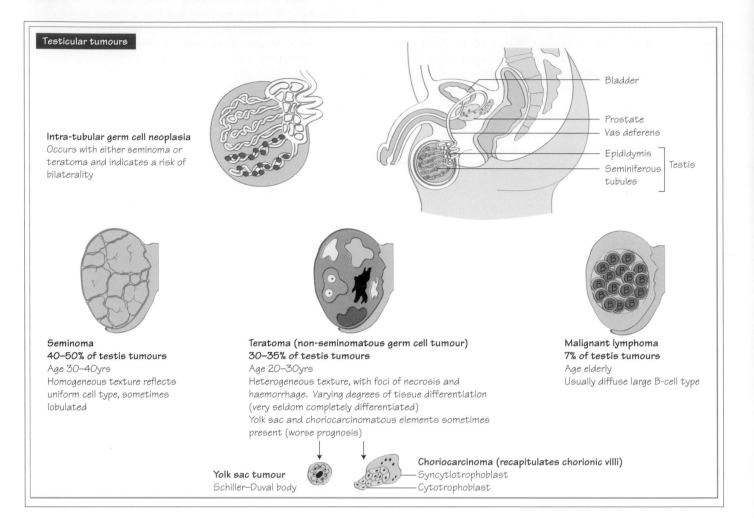

Testicular tumours

Intra-tubular germ cell neoplasia
Occurs with either seminoma or teratoma and indicates a risk of bilaterality

Bladder

Prostate
Vas deferens

Epididymis
Seminiferous tubules ⎤ Testis

Seminoma
40–50% of testis tumours
Age 30–40yrs
Homogeneous texture reflects uniform cell type, sometimes lobulated

Teratoma (non-seminomatous germ cell tumour)
30–35% of testis tumours
Age 20–30yrs
Heterogeneous texture, with foci of necrosis and haemorrhage. Varying degrees of tissue differentiation (very seldom completely differentiated)
Yolk sac and choriocarcinomatous elements sometimes present (worse prognosis)

Malignant lymphoma
7% of testis tumours
Age elderly
Usually diffuse large B-cell type

Yolk sac tumour
Schiller–Duval body

Choriocarcinoma (recapitulates chorionic villi)
Syncytiotrophoblast
Cytotrophoblast

Systems pathology

Definition

Testicular cancer comprises several malignant tumours which are derived from the tissues of the testis.

Epidemiology

The incidence is seven per 100 000 per year. Testicular cancer is the commonest malignant tumour in males aged 25–34 years. Presentation in general is usually between 20 and 40 years. The disease is rarer in men of African descent. There is an increased incidence in higher socioeconomic groups.

Risk factors

The main known risk factor is cryptorchidism, although this is implicated in only 10% of cases. The risk of cancer in an undescended testis is elevated by up to 40 times. This risk is reduced if orchidopexy is performed before the age of 8 years. In cases of unilateral maldescent, the normally descended testis is also at an elevated risk, albeit not as great as that of the maldescended testis. This implies a more complex problem in the development of the genitourinary system that has effects beyond simple mechanical descent.

Pathology

Most testicular tumours are derived from germ cells. These germ cell neoplasms are classified into seminomatous and non-seminomatous types.

Seminoma

This is a form of germ cell malignancy and accounts for 40–50% of testicular cancers. Its peak age is 30–40 years.

A seminoma is a well-defined, circumscribed mass that is usually unilateral. The tumour has a homogenous light grey cut surface that is often likened to a potato. Haemorrhage and necrosis are unusual and their presence should raise suspicions of a non-seminomatous component.

The tumour is formed by large cells that are derived from the seminiferous epithelium. The cells have abundant clear cytoplasm and a large, centrally positioned nucleus. The cells are arranged in aggregates that are separated by a delicate fibrovascular stroma in which abundant lymphocytes can feature. Scattered syncytiotrophoblast-like giant cells are found in 25% of cases and are responsible for a mildly elevated human chorionic gonadotrophin. However, in a pure seminoma, accompanying cytotrophoblast is not encountered. A granulomatous reaction may also be present.

Spermatocytic seminoma is an unusual variant (approximately 5%) that occurs in men over 65 years and features large, medium and small cells.

Non-seminomatous germ cell tumours (NSGCTs)

Historically, these tumours are regarded under the general term of teratoma, although pure mature teratoma of the testis is rare. Further confusion in the nomenclature arises from overlapping British and American systems and the fact that many NSGCTs feature more than one component subtype.

NSGCTs constitute 30–35% of testicular cancers and present approximately a decade earlier than seminomas.

Several different subtypes of tumour fall under the term of NSGCT. Tumours that are a mixture of two or more of these elements are more common that monotypic forms. Of all testicular tumours, combined immature teratoma and embryonal carcinoma accounts for 25%, with embryonal carcinoma in combination with seminoma comprising 15% and embryonal carcinoma plus immature teratoma plus seminoma constituting another 15%.

- The immature teratoma (malignant teratoma intermediate) features various types of tissue that are in immature stages of development.
- Embryonal carcinoma (malignant teratoma undifferentiated) is composed of sheets of large, pleomorphic, mitotically active, abnormal, primitive cells. Necrosis is common. It is frequently associated with an immature teratoma.

The two other patterns that can be found in an NSGCT are choriocarcinoma and yolk sac tumour. Neither of these tends to be present as the sole component of an NSGCT.

- Choriocarcinoma requires the presence of both syncytiotrophoblast and cytotrophoblast components and behaves in a highly malignant fashion.
- The pure form yolk sac tumour is the commonest childhood testicular neoplasm but in adults is found as part of a neoplasm that has several components. The tumour displays a myriad of growth patterns. A characteristic pattern is the Schiller–Duval body in which a blood vessel is lined by the tumour cells and is situated in a cystic space that is also lined by the tumour cells.

Unlike seminomas, NSCGTs are poorly demarcated, have a variegated cut surface and show haemorrhage and necrosis. Examination of these areas microscopically is important as they can contain the highest grade components.

Intratubular germ cell neoplasia

This is a precursor lesion that is associated with seminoma and NSGCTs but not spermatocytic seminoma. Abnormal germ cells are situated within the seminiferous tubules. The lesion can be found in the ipsilateral testis adjacent to a malignant tumour or in the contralateral testis.

Sex cord stromal tumours

Sex cord stromal tumours are uncommon and comprise only approximately 5% of testicular tumours. Their age range is broader than the germ cell tumours. The three main types are Sertoli cell tumour, Leydig cell tumour and granulosa cell tumour. Prediction of biological behaviour can be difficult, although Leydig cell tumours are almost always benign.

Lymphoma

Primary lymphoma of the testis is responsible for 7% of testicular tumours and tends to occur in older males aged 60–70 years. The most common type is diffuse large B cell lymphoma.

Pattern of spread

Malignant tumours initially invade the structures of the testis and are then resisted by the tunica albuginea such that invasion of the scrotum is rare. The tumour may permeate the spermatic cord. Lymphatic spread is to the para-aortic lymph nodes.

Seminomas show haematogenous dissemination late, whereas this process occurs early in NSCGTs. The lungs and liver are the main sites, with the brain, bone and skin also susceptible.

Prognosis

Seminomas have an excellent overall cure rate of over 90%. Stage 1 NSGCT has a 95% cure rate and, even with disseminated disease, the sensitivity of the tumour to chemotherapy yields long disease-free intervals.

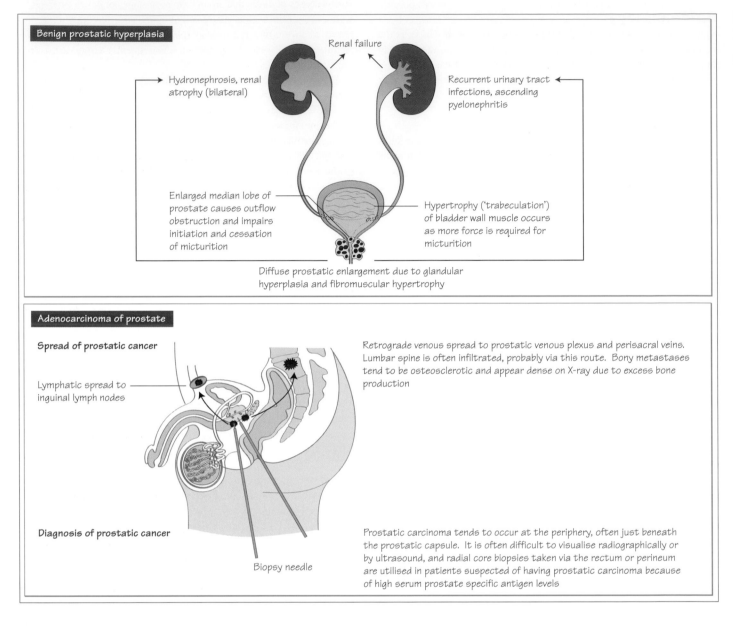

Benign prostatic hyperplasia

Renal failure

Hydronephrosis, renal atrophy (bilateral)

Recurrent urinary tract infections, ascending pyelonephritis

Enlarged median lobe of prostate causes outflow obstruction and impairs initiation and cessation of micturition

Hypertrophy ('trabeculation') of bladder wall muscle occurs as more force is required for micturition

Diffuse prostatic enlargement due to glandular hyperplasia and fibromuscular hypertrophy

Adenocarcinoma of prostate

Spread of prostatic cancer

Lymphatic spread to inguinal lymph nodes

Retrograde venous spread to prostatic venous plexus and perisacral veins. Lumbar spine is often infiltrated, probably via this route. Bony metastases tend to be osteosclerotic and appear dense on X-ray due to excess bone production

Diagnosis of prostatic cancer

Biopsy needle

Prostatic carcinoma tends to occur at the periphery, often just beneath the prostatic capsule. It is often difficult to visualise radiographically or by ultrasound, and radial core biopsies taken via the rectum or perineum are utilised in patients suspected of having prostatic carcinoma because of high serum prostate specific antigen levels

Systems pathology

Prostate cancer

Epidemiology

The incidence of prostate cancer is closely related to age, being rare under 50 years. The prevalence of the disease can reach considerable levels at older ages, with some autopsy studies suggesting that it is present in up to 40% or more males over 50 years.

Prostate cancer is rare in Japan and is more common in Afro-Caribbeans, with the incidences being three per 100 000 per year and 130 per 100 000 per year, respectively. The incidence in males in the UK is 95 per 100 000 per year.

Risk factors

Testosterone is the main factor that promotes the development of prostate cancer. The disease is rare in castrated men and those with cirrhosis.

There is an eight times increased risk in men who have a first degree relative who has breast cancer.

Pathology

The tumour can be difficult to discern macroscopically, with perhaps only 10% being clearly visible. This has implications for how a radical prostatectomy specimen is handled by a pathologist.

The tumours usually develop at the periphery of the gland, unlike benign prostatic hyperplasia which is a more central disease.

Prostatic cancers are almost always adenocarcinomas and in general have features that are common to adenocarcinomas in general. However, the grading is more complex than most adenocarcinomas and employs the Gleason method. Five patterns of prostatic adenocarcinoma are described in the Gleason system, with one equating to the most well-differentiated and five to the most poorly differentiated. If the carcinoma has two different patterns of growth a grade is assigned to each and these are added to yield the Gleason score, which ranges from 2 to 10. If only one pattern is found, the grade is doubled to give a score. Scores 2–4 are broadly equivalent to well differentiated, 5–7 to moderate (although 7 is prognostically discrete) and 8–10 to poorly differentiated.

Pattern of spread

Growth of the tumour within the gland may cause urethral obstruction. Local spread can also involve the rectum or bladder neck. Lymphatic spread is to local lymph nodes.

Retrograde venous spread reaches the lumbar spine but more widespread haematogenous dissemination also occurs and shows a predilection for the bones. The metastases are frequently osteosclerotic.

Staging

The TNM classification is used (see Chapter 28). Lower stages relate to the mechanism by which the tumour was discovered (transurethral resection of the prostate versus core biopsies), with progression through the structure of the prostate distinguishing the higher stages. Core biopsies from the periphery of the prostate are more likely to identify carcinoma at an early stage. If cancer is present in tissue reamed from the prostatic urethra it will be more advanced.

Prognosis

Despite being a malignant tumour, prostatic carcinoma can behave in a remarkably indolent fashion and even those with disseminated disease can have an unusually long survival for a stage 4 tumour. The overall 5-year survival is around 70–75%.

Screening

Despite the frequency of prostate cancer, a screening programme has yet to be developed. Prostate-specific antigen (PSA) levels are not particularly sensitive and while raised in many people with prostate cancer, they are often those with advanced disease. Furthermore, PSA can be elevated in benign enlargement of the prostate and in inflammation. In addition, the frequently good survival of patients with high stage prostatic carcinoma means that it is not clear what treatment should be offered to patients discovered by screening given that the most likely treatment, radical prostatectomy, has significant attendant morbidity, such as impotence and/or incontinence.

Benign prostatic hyperplasia

Definition

Benign prostatic hyperplasia is excessive growth of the prostatic glandular and fibromuscular tissue.

Epidemiology

The condition becomes more common with increasing age, reaching a prevalence of 75% or more in men over 80 years of age.

Pathogenesis

Testosterone is the basic underlying factor, but the precise mechanism by which the condition is produced is not known.

Pathology

In contrast to prostatic carcinoma, benign prostatic hyperplasia commences in the central portion of the gland in the periurethral tissue. The affected tissue has a firm consistency.

There is an increase in the glandular and stromal elements of the prostate. The relative proportion contributed by the two elements may vary between individuals or within an individual at different stages of the disease. The glands retain their arrangement in lobules and still have a basally located layer of myoepithelial cells but can have somewhat undulating luminal contours. Inspissated secretions form structures known as corpora amylacea.

Clinical correlations

The urethra is compressed, leading to difficulty in micturition and the symptoms of a poor stream and incomplete emptying. The increased resistance to the flow of urine causes hypertrophy of the bladder, which may develop a trabeculated surface. In severe cases, the pressure can dilate the ureters and even result in hydronephrosis.

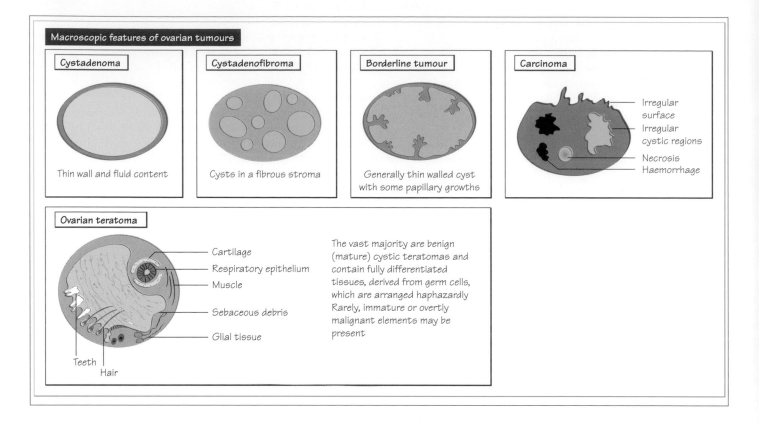

Macroscopic features of ovarian tumours

Cystadenoma
Thin wall and fluid content

Cystadenofibroma
Cysts in a fibrous stroma

Borderline tumour
Generally thin walled cyst with some papillary growths

Carcinoma
Irregular surface
Irregular cystic regions
Necrosis
Haemorrhage

Ovarian teratoma
Cartilage
Respiratory epithelium
Muscle
Sebaceous debris
Glial tissue
Teeth
Hair

The vast majority are benign (mature) cystic teratomas and contain fully differentiated tissues, derived from germ cells, which are arranged haphazardly Rarely, immature or overtly malignant elements may be present

General epidemiology

The incidence of ovarian cancer is 22 per 100 000 per year, with the tumours tending to present between 60 and 70 years. Malignant tumours develop at a later age than benign tumours. Ovarian cancer tends to be seen in industrialised countries, with the exception of Japan.

Epithelial tumours

Epithelial tumours account for the majority of ovarian tumours. There is debate as to the origin of the epithelium as the ovary does not intrinsically possess epithelium. One suggestion is that the epithelium is of peritoneal derivation.

The three main epithelial subtypes are serous, mucinous and endometrioid. Less common are transitional cell and clear cell.

Epithelial tumours may be benign, borderline or malignant (Table 73.1). The borderline category encompasses tumours that have properties intermediate between those of straightforward benign and malignant tumours and is of most relevance in serous and mucinous tumours. The other epithelial variants tend not to yield tumours in this category. There are usually relatively subtle architectural and cytological changes at the microscopic level, although fully developed malignant changes are still not manifested. The prognosis of borderline tumours is very good.

Cystadenoma

A cystadenoma is the typical benign tumour of the serous and mucinous subtypes. It forms a mass that can range from small to huge. Serous

tumours contain thin, clear fluid, while mucinous tumours feature thick, tenacious material.

The wall of the cyst is thin and while the cyst can be unilocular or multilocular, both its external and internal surfaces are smooth. Serous tumours in particular may resemble a water balloon.

A cystadenofibroma shows abundant fibrous tissue within the wall of the cyst and adenofibromas demonstrate predominantly fibrous tissue in which there are small glandular structures formed by bland cells.

Brenner tumour

Brenner tumour is the eponym for the benign variant of the ovarian transitional cell tumour. The cells resemble those of normal urothelium. One-third of Brenner tumours are only discovered on microscopic examination of an ovary. In one-quarter of cases there is another ovarian tumour associated with the Brenner tumour; in two-thirds this is of mucinous type.

Borderline tumours

Reliable distinction is not possible macroscopically, but suspicion can be raised by tumours that have small papillary formations on their internal surface. Microscopic attention must focus diligently on these regions as borderline changes can be focal.

Malignant tumours

All five types contribute malignant variants, with the endometrioid and clear cell types tending only to have malignant tumours.

Table 73.1 Comparison of aspects of ovarian epithelial tumours

	Proportion of ovarian tumours	Benign	Borderline	Malignant
Serous	30%	60%	10%	30%
Mucinous	15%	75%	10%	15%
Endometrioid	2–4%	Rare	Rare	Most
Transitional	1–2%	90%	5%	5%
Clear cell	2%	Rare	Rare	Most

The tumours are usually large and can be partially cystic. However, the partially cystic tumours will include a significant proportion of a solid component. The solid element of the tumour has a variegated cut surface in which regions of haemorrhage and necrosis are frequent. The capsule of the ovary may be breached by the tumour, leaving an irregular surface.

Mucinous tumours are distinguished microscopically by the presence of mucin vacuoles within the cells. Endometrioid tumours appear similar to endometrial endometrioid adenocarcinoma. Serous tumours comprise columnar cells, often arranged in papillae that feature laminated calcified formations known as Psammoma bodies.

Germ cell tumours
Teratomas
Approximately 90% of ovarian teratomas are benign (mature) and consist of fully differentiated tissues. This contrasts with testicular teratomas, which are almost always malignant (immature).

The mature teratoma is also known as a dermoid cyst and contains tissue from all three embryonal layers. It is the most common ovarian tumour between 18 and 30 years and accounts for 20–50% of ovarian tumours.

The tumour is a cystic mass that is frequently filled with malodorous, soft yellow material that is the result of accumulation of the keratin and sebaceous secretions produced by the skin – a frequent component of tumour. Hair is also a common constituent. The wall is usually thin, but can include teeth.

Struma ovarii is a variant of a mature teratoma in which the teratoma is formed only by thyroid follicles. These can be active and produce hyperthyroidism.

Immature teratomas are much rarer in the ovary and tend to occur under 20 years. They contain immature tissue, frequently neural.

Dysgerminoma
This is analogous to seminoma of the testis. Although the commonest ovarian malignant germ cell tumour (the others being yolk sac tumour, choriocarcinoma and embryonal carcinoma), it constitutes only 1% of all ovarian cancers, but 20–30% of those encountered during pregnancy. Most develop in the second and third decades.

Sex cord and stromal tumours
These tumours are derived from the various stromal and oocyte supporting elements of the ovary and are a diverse group. A detailed discussion of the various subtypes is not possible within this book, but the main basic aspects are that the tumours are rare, account for a small minority of all ovarian neoplasms and that it can be difficult to predict their biological behaviour from conventional histological parameters.

The types include
- Adult granulosa cell.
- Juvenile granulosa cell.
- Fibroma – benign.
- Thecoma – benign.
- Sertoli cell.
- Leydig cell.
- Sertoli–Leydig cell.
- Mixed variants.

Secondary neoplasms
The ovary can also demonstrate metastatic deposits. The classic example is the Krukenberg tumour in which there is transcoelomic spread of a gastric adenocarcinoma, usually of signet ring cell type, across the peritoneal cavity, to the ovary. Confusion can exist in this case with a primary ovarian clear cell carcinoma.

Secondary tumours tend to involve the surface of the ovary, with less penetration into the underlying stroma. Primary tumours often have more bulky parenchymal disease. Bilateral deposits suggest a secondary tumour, but primary ovarian tumours may either be bilateral, or show contralateral metastases.

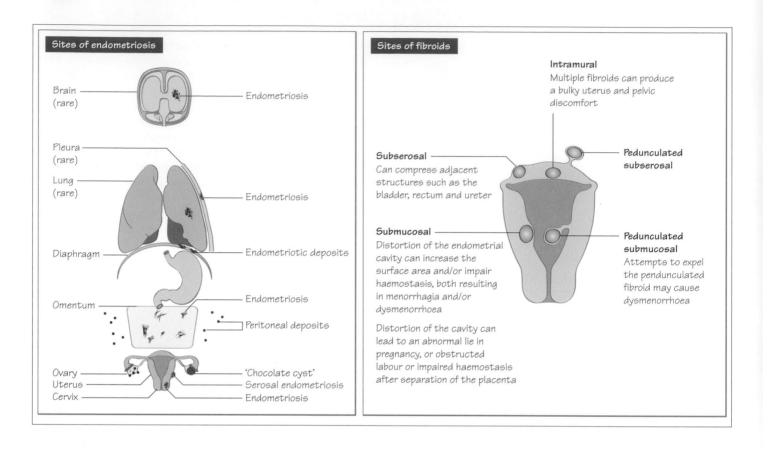

Sites of endometriosis

Brain (rare) —— Endometriosis

Pleura (rare)

Lung (rare) —— Endometriosis

Diaphragm —— Endometriotic deposits

Omentum —— Endometriosis

—— Peritoneal deposits

Ovary —— 'Chocolate cyst'
Uterus —— Serosal endometriosis
Cervix —— Endometriosis

Sites of fibroids

Intramural
Multiple fibroids can produce a bulky uterus and pelvic discomfort

Subserosal
Can compress adjacent structures such as the bladder, rectum and ureter

Pedunculated subserosal

Submucosal
Distortion of the endometrial cavity can increase the surface area and/or impair haemostasis, both resulting in menorrhagia and/or dysmenorrhoea

Distortion of the cavity can lead to an abnormal lie in pregnancy, or obstructed labour or impaired haemostasis after separation of the placenta

Pedunculated submucosal
Attempts to expel the pendunculated fibroid may cause dysmenorrhoea

Fibroids
Definition
Fibroids are benign smooth muscle tumours (leiomyomas) of the uterus.

Epidemiology
Fibroids affect approximately 5% of women, although they may be asymptomatic in two-thirds of cases. The tumours are oestrogen dependent and are more common with increasing age within the reproductive years. Fibroids are more common in non-Caucasians.

Pathology
Fibroids can be classified depending on their location into submucosal, intramural and subserosal. Any combination of these types can coexist in the same uterus. The serosal type can become pedunculated and, in rare circumstances, may attach to adjacent tissue, such as the broad ligament, loose their peduncle and be referred to as a parasitic leiomyoma.

Myometrial leiomyomas are circumscribed tumours that can range in size from under a millimetre to many centimetres across. They typically have a whorled, light grey, cut surface. Larger and older fibroids may show calcification, hyalinisation or even cystic change.

Microscopically, fibroids are composed of interlacing fascicles of smooth muscle cells. These are spindle-shaped cells that lack atypical features.

Red degeneration is a particular complication of pregnancy in which a fibroid undergoes infarction.

Complications
• Distortion of the endometrial cavity can produce menorrhagia, in part by increasing the surface area of the endometrium. Dysmenorrhoea can occur.
• Pressure of a fibroid on the bladder or rectum can cause symptoms of frequency or obstruction.
• Obstetric complications usually reflect the mechanical effects of the fibroid in relation to the shared space with the foetus and include infertility, spontaneous abortion, premature labour, malpresentation and post-partum haemorrhage.

Adenomyosis
Definition
Adenomyosis is the presence of endometrial tissue within the myometrium.

Pathology
Both endometrial glands and stroma are found misplaced within the myometrium and they remain responsive to oestrogen and progesterone and, while they can show endometrial cycling, they are often of the basal type and are relatively inactive.

The degree of adenomyosis can vary greatly, in some cases being very focal and an incidental finding in a uterus removed for another reason; while at the opposite end of the spectrum there can be diffuse adenomyosis which occupies most of the myometrium. Established cases have a large, bulky uterus, the cut surface of which can feel boggy.

Complications

Adenomyosis may be asymptomatic, but can cause dysmenorrhoea or menorrhagia.

Endometriosis

Definition

Endometriosis is the presence of endometrial tissue in a site distant from the uterus.

Epidemiology

Endometriosis is present in around 5% of women, but this figure rises to 30–40% of those who are subfertile.

Pathogenesis

Many of the sites affected by endometriosis can be explained by retrograde menstruation in which shed endometrium enters the pelvis and abdomen via the fallopian tubes. However, this process does not explain some of the more distant sites, nor why only some women are affected. More complex theories involve impaired immune responses.

Pathology

A wide variety of locations may exhibit endometriosis. Common sites include the fallopian tubes, the ovaries, broad ligament, pouch of Douglas, bowel, peritoneum and omentum. Distant sites include the pleura and even the brain. Laparotomy and laparoscopy scars are also recognised sites.

Endometriosis is typically described as small blue nodules, but can produce larger lesions. Fibrous adhesions may develop in association with deposits of endometriosis.

Ovarian endometriosis has a tendency to be cystic. The cyst is lined by the endometriotic tissue and repeated episodes of haemorrhage cause altered blood to accumulate within the cystic cavity. The term chocolate cyst is employed to describe this appearance.

Foci of endometriosis initially contain both endometrial glands and stroma. However, as older lesions can show loss of one or other of these components, the diagnosis can be made if at least any two of endometrial glands, endometrial stroma or evidence of haemorrhage are present. The last criterion is permitted because the endometriotic foci remain hormonally responsive and therefore follow the changes of the menstrual cycle. This process of repeated haemorrhage can lead to fibrosis as well as explaining some of the painful aspects of endometriosis.

Complications

Endometriosis is found in 30–40% of women who have reduced fertility. The exact mechanism that links the two entities is uncertain. In some women, fibrosis around the fallopian tubes and ovaries may disrupt release of the oocyte and its progression along the fallopian tube, but assorted other variables are likely to be involved.

While dysmenorrhoea is a common symptom of endometriosis, the location of the disease outside the endometrium and myometrium means that menorrhagia is not a feature.

The pelvic fibrosis that can accompany endometriosis may tether the ovaries close to the vaginal fornices, leading to dyspareunia. The uterus can also be fixed in an unusual position. Deposits of endometriosis on other organs can also produce symptoms, some relating to micturition or defaecation.

Salpingitis

Salpingitis is inflammation of the fallopian tube and may be acute or chronic. Acute salpingitis occurs in sexually transmitted diseases such as gonorrhoea and chlamydia. The pathological changes are those of the acute inflammatory process. Chronic salpingitis follows suboptimal resolution of acute salpingitis. The fallopian tube is distended and partially obstructed, leading to accumulation of fluid (hydrosalpinx). Scattered plasma cells are present within the wall of the fallopian tube. Progression of acute salpingitis to chronic salpingitis can therefore lead to reduced fertility.

Tuberculosis may also produce a salpingitis.

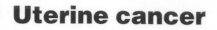

Uterine cancer

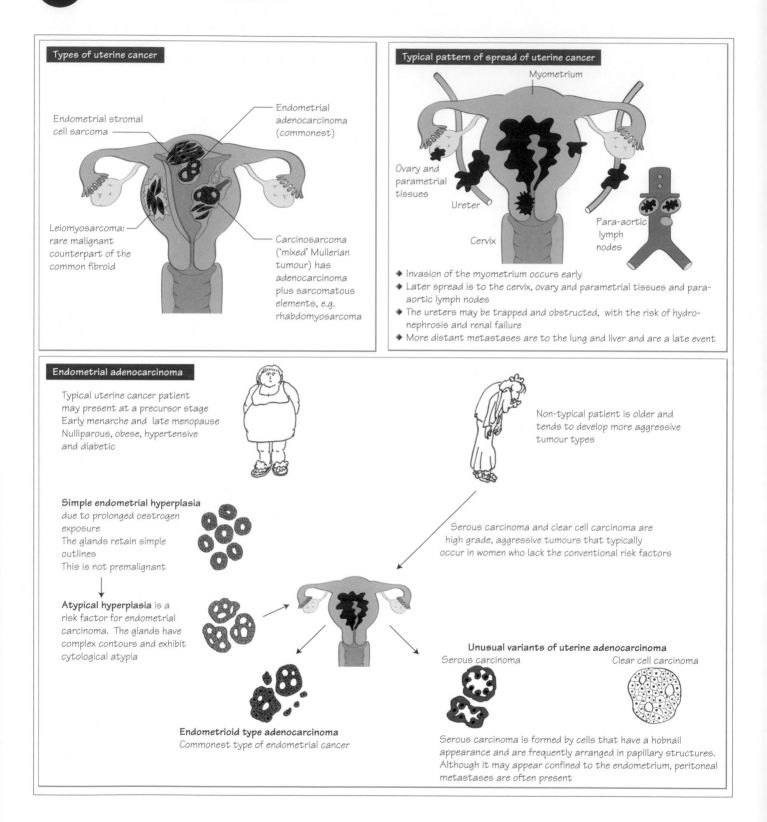

Types of uterine cancer

Endometrial stromal cell sarcoma

Endometrial adenocarcinoma (commonest)

Leiomyosarcoma: rare malignant counterpart of the common fibroid

Carcinosarcoma ('mixed' Mullerian tumour) has adenocarcinoma plus sarcomatous elements, e.g. rhabdomyosarcoma

Typical pattern of spread of uterine cancer

Myometrium

Ovary and parametrial tissues

Ureter

Cervix

Para-aortic lymph nodes

◆ Invasion of the myometrium occurs early
◆ Later spread is to the cervix, ovary and parametrial tissues and para-aortic lymph nodes
◆ The ureters may be trapped and obstructed, with the risk of hydronephrosis and renal failure
◆ More distant metastases are to the lung and liver and are a late event

Endometrial adenocarcinoma

Typical uterine cancer patient may present at a precursor stage Early menarche and late menopause Nulliparous, obese, hypertensive and diabetic

Non-typical patient is older and tends to develop more aggressive tumour types

Simple endometrial hyperplasia due to prolonged oestrogen exposure
The glands retain simple outlines
This is not premalignant

Serous carcinoma and clear cell carcinoma are high grade, aggressive tumours that typically occur in women who lack the conventional risk factors

Atypical hyperplasia is a risk factor for endometrial carcinoma. The glands have complex contours and exhibit cytological atypia

Unusual variants of uterine adenocarcinoma

Serous carcinoma

Clear cell carcinoma

Endometrioid type adenocarcinoma
Commonest type of endometrial cancer

Serous carcinoma is formed by cells that have a hobnail appearance and are frequently arranged in papillary structures. Although it may appear confined to the endometrium, peritoneal metastases are often present

Systems pathology

 Pathology at a Glance. By C.J. Finlayson and B.A.T. Newell. Published 2009 by Blackwell Publishing. ISBN: 978-1-4051-3650-1

Endometrial carcinoma

Definition
Endometrial carcinoma is a malignant tumour of the endometrial epithelium.

Epidemiology
The incidence is 20 per 100 000 per year. The disease tends to affect post-menopausal women. The highest incidence is in the USA and the lowest is in Japan.

Risk factors
Two distinct groups of women develop endometrial cancer. One comprises the traditional cohort of women who had an early menarche, late menopause, are nulliparous, obese, hypertensive and diabetic. In this group, the underlying process is one of oestrogenic stimulation of the uterus. The other group, which has more recently been defined, lacks these risk factors and is composed of older women who tend to have more aggressive subtypes of endometrial carcinoma.

Precursor lesion
The precursor lesion of endometrial hyperplasia is found in the group of women whose carcinoma is related to oestrogen exposure. In endometrial hyperplasia the mass of the endometrium is increased. It can result from prolonged oestrogen exposure. In simple endometrial hyperplasia, the quantity of endometrium is increased but the glands retain simple outlines and lack abnormal cytological features. Simple hyperplasia without atypia is not pre-malignant. By contrast, atypical hyperplasia is a risk factor for endometrial carcinoma. The glands possess complex contours and exhibit cytological atypia. (Note that architecturally simple hyperplasia may rarely display cytological atypia and this is then considered as atypical hyperplasia.)

Pathology
Several subtypes of endometrial carcinoma exist. The majority of cases are endometrioid adenocarcinomas and are the type encountered in women who have the traditional risk factors given above.

The carcinoma may be a nodule, plaque or polypoid mass that fills and distorts the uterine cavity. Ulceration, haemorrhage and necrosis may be seen. Invasion of the myometrium is frequently discernible macroscopically.

The tumour is composed of glands that resemble those of the endometrium. This distinction becomes important when considering some of the other variants. The proportion of the tumour that forms glands as opposed to solid sheets is critical in grading. The higher the proportion of sheets, the higher the grade.

Whereas invasion of the myometrium occurs early, further spread is a later event, possibly because the myometrium acts as a delaying barrier. However, the carcinoma eventually spreads to the parametrial tissues and para-aortic lymph nodes. More distant metastases are to the lung and liver and are a late event.

Serous carcinoma and clear cell carcinoma are high grade, aggressive tumours that are found in the second group of women (those who lack the conventional risk factors). Serous carcinoma is formed by cells that have a hobnail appearance and are frequently arranged in papillary structures. The carcinoma may frequently appear to involve only the endometrium, with minimal myometrial invasion, but nevertheless tends to be associated with widespread peritoneal metastases at the time of presentation. Clear cell carcinomas have a variety of growth patterns.

Staging
The TNM classification is employed (see Chapter 28). The depth of myometrial invasion is the key parameter for separating the early stages, with progressive involvement of other pelvic organs defining the higher stages.

Prognosis
Endometrioid adenocarcinoma tends to present as stage 1, in which the 5-year survival can be in the region of 90%. Serous and clear cell carcinomas have a much worse prognosis. The general 5-year survival is around 75%.

Carcinosarcoma
Carcinosarcoma is a rare tumour of the uterus that is also known as mixed Mullerian malignant tumour. It is an aggressive cancer that shows both malignant epithelial and malignant mesenchymal elements. The mesenchymal elements can either be homologous and derived from tissue found in the uterus, such as leiomyosarcoma, or be heterologous, such as chondrosarcoma. Metastases tend to be formed of the epithelial elements only.

Leiomyosarcoma
Leiomyosarcoma encompasses only 1–2% of uterine malignant tumours and tends to present around 50 years.

The tumour is large and usually solitary. Regions of haemorrhage and necrosis may be evident macroscopically. The presence of necrosis of tumour cells is a crucial diagnostic feature microscopically. The tumour cells also have a high level of mitotic activity and exhibit nuclear abnormalities.

Endometrial stromal sarcoma
The stroma of the endometrium can form tumours, although these are much rarer than their epithelial counterparts.

Changes in terminology have occurred recently and the division into high and low grade variants has been abandoned. Tumours designated as endometrial stromal sarcomas now tend all to be low grade entities, with the higher grade variants reclassified into a more general sarcoma category.

The cells of endometrial stromal sarcoma resemble normal endometrial stroma and nuclear atypia can be very limited. A rich network of small blood vessels within the tumour can be a useful clue to the diagnosis but the crucial parameter is invasion of the myometrium and an irregular border to the tumour. This border is critical as it is essential in distinguishing the sarcoma from the benign alternative of endometrial stromal nodule.

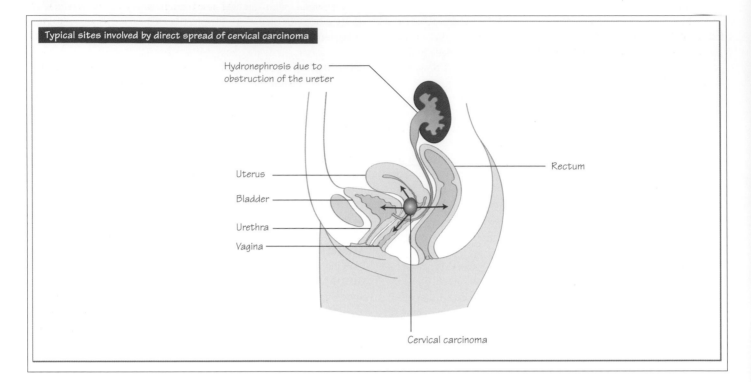

Typical sites involved by direct spread of cervical carcinoma

Hydronephrosis due to obstruction of the ureter

Uterus

Bladder

Urethra

Vagina

Rectum

Cervical carcinoma

Systems pathology

Definition

Cervical cancer is a malignant tumour of the cervix of the uterus.

Epidemiology

The incidence is 10 per 100 000 per year and the disease causes approximately 2000 deaths per year in the United Kingdom. Presentation is usually between the ages of 30 and 50 years.

Risk factors

The most important risk factor is the human papilloma virus (HPV), specifically the high risk subtypes 16, 18, 31 and 33. Acquisition and persistence of these subtypes is an integral aspect of the development of cervical squamous cell carcinomas. Most of the other risk factors below operate by increasing this exposure:

- Early age at first intercourse.
- Frequency of intercourse.
- Multiple sexual partners.
- Smoking.

Precursor lesions

The cervical screening programme is based on the existence of an identifiable precursor lesion for cervical carcinoma, cervical intraepithelial neoplasia (CIN). CIN is a disordered proliferation of the cervical epithelium, in the absence of invasion of the subepithelial tissues. It is divided into three grades 1 to 3, which correlate with mild, moderate and severe dysplasia. In basic terms, as the grade increases, the proportion of the epithelium that is occupied by cells that fail to mature increases and the degree of cytological atypia rises. The latter of these features permits the grades of CIN to be predicted by cervical cytology, in which only the cytological characteristics of the cells, not the architecture, are apparent.

As a consequence of the screening programme, the incidence of squamous cell carcinoma of the cervix has fallen, while that of CIN has increased, as would be expected by shifting the time of diagnosis to an early stage of the disease.

Note that the progression of CIN to invasive cervical carcinoma is not inevitable. CIN may regress, especially low grade CIN and even CIN 3 does not automatically evolve into invasive carcinoma.

Pathology

Cervical cancers are almost always carcinomas. At least 70% are squamous cell carcinomas, with adenocarcinomas accounting for most of the remainder. Although the HPV risk factor was initially described for squamous cell carcinoma, around 90% of cervical adenocarcinomas are also positive for HPV.

Squamous cell carcinomas arise from the transformation zone, which is the junctional region between the glandular epithelium of the endocervix and the squamous epithelium of the ectocervix. This location is visible on colposcopic examination and in established cases the tumour is visible as a polypoid or friable mass. However, since the advent of the screening programme, many cervical cancers are detected at a much earlier stage, in which they produce more subtle lesions at colposcopy.

The histology of squamous cell carcinoma is that of a standard squamous cell carcinoma.

Adenocarcinomas tend to develop within the endocervical canal. This means that they are often not visible at colposcopy and can therefore be more difficult to recognise. A precursor lesion is described, cervical glandular intraepithelial neoplasia. Although the screening programme was not designed to address cervical adenocarcinoma, in part because the bulk of the glandular tissue is further up the cervical canal than that intended to be sampled by a screening smear, glandular abnormalities can nevertheless be detected.

Pattern of spread

The initial spread is locally, with extension first to the vagina and uterus, then to the pelvic side wall and the other pelvic organs, particularly the bladder and rectum. Local spread can also cause obstruction to one or both ureters, causing hydronephrosis.

Distant spread can involve the lungs.

Staging

The TNM system is employed (see Chapter 28). The later stages are determined by the degree of local spread given above. Stage 1 is divided and subdivided depending upon the dimensions of the tumour. These measurements are often derived from long loop excisions of the transformation zone (LLETZs) and can be compromised if a LLETZ specimen is submitted as multiple pieces.

Prognosis

The prognosis tends to follow the stage, with stage 1 disease having a better than 80% 5-year survival rate. The prognosis is worse for adenocarcinoma, or for those patients aged under 40 years. Pilot studies indicate that HPV vaccination will protect most recipients against the development of both squamous and adenocarcinoma of the cervix.

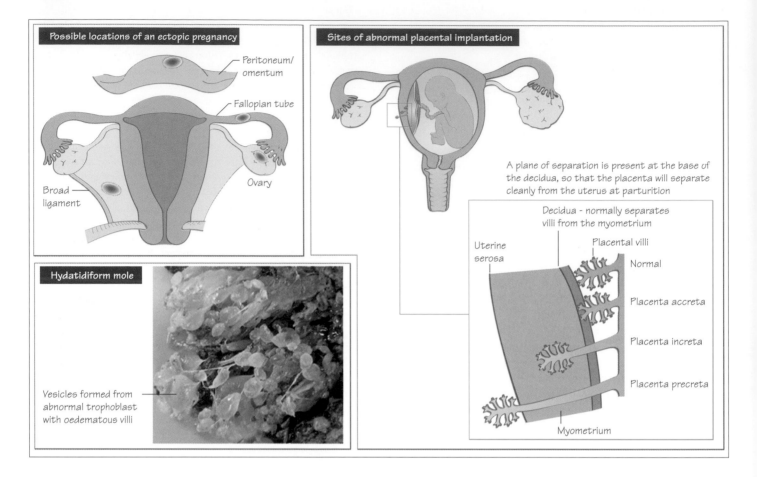

Possible locations of an ectopic pregnancy

Peritoneum/omentum

Fallopian tube

Ovary

Broad ligament

Sites of abnormal placental implantation

A plane of separation is present at the base of the decidua, so that the placenta will separate cleanly from the uterus at parturition

Decidua - normally separates villi from the myometrium

Placental villi

Uterine serosa

Normal

Placenta accreta

Placenta increta

Placenta precreta

Myometrium

Hydatidiform mole

Vesicles formed from abnormal trophoblast with oedematous villi

Complete hydatidiform mole

Definition

A complete hydatidiform mole is an abnormal diploid conceptus in which the foetus is absent, the placental tissue is abnormal and all the genetic material is derived from the father.

Epidemiology

A hydatidiform mole affects approximately one in 2000 pregnancies. The condition is more common at the extremes of maternal age. There is a geographic variation that may reflect the decreased incidence in whites. Regions with an increased incidence include the Far East and Africa. A previous hydatidiform mole increases the likelihood of a further mole.

Pathology

A complete hydatidiform mole has a diploid chromosomal composition, being 46XX in 85% of cases and 46XY in the remaining 15%. Both sets of chromosomes are of paternal derivation. It is believed that imprinting causes the fertilised ovum to develop in an abnormal fashion and that the gestation results from the fertilisation of an ovum with an absent nucleus by two sperm or by a single sperm that has a diploid nucleus.

Macroscopically, the mole consists of numerous distended placental villi that resemble a bunch of grapes. This placental mass is large for dates and fills the uterine cavity. No foetus is present.

The microscopic hallmark of a complete hydatidiform mole is abnormal proliferation of the trophoblast. Most to all villi are affected by this in a complete mole, and the abnormal proliferation takes the form of multilayering of the trophoblast and the formation of exuberant projections of trophoblast. This proliferation affects the entire circumference of each villus. In addition, there are also changes to the stroma of the villi. Marked oedema is observed, yielding the formation of large, centrally located, fluid-filled cisterns. Foetal vessels are absent from the villi, as are foetal nucleated red cells.

Complications

As the mole is an abnormally large mass of placental tissue, with excess trophoblast, there is excessive production of human chorionic gonadotrophin (HCG). In around 3% of cases, this is sufficient to produce hyperthyroidism, due to a thyroid-stimulating hormone (TSH) like action of HCG.

An invasive mole is encountered in 5–10% of cases and is a variant in which the villi invade into the myometrium and may potentially reach the serosa or beyond.

Choriocarcinoma arises in 2–3% and is discussed below.

Partial hydatidiform mole

A partial mole is also an abnormal conceptus that has some of the features of a complete mole, but these are not as developed. One of the critical distinctions is that a complete mole is triploid and that fetal tissue may be found.

Abnormal trophoblastic proliferation is present, but is not as marked as in a complete mole. Only some villi are affected and, of the involved villi, only part of the circumference may show abnormal proliferation. Cistern formation is present and is only seen in a proportion of the villi. Unlike a complete mole, normal villi may be readily identified.

Choriocarcinoma is considerably rarer in a partial mole than a complete mole.

Choriocarcinoma

Choriocarcinoma is a malignant tumour of the trophoblast that affects one in 40 000 pregnancies. The majority of cases of choriocarcinoma occur after a complete mole (70%), with 20% being after an abortion and 10% following an otherwise normal pregnancy. Interestingly, the risk is 10 times greater in a woman with blood group A who is fertilised by a male of blood group O.

Pathology

Care should be taken with the term choriocarcinoma as it may be encountered outside the obstetric context. Primary choriocarcinomas of the ovary may develop and are unrelated to gestation. In addition, the testis can also produce a choriocarcinoma.

In the obstetric situation, a choriocarcinoma is derived from the gestational tissue and is therefore of a different genetic composition from the mother. The tumour exists as a large, irregular, haemorrhagic mass in the uterus that invades into and through the myometrium. The interval between the pregnancy and the development of the choriocarcinoma may be years.

The tumour is composed of both cytotrophoblastic and syncytiotrophoblastic elements. These infiltrate through the uterine wall, often with extensive invasion of vascular spaces. The combination of both trophoblastic elements is vital for the diagnosis. Villi are not seen.

Distant metastases occur early and are haematogenous. Common sites are the lungs, brain and liver.

Prognosis

The tumour is often highly sensitive to chemotherapy.

Placenta creta

Normally, a layer of decidua separates the chorionic villi from the myometrium. In the various forms of placenta creta, the villi are directly applied to the myometrium. The mildest form is placenta accreta, in which the villi adhere to the adluminal aspect of the myometrium but do not penetrate any deeper. In placenta increta, the villi permeate into the myometrium; while in placenta percreta, the villi reach the serosa of the uterus.

Clinically, this abnormal interface is associated with an abnormally adherent placenta and therefore with a retained placenta.

Ectopic pregnancy

An ectopic pregnancy is one that develops outside the uterine cavity. The most common site is the fallopian tube, typically the outer third. Other locations include the ovary, the broad ligament and peritoneum.

Pathologically, the key finding in material from an ectopic pregnancy is the presence of villi, or at least trophoblast.

Ectopic pregnancy may be predisposed to by any condition that impedes the passage of the ovum or zygote along the fallopian tube. Such conditions include chronic pelvic inflammatory disease and salpingitis isthmica nodosum, in which there is narrowing and diverticulum formation in the proximal portion of the fallopian tube.

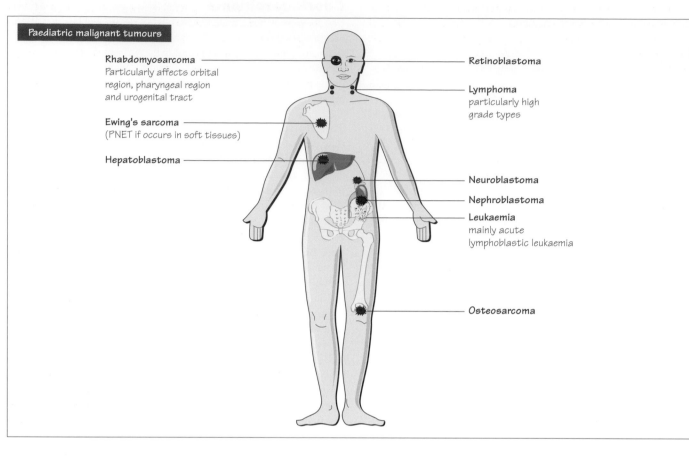

Paediatric malignant tumours

Rhabdomyosarcoma
Particularly affects orbital
region, pharyngeal region
and urogenital tract

Ewing's sarcoma
(PNET if occurs in soft tissues)

Hepatoblastoma

Retinoblastoma

Lymphoma
particularly high
grade types

Neuroblastoma

Nephroblastoma

Leukaemia
mainly acute
lymphoblastic leukaemia

Osteosarcoma

Many of the common tumours that are encountered in adults, particularly carcinomas, are rare in children. However, there are various tumours that can affect both children and adults, as well as those that are more common in childhood, or seen only in childhood. The group of tumours that are specific to childhood is diverse and affects a multitude of organ systems, but several of the more important entities can be considered under the designation of small round blue cell tumours (SRBCTs).

Common pathology

Although some SRBCTs can develop spontaneously, there is often an underlying predisposing factor, which is usually genetic. The descriptive term of SRBCT encapsulates the characteristic appearance of the tumour cells that are typical of these tumours. While various types of SRBCTs possess features that assist in distinguishing them from other SRBCTs, pathological diagnosis typically requires the integration of data from immunohistochemistry and cytogenetic studies with the microscopic morphology and the anatomical distribution of the tumour.

The tumours that fall in the SRBCT category include Ewing's sarcoma/primitive neuroectodermal tumour (PNET), nephroblastoma, neuroblastoma, lymphoma/leukaemia, retinoblastoma and certain forms of rhabomyosarcoma. Childhood lymphomas tend to be high grade, such as Burkitt-like lymphoma. Childhood leukaemia is most commonly acute lymphoblastic leukaemia; both chronic lymphocytic leukaemia and chronic myeloid leukaemia are unusual in children.

One of the most important aspects of all childhood malignancies, whether or not they fall into the SRBCT category, is the increased risk of a second malignancy later in life due to the effects of chemotherapy and radiotherapy on DNA. In children who survive their paediatric cancer, there are several remaining decades in which the mutations that may result from treatment can be added to by subsequent sporadic mutations.

Nephroblastoma

Nephroblastoma is also known as Wilm's tumour and is a malignant renal tumour that is derived from the renal blastema. It has an incidence of six per 100 000 per year and accounts for 7% of childhood cancers. The tumour normally presents before 5 years.

The predisposing factors centre around chromosome 11 and include the aniridia Wilm's syndrome and Beckwith–Wiedmann syndrome. At least two Wilm's tumour genes (WT1 and WT2) are situated on chromosome 11. Inherited mutation of these genes can predispose to nephroblastoma and nephroblastomas characteristically have an abnormal WT1 or WT2.

Macroscopically, the tumour is well circumscribed and large. The cut surface features cystic change, haemorrhage and necrosis.

Nephroblastomas have three components: blastema, mesenchyme and epithelium. The blastema is the small round blue cell element. The mesenchyme is a spindle cell stroma. The epithelial part forms tubular and glomerular structures. The proportions of the three components vary between tumours.

Local spread is by direct invasion into adjacent organs. Local lymph node metastases may develop. Distant metastases are to lungs and liver.

The long-term survival is around 90%.

Neuroblastoma

A neuroblastoma is a malignant tumour that arises from sympathetic neuroblasts. The incidence is 10 per 100 000 per year. The tumour tends to present around 2 years and is rare beyond 6 years. Neuroblastomas can be familial and are associated with the Beckwith–Wiedmann syndrome.

A neuroblastoma may arise anywhere in the sympathetic nervous system, but the majority are retroperitoneal and the adrenal is the most common site, probably due to the large concentration of sympathetic tissue within it.

The tumour is large and soft and frequently has regions of haemorrhage, necrosis or calcification. The constituent small round blue cells may form Homer–Wright rosettes in which the nuclei of the cells are arranged as a peripheral ring around a centre of neurofibrillary material.

Approximately 75% have metastasised at presentation, with common sites being the liver, bone and bone marrow, skin, ovary and orbit.

While the 5-year survival can be 90% in stage 1 disease, it may be as low as 20% in most stage 4 tumours (although a certain subcategory of stage 4 disease has a better prognosis). Neuroblastomas that express the Trk receptor have a better prognosis.

The ganglioneuroblastoma is closely related to the neuroblastoma and may most simply be considered as a neuroblastoma in which there is evidence of differentiation towards mature ganglion cells. These tumours have a better prognosis than neuroblastomas.

Retinoblastoma

Retinoblastomas are malignant tumours of the retina. The incidence is five per 100 000 per year. The presentation is usually between 16 months and 2 years and is frequently in the form of strabismus or a white pupillary reflex (rather than the red one that is commonly seen in flash photography).

Around 40% of retinoblastomas are familial and are due to a mutation in the retinoblastoma gene on chromosome 13q14. Both alleles need to be mutated for the tumour to develop. One defective allele is usually inherited as a consequence of mutation in a germ cell. An acquired mutation in the second allele then leads to the tumour. Most sporadic (non-inherited) retinoblastomas also display mutation of both retinoblastoma genes.

The tumour is bilateral in around 30% of all cases, but in 90% of familial cases. In some instances, the pineal gland is affected by a neoplasm with similar features, resulting in the term trilateral retinoblastomas.

Despite their location, retinoblastomas can often reach a relatively large size before presenting and are an irregular, white, partially necrotic mass that can detach the retina. The small round blue cells grow in sheets and may also be arranged in formations known as Flexner–Wintersteiner rosettes and fleurettes.

Spread is by direct extension along the optic nerve into the brain. Distant metastases may or may not occur, but when present tend to involve bones. Even in the absence of distant metastases, the ability of the tumour to invade the brain often requires treatment by enucleation of the eye.

The cure rate is around 90%.

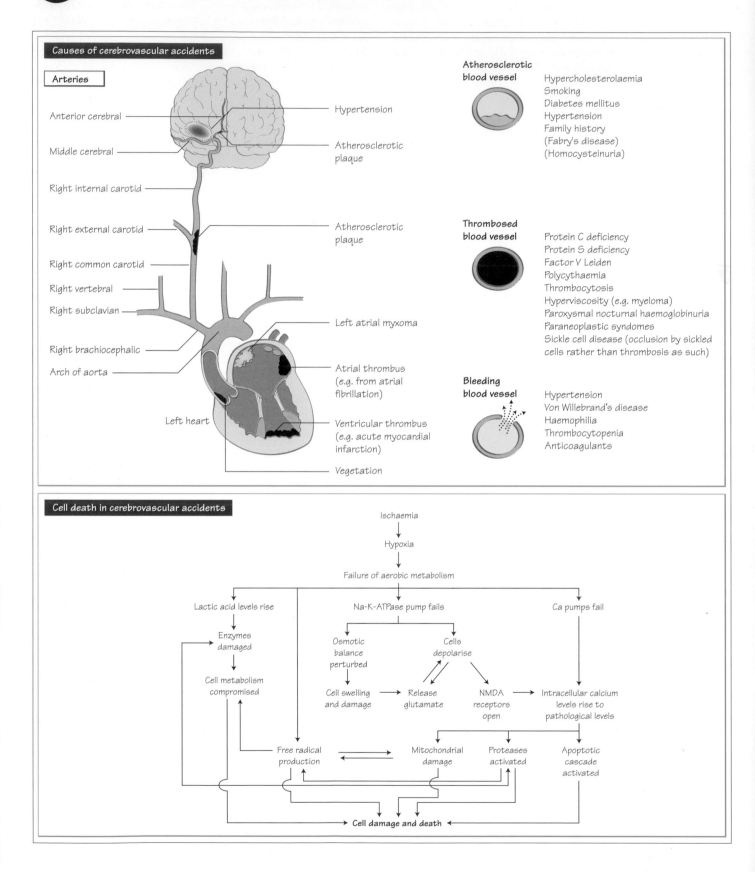

Causes of cerebrovascular accidents

Arteries

Anterior cerebral

Middle cerebral

Right internal carotid

Right external carotid

Right common carotid

Right vertebral

Right subclavian

Right brachiocephalic

Arch of aorta

Left heart

Hypertension

Atherosclerotic plaque

Atherosclerotic plaque

Left atrial myxoma

Atrial thrombus (e.g. from atrial fibrillation)

Ventricular thrombus (e.g. acute myocardial infarction)

Vegetation

Atherosclerotic blood vessel

Hypercholesterolaemia
Smoking
Diabetes mellitus
Hypertension
Family history
(Fabry's disease)
(Homocysteinuria)

Thrombosed blood vessel

Protein C deficiency
Protein S deficiency
Factor V Leiden
Polycythaemia
Thrombocytosis
Hyperviscosity (e.g. myeloma)
Paroxysmal nocturnal haemoglobinuria
Paraneoplastic syndomes
Sickle cell disease (occlusion by sickled cells rather than thrombosis as such)

Bleeding blood vessel

Hypertension
Von Willebrand's disease
Haemophilia
Thrombocytopenia
Anticoagulants

Cell death in cerebrovascular accidents

Ischaemia

Hypoxia

Failure of aerobic metabolism

Lactic acid levels rise

Na-K-ATPase pump fails

Ca pumps fail

Enzymes damaged

Cell metabolism compromised

Osmotic balance perturbed

Cells depolarise

Cell swelling and damage → Release glutamate

NMDA receptors open → Intracellular calcium levels rise to pathological levels

Free radical production

Mitochondrial damage

Proteases activated

Apoptotic cascade activated

Cell damage and death

176 *Pathology at a Glance.* By C.J. Finlayson and B.A.T. Newell. Published 2009 by Blackwell Publishing. ISBN: 978-1-4051-3650-1

Systems pathology

Definition

A cerebrovascular accident (CVA) is a focal neurological deficit that persists for more than 24 hours and is due to a vascular cause.

Epidemiology

The incidence in the general population is 150 per 1 000 000 per year but in those over 75 it is 1000 per 100 000 per year; 80% of strokes occur over the age of 60 years. Males are affected slightly more often than females.

Types

A CVA is either thrombotic (50%), where the occlusion of the blood vessel occurs locally, embolic (30%), where the occlusive agent originates at a distant site, or haemorrhagic (20%). Thromboembolic strokes are also referred to as ischaemic CVAs.

Risk factors

The risk factors for thrombotic and embolic strokes overlap as thrombosis is usually secondary to atherosclerosis and many embolic strokes are due to emboli derived from carotid artery atheroma. Once the carotid arteries are excluded, the next most common source of emboli is the heart. Therefore any process that induces intraventricular or intra-atrial thrombosis, or generates friable lesions on the valves, is a potential source of an embolic CVA.

The risk factors centre round those that are involved in the processes of atherosclerosis, hypertension and coagulation disturbances.

Pathophysiology

The brain is highly dependent on aerobic metabolism and is therefore particularly sensitive to hypoxia, such that irreversible neuronal damage can occur after only a few minutes.

Hypoxia results in failure of the $Na^+/K^+/ATPase$ system, leading to neuronal depolarisation and osmotic damage. Depolarisation also causes massive opening of the calcium channels and this abnormal influx of calcium ions – rather than the normal physiologically controlled opening in usual neurotransmission and neuronal excitation – triggers harmful intracellular cascades and mitochondrial damage, processes that rapidly become irreversible. In addition, the depolarisation results in neuronal firing, which can exacerbate the depolarisation consequences elsewhere. The whole process is known as excitotoxicity as the damage is a consequence of neuronal excitation (depolarisation).

Neurones on the periphery of the infarct are in a parlous state, at a point of critical ischaemia. This occurs when oxygen delivery is around 30% of normal (interestingly, this is approximately that delivered by good basic cardiopulmonary resuscitation). In this state, neurones enter a form of partial shutdown whereby they maintain their membrane potential but fail to produce action potentials. Any further ischaemia can hurl the neurones into the abyss of cell death. The region of the brain in this precarious predicament is called the ischaemic penumbra. The stroke itself would be the umbra.

Oedema is part of an ischaemic infarct. The oedema produces swelling, so a large ischaemic infarct can behave as a space-occupying lesion. A haemorrhagic infarct is also well placed to act as a space-occupying lesion.

The CVA also deranges cerebral blood flow autoregulation. This is normally tightly locally regulated. After a CVA, this autoregulation is lost and blood flow becomes critically dependent on systemic arterial pressure. Therefore, well meaning but poorly informed attempts to lower apparent hypertension can plummet the cerebral blood flow and extend a CVA. Conversely, rampant hypertension is not ideal after a haemorrhagic CVA, so a difficult balance may have to be achieved.

Gross features

An ischaemic infarct may initially appear only as a region of softening of the brain, something that is better appreciated after fixation in formalin. The CVA may also be pale and show a loss of the usual definition between the grey and white matter. Haemorrhage can occur into an infarct.

Haemorrhagic strokes are described as massive if they are over 2 cm and small if they are 1–2 cm. Slit haemorrhages occur at the junction of the grey and white matter. Petechial haemorrhages can occur. It is important when looking at a fixed specimen to remember that blood turns black on exposure to formalin. Haemorrhagic CVAs tend to affect, in decreasing order, the internal capsule, the central white matter, thalamus, cerebellar hemispheres and pons.

Over the ensuing weeks, the infarct becomes shrunken and cystic.

Lacunar infarcts are small cavities that occur in the white matter of the cerebral hemispheres.

Microscopic features

Neuronal necrosis is present and there is pallor of myelin staining. Oedema can be present in and around the CVA. Axons that cross the infarct show Wallerian degeneration. After a few days, the necrotic tissue degenerates and is removed by macrophages. Due to the high water and fat content of the brain, the process is one of liquefactive necrosis. This loss of cellular elements and the presence of a glial proliferative response, rather than fibrosis, results in the macroscopic shrinkage and cystic change mentioned above. In haemorrhagic strokes, haemosiderin deposition may be present.

Clinical correlations

The neurological deficit that occurs will depend on the region of the brain that is involved (see Chapter 82). This is usually approached in terms of the right and left side and vascular territories.

The anterior circulation territory is supplied by the internal carotid artery, with its division into the anterior cerebral artery, middle cerebral artery and the superior and inferior subdivisions of this, together with the deep penetrating arteries that supply the cerebral white matter. The posterior circulation originates from the vertebral arteries. These unify to give the basilar artery, which bifurcates to yield the posterior cerebral arteries. The posterior circulation includes assorted brainstem and cerebellar arteries, which can give very precise CVA syndromes.

Due to the organisation of the brain, small CVAs, such as lacunar infarcts, can have devastating effects, especially those in the internal capsule or brainstem.

Systems pathology

Stroke syndromes

Artery	Division	Structure damaged	Clinical consequences
Anterior cerebral artery	n/a	Primary motor cortex, leg and foot region Primary sensory cortex, leg and foot region Higher motor regions Frontal eye fields Frontal lobes Frontal lobes	Contralateral upper motor neurone paralysis of leg and foot Contralateral sensory loss in foot and leg Motor apraxia Deviation of eyes to side of lesion Emergency of primitive reflexes such as grasp and suckling Incontinence
Middle cerebral artery	Superior	Primary motor cortex Primary sensory cortex Superior part of optic radiation Broca's area (dominant hemisphere) Wernicke's area (dominant hemisphere) Both speech areas (dominant hemisphere)	Contralateral hemiparesis Contralateral sensory loss Contralateral homonymous inferior quadrantinopia Expressive dysphasia Receptive dysphasia Global aphasia
	Inferior	Wernicke's area Inferior part of optic radiation Whole of optic radiation	Receptive dysphasia Contralateral homonymous superior quadrantinopia Contralateral homonymous hemianopia
	Whole territory	Primary motor cortex Primary sensory cortex Whole of optic radiation Both speech areas (dominant hemisphere) Higher sensory areas Higher areas (non-dominant hemisphere) Higher areas (dominant hemisphere)	Contralateral hemiparesis Contralateral sensory loss Contralateral homonymous hemianopia Global aphasia Sensory agnosia Impaired judgement of distance and visual illusions, contralateral neglect Acalculia, alexia and right-left confusion
Posterior cerebral artery	Peripheral	Primary visual cortex Higher visual areas Medial temporal lobe Temporal lobe	Contralateral homonymous hemianopia Achromatopsia, oculomotor apraxia, impaired processing of visual data Prosopagnosia Memory defect
	Central	Thalamus Thalamus and deep white matter Cerebral peduncle	Sensory loss Spontaneous pain Dysaesthesia Hemiparesis Intention tremor Choreoathetosis Cerebellar ataxia Contralateral hemiplegia
Middle or posterior cerebral arteries	Perforating branches (Lacunar infarcts)	Anterior limb of internal capsule Posterior limb of internal capsule	Contralateral hemiplegia Contralateral dense sensory loss
Vertebrobasilar arteries	Medial medulla oblongata territory	Pyramidal tract Hypoglossal nerve and nucleus Medial lemniscus	Contralateral hemiparesis sparing the face Ipsilateral lower motor neurone lesion of the tongue Contralateral impaired fine touch and conscious proprioreception
	Lateral medulla oblongata territory	Vestibular nerve nuclei Spinocerebellar tracts and cerebellar peduncles Spinothalamic tract Spinothalamic tract Vagus nerve nucleus Sympathetic fibres	Vertigo, nausea and vomiting, nystagmus Ataxia Contralateral impaired contralateral sensation for the body Contralateral impaired ipsilateral sensation for the face Ipsilateral vocal cord palsy, loss of gag reflex, dysphagia, dysarthria Ipsilateral Horner's syndrome
	Basilar artery	Bilateral pyramidal tracts Bilateral long sensory tracts Both occipital cortices Reticular activating system Overall	Bilateral hemiparesis Bilateral sensory loss Bilateral homonymous hemianopias Loss of consciousness Locked in syndrome
	Assorted territories in pons and midbrain	Pyramidal fibres Spinothalamic fibres Posterior column fibres (medial lemniscus) Cerebellar peduncles Projections from cerebral cortex to cerebellum Cerebellar pathways Vestibular nuclei Cranial nerve nuclei (3rd to 9th)	Contralateral hemiparesis Contralateral loss of pain and temperature sensation Contralateral loss of fine touch and temperature sensation Ipsilateral ataxia Contralateral ataxia Nystagmus, vertigo Nystagmus, vertigo, nausea and vomiting Motor and/or sensory palsies

Key: Blue = Motor; Purple = Sensory; Red = Cerebellar; Green = Visual; Black = Miscellaneous

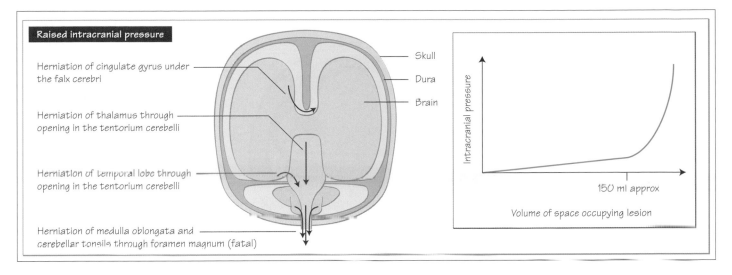

Raised intracranial pressure

Herniation of cingulate gyrus under the falx cerebri

Herniation of thalamus through opening in the tentorium cerebelli

Herniation of temporal lobe through opening in the tentorium cerebelli

Herniation of medulla oblongata and cerebellar tonsils through foramen magnum (fatal)

Skull

Dura

Brain

Intracranial pressure

150 ml approx

Volume of space occupying lesion

Definition

Normal intracranial pressure is 2–12 mmHg. A raised intracranial pressure is an intracranial pressure above 15 mmHg.

Causes

Intracranial pressure is increased by any process that increases the volume of material within the cranial cavity. This can be due to a tumour, haemorrhage, oedema (either related to a tumour, cerebrovascular accident or metabolic process) or an increased volume of cerebrospinal fluid (CSF).

Pathophysiology

The intracranial cavity is a rigid space that is enclosed by bone, which will not yield to any increase in pressure arising from an organic process within the cranial cavity. Some other form of release mechanism therefore has to take place.

Initially, a rise in intracranial pressure is countered by compression of the ventricular system and a decrease in the volume of cerebrospinal fluid. The ventricular system and CSF provide a volume of approximately 100–150 ml that can be sacrificed in order to prevent a rise in intracranial pressure.

Herniation

Once the ventricular system has been collapsed as far as possible, intracranial pressure rises rapidly. Pressure is transmitted to the brain, which is not well placed to withstand it and several processes occur.

Most causes of a raised intracranial pressure will affect one side more than the other and are supratentorial in location. Once a critical pressure is reached, it will produce a 'midline shift', in which the cerebral hemisphere on the side of the lesion is pushed across the midline towards the contralateral side, such that midline structures are noted on imaging to have deviated. The movement of cerebral structures past a less mobile structure into an abnormal position is referred to as herniation. Several types of herniation can occur:
• The cingulate gyrus can herniate under the falx cerebri.
• The median temporal lobe may move into the opening in the tentorium.

• The thalamic region can move down through the central space in the tentorium,

Such movements of the relatively delicate substance of the brain are dangerous in themselves, but also herald the ultimate, catastrophic consequence of an unrelieved elevation of intracranial pressure. When all other mechanisms have been overwhelmed, the only point of give in the cranial cavity is the foramen magnum and the forcing of the brainstem and tonsils of the cerebellum out through it. This is known as coning and is almost invariably fatal.

Vascular compression

In addition to compression and herniation of the brain itself, the increase in intracranial pressure can compress blood vessels and thus interfere with perfusion of the brain. In general, if the intracranial arterial pressure is less than 40–60 mmHg higher than the intracranial pressure, cerebral perfusion will be compromised and ischaemic damage will develop.

Asymmetrical pupils

Much emphasis is often placed on asymmetrical pupils in the context of raised intracranial pressure and head injury in particular. This is due to the fact that herniation of the median temporal lobe compresses the oculomotor nerve. As the sympathetic fibres run on the outside of the nerve, they are the first to suffer under the compression. Hence, the ipsilateral pupil dilates even though extraocular movements are unaffected. If a pupil does dilate (often referred to as 'blowing a pupil') in a head injury, this is a very serious sign because herniation of the median temporal lobe means that coning is imminent.

However, the emphasis of the significance of a blown pupil is often misplaced, in that some individuals proceed on the mistaken assumption that if the pupils are symmetrical, the situation inside the patient's skull is not serious. This reasoning is incorrect. All the absence of a dilated pupil means is that one particular catastrophic process has not yet occurred. Others (such as ischaemia) may be ongoing and, once a pupil does blow, the opportunity to prevent a serious neurological deficit may have been irretrievably lost. Therefore, treat asymmetrical pupils very seriously, but do not be lulled into a false sense of security if they are symmetrical.

Systems pathology

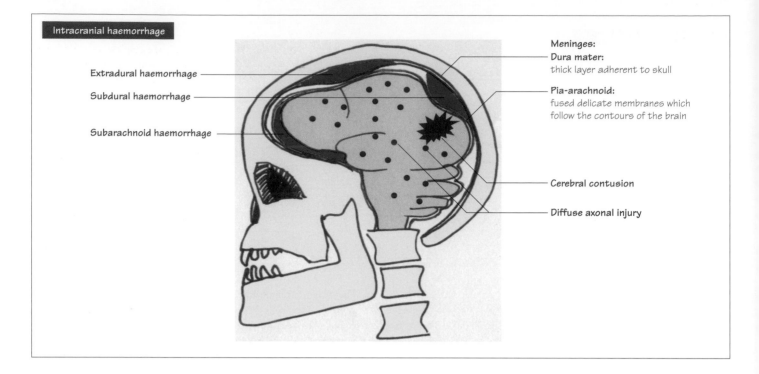

Intracranial haemorrhage

Meninges:
Dura mater:
thick layer adherent to skull

Pia-arachnoid:
fused delicate membranes which
follow the contours of the brain

Extradural haemorrhage

Subdural haemorrhage

Subarachnoid haemorrhage

Cerebral contusion

Diffuse axonal injury

Intracranial haemorrhage is bleeding that occurs inside the cranial cavity. There are many causes:
- Trauma:
  - Extradural haemorrhage.
  - Chronic subdural haemorrhage.
  - Acute subdural haemorrhage.
  - Cerebral contusions.
- Subarachnoid haemorrhage.
- Arteriovenous malformation.
- Cerebrovascular accident.
- Tumour.

In basic terms, a volume of blood that accumulates inside the skull acts as a space-occupying lesion and its effects therefore include those of raised intracranial pressure.

Extradural haemorrhage

Extradural haemorrhage occurs in the extradural space, which exists between the inside of the skull and the outer surface of the dura. Extradural haemorrhage is usually caused by bleeding from an artery. The classic example is the middle meningeal artery. This lies on the inner surface of the thinnest part of the temporal bone (squamous region) and is therefore more vulnerable to trauma than many of the other arteries that run over the meninges.

The attachment of the dura to the inside of the skull is quite tough and requires a degree of pressure to separate the dura from the bone. This separation is necessary if the volume of blood is to expand. Therefore, after the initial trauma that ruptures the artery, there is an interval where the patient is relatively free of symptoms. However, once the dura separates and the clot expands, the effects of rapidly rising intracranial pressure supervene. Although the middle meningeal artery is vulnerable,

the degree of trauma necessary to damage it or any related artery is usually sufficient to cause unconsciousness. Typically, the period of unconsciousness is brief.

Chronic subdural haemorrhage

This occurs between the dura and pia mater. The bleeding is from one of the veins that bridges the space between the skull and the meningeal layers. These are more fragile than the dural arteries. However, they are normally protected by the snug fit of the brain inside the skull and their anatomy means that a shearing force is necessary to damage them. Therefore, conditions in which there is atrophy of the brain, such as dementia, render these vessels more susceptible. Under such circumstances, the trauma that damages them is often minor and not associated with a loss of consciousness.

In addition, the rate of blood flow is often very slow, so the clot only attains an appreciable size over a period of weeks to months. The blood flow is also at venous rather than arterial pressure, so the haemorrhage may be more readily contained by simple mechanical factors. This slower process affords the brain greater opportunity to adapt to the increase in intracranial pressure. Nevertheless, this adaptation is not without problems as the function of the brain can be compromised such that a chronic subdural haematoma can masquerade as dementia, or exacerbate pre-existing dementia.

Acute subdural haemorrhage

As with a chronic subdural haemorrhage, this is caused by damage to the bridging veins, although it is typically of a greater degree. It is associated with the types of trauma that produce an extradural haemorrhage, with which it often coexists.

Subarachnoid haemorrhage

This is a haemorrhage that occurs beneath the arachnoid mater and therefore lies on the surface of the brain itself. The incidence is 4–5 per 100 000 per year.

Pathology

Subarachnoid haemorrhages are arterial, from the cerebral arteries of the circle of Willis, usually as the result of rupture of a pre-existing abnormality. In approximately 70–90% of cases, the abnormality is a saccular aneurysm on the circle of Willis. These are situated at the points of division of the arterial network and are also often known as berry aneurysms. Although the posterior communicating artery is the most often mentioned, it is actually the anterior communicating artery that is the most common location of a berry aneurysm. Rather perturbingly, berry aneurysms are found in around 5% of all autopsies.

Most of the remaining cases of subarachnoid haemorrhage are due to arteriovenous malformations.

Rupture of the aneurysm or malformation is spontaneous, without a history of trauma, although hypertension may be contributory. The blood emerges at arterial pressure and spreads over the surface of the brain, producing an irritant effect that initially manifests as a severe headache and often very quickly proceeds to unconsciousness. The onset of unconsciousness can occur within seconds.

Complications

There are three main complications of a subarachnoid haemorrhage and these contribute significantly to the morbidity and mortality.

• Rebleeding occurs in 10–30% in the first 3 weeks and is fatal in 60%.
• Vasospasm affects 30% and can cause severe neurological deficits. The precise cause is uncertain but one possibility is that the blood clot around the arteries on the base of the brain prevents the cerebrospinal fluid (CSF) from supplying nutrients to the vessel. This deprives the smooth muscle of the vessel of adenosine triphosphate (ATP), which inhibits relaxation of the vessel while breakdown products from the clot induce vasoconstriction.
• Hydrocephalus is caused by obstruction to the flow of CSF by the blood clot.

Prognosis

The prognosis is not good. Over 10% die in the first 24 hours and at least another 25% die within 3 months. Of the remaining 65%, over half have severe residual neurological deficits. Hence, only around 30% have a good outcome.

Cerebral contusions

Cerebral contusions are haemorrhage into the substance of the brain as a result of trauma and are therefore bruises. Contusions can occur not only in the brain that lies under the part of the skull that received the impact of the trauma, but on the opposite side. This is the coup and contra-coup pattern of injury and occurs because the brain is not entirely snug inside the skull. Instead, there is some movement such that the brain opposite the site of injury can strike the inside of the skull. Furthermore, rapid acceleration and deceleration induces negative pressures that can tear vessels and produce haemorrhage.

Diffuse axonal injury

Although not a form of haemorrhage, diffuse axonal injury (DAI) is mentioned here as it is a serious consequence of heavy trauma. DAI affects the axons of the white matter in a diffuse pattern throughout the brain and therefore produces global damage. DAI is one of the main causes of the persistent vegetative state.

The underlying mechanism of injury is shearing and stretching of the axons, but the mechanical process alone is not responsible for the axonal damage. Instead, the mechanical deformation induces changes in ion channels, the cytoskeleton of the axon and metabolic pathways that culminate in damage.

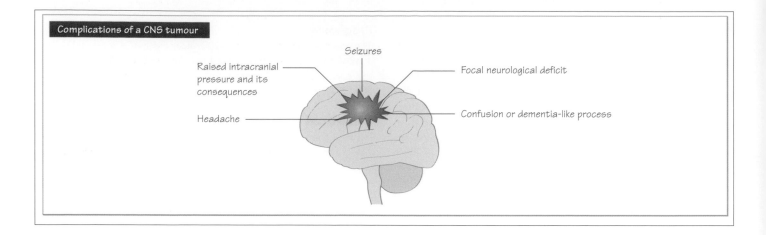

Complications of a CNS tumour

Raised intracranial pressure and its consequences — Seizures — Focal neurological deficit

Headache — Confusion or dementia-like process

Primary tumours

Definition

A primary tumour of the central nervous system (CNS) is a neoplasm that arises from the tissue of the CNS. Multiple types exist.

Epidemiology

Primary tumours of the CNS have an incidence of 15 per 100 000 per year. All ages can be affected, although the individual subtypes affect specific ages. Importantly, primary malignant tumour of the CNS is the second commonest malignancy in children under 15 years. The male to female ratio can vary with the tumour subtype.

General pathology

A tumour within the CNS will behave as a mass lesion. Hence it has the potential to cause localising signs that are related to its position and to produce features that are secondary to raised intracranial pressure. Both of these phenomena can be exacerbated by the oedema that can develop in the tissue around the tumour.

The division of tumours into benign and malignant, which operates elsewhere in the body, requires a different emphasis in the CNS. It is extremely rare for even the most high grade tumour to metastasise outside the CNS. Conversely, a tumour that is histologically bland can have disastrous consequences if it is in the wrong location, for example a posterior fossa meningioma. Nevertheless, the designations of benign and malignant are still used.

Grading of gliomas

Gliomas are tumours of glial cells and are graded as follows:
• Score one point for each of pleomorphism, mitoses, necrosis and endovascular proliferation.
• Grade = score + 1, up to a maximum of four.

Necrosis and endovascular proliferation are unusual in low grade tumours.

Tumour types

Astrocytoma

An astrocytoma is a grade 2 tumour derived from astrocytes and is one of the gliomas. Astrocytes have a variety of functions, not all of which

are understood, but it is believed that they provide assorted forms of metabolic support for the neurones.

Astrocytomas primarily occur in the third and fourth decades and account for approximately 10% of primary CNS tumours. Astrocytomas tend to be found in the white matter of the cerebral hemispheres, but can be encountered in a wide range of other locations. The margins of the tumour are indistinct and it tends to permeate the adjacent tissue. This can make obtaining surgical excision difficult to impossible.

Microscopically, the tumour is recognised by an increased density in the cellularity of astrocytes, coupled with an abnormal architecture and permeating pattern of growth.

Anaplastic astrocytoma

This is often derived from an astrocytoma and is a grade 3 glioma. In relation to this, the typical age of presentation is a few years later than for a grade 2 astrocytoma. The tumour is more pleomorphic than a grade 2 astrocytoma and the prognosis is worse.

Glioblastoma multiforme

A glioblastoma multiforme is a grade 4 glioma and is highly malignant. It may arise from transformation from one of the lower grade astrocytomas (see above), or develop without a precursor lesion. The main age of presentation is greater than the lower grade lesions. Its macroscopic appearance of relative circumscription is illusory as it is highly invasive and can spread from one hemisphere to the other across the corpus callosum. Survival is measured in months.

Pilocytic astrocytoma

A pilocytic astrocytoma is a specific lesion found in the cerebellum, optic nerve, optic chiasm and third ventricle region of young people and is a grade 1 glioma. The tumour cells have very long, slender, bipolar processes and are arranged in a fascicular and microcystic pattern. The tumour has a rich vascular background that includes Rosenthal fibres, which at the most simple level are characteristically shaped extracellular blobs. Assuming surgery is possible, the prognosis is good.

Oligodendroglioma

Oligodendrocytes are the cells that myelinate CNS axons. Hence,

182 *Pathology at a Glance.* By C.J. Finlayson and B.A.T. Newell. Published 2009 by Blackwell Publishing. ISBN: 978-1-4051-3650-1

oligodendrogliomas predominantly affect the white matter of the cerebral hemispheres. The tumour occurs in the young and middle aged. Oligodendrogliomas are well circumscribed, gelatinous and may be cystic. Microscopically, there are sheets of uniform cells that have a clear halo, which leads to talk of a fried egg appearance. Most are grade 2, but anaplastic (grade 3) variants exist.

Ependymoma

Ependymomas may be located intracranially, in which case they usually affect children, or found in the spinal cord, where adults are the main age group. Given their derivation from ependymal cells, the tumours are typically positioned in the region of the ventricles, particularly the fourth; spinal cord tumours are mainly situated in the filum terminale. The cells form rosette-like structures.

Choroid plexus papilloma

This is another ventricle-based tumour and one that also predominantly affects children. The malignant variant is the choroid plexus carcinoma.

Meningioma

The meninges can also give rise to tumours. These present in middle age and are more common in females. The tumours are based on the dura, particularly near the superior sagittal sinus, over the cerebral convexities or the falx cerebri. While meningiomas tend to compress rather than invade brain, they can invade bone, although interestingly this does not invoke a designation of malignancy.

The grading system described above does not translate strictly across to meningeal tumours but typical and atypical meningiomas exist. Multiple microscopic appearances are described.

Secondary tumours

Secondary tumours of the CNS are more common than primary tumours. Many malignant neoplasms can metastasise to the brain, but those with a particular propensity include lung, colon and breast.

Vasogenic oedema can be a particular problem with secondary tumours and as with metastases elsewhere in the body, they may be multiple.

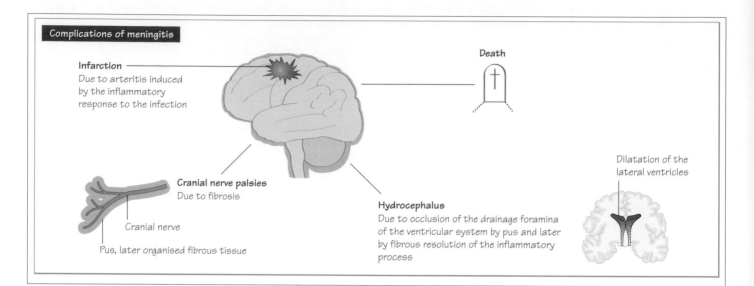

Complications of meningitis

Infarction
Due to arteritis induced by the inflammatory response to the infection

Death

Cranial nerve palsies
Due to fibrosis

Cranial nerve

Pus, later organised fibrous tissue

Hydrocephalus
Due to occlusion of the drainage foramina of the ventricular system by pus and later by fibrous resolution of the inflammatory process

Dilatation of the lateral ventricles

Bacterial meningitis

Definition
Bacterial meningitis is a bacterial infection of the pia and arachnoid mater and cerebrospinal fluid (CSF).

Epidemiology
The incidence is five per 100 000 per year. Children and the elderly are the main groups affected.

Risk factors
The risk factors reflect either a general susceptibility to infection or a specific disorder that renders the meninges vulnerable. The former include:
- Overcrowding and poverty.
- Alcoholism.
- Immunosuppression.
- Diabetes mellitus.
  The latter feature:
- Otitis media.
- Sinusitis.
- Mastoiditis.
- Head injury.
- CSF shunts.

Microbiology
A variety of bacteria can cause meningitis. There are three main agents:
- *Streptococcus pneumoniae*: this covers all ages, but is the commonest agent in older age groups.
- *Neisseria meningitidis* (meningococcus): this is the commonest cause in the UK and has peaks around 6 months and in teenagers.
- *Haemophilus influenzae*: this has the youngest target population, specifically 6 months to 4 years.
Other organisms can also cause meningitis. Neonatal infections are usually due to *Escherichia coli*, group B streptococci or *Listeria monocytogenes*.

Skin commensal staphylococci tend to be the causative bacteria in patients with CSF shunts.

Pathology
Spread of the bacteria to the meninges is usually haematogenous, with the three main causative agents normally being present in the nasopharynx. Direct spread is less common.

As is expected from a bacterial infection, bacterial meningitis generates an acute inflammatory response. This includes the production of pus, which accumulates in the subarachnoid space, particularly in the sulci and the base of the brain. The inflammation also causes arteritis and phlebitis. This can lead to vascular necrosis and thrombosis, with subsequent infarction.

Delayed treatment allows fibrous organisation of the inflammatory exudate to occur, which may result in obliteration of the outflow foramina for CSF and hydrocephalus. Cranial nerve palsies may also develop from this process of fibrosis. Early treatment prevents the infection from reaching a level that can be succeeded by fibrosis.

Other forms of meningitis
- **Tuberculous meningitis**: tuberculosis (TB) may cause meningitis; it presents with a subacute rather than an acute time course. The exudate in tuberculous meningitis is very rich in proteins and is therefore very viscous. This can make patients particularly prone to developing the fibrotic complications of cranial nerve palsies and hydrocephalus.
- **Cryptococcal meningitis**: this is a fungal meningitis that is the most common form of the disease in AIDS. As with tuberculous meningitis, the course is subacute.
- **Viral meningitis**: many viral illnesses are associated with viral infection of the meninges. The condition is mild.

Encephalitis
Unlike meningitis, encephalitis is inflammation of the substance of the brain itself. In further contrast with meningitis, encephalitis without further specification is a viral illness.

Systems pathology

While mild encephalitis may be an aspect of many viral infections, serious disease is rare. In the United Kingdom, the causative agent of serious encephalitis is virtually always herpes simplex. However, other aggressive viruses are found in other countries and may be missed if a history of travel is not obtained.

The basic process is one of inflammation. As would be expected from a disease that affects the brain itself and is generalised, the clinical features are those of global cerebral dysfunction. However, herpes simplex encephalitis exhibits a propensity to infect the temporal lobes, where it may produce massive destruction – in extreme cases leading to obliteration of both temporal lobes. This can wreak havoc with the hippocampal gyri and destroy the ability to transfer memories from short term to long term.

Brain abscess

Brain abscesses are rare lesions that tend to present in the fourth decade and have a male : female ratio of 2 : 1. Around 90% are secondary to an infection elsewhere in the body, of which 40% are situated in the paranasal sinuses and middle ear systems. Involvement of the brain by these routes is either due to direct extension via osteomyelitis or by phlebitis. A further 33% are due to haematogenous spread from more distant sites, particularly the lungs in bronchiectasis. Most of the remainder are cardiac in origin, being derived either from bacterial endocarditis or congenital cardiac disease.

Brain abscesses are usually solitary, with the frontal lobe being the most frequent location. Initially, there is a localised accumulation of an acute inflammatory exudate, as would be expected with an abscess. Vessels in the vicinity can show thrombosis and there is necrosis of the involved brain parenchyma. With persistence of the abscess, there is a granulation tissue response at the periphery, followed by fibrosis. In the adjacent brain parenchyma, there is oedema, together with a chronic inflammatory cell infiltrate and reactive proliferation of the glia.

Although the process is focal and frequently features localising signs and symptoms, there may be general disturbances of neurological function, as well as raised intracranial pressure.

Other infections

A few other neurological infections can be mentioned briefly.

Tetanus: Tetanus is caused by the toxin of *Clostridium tetani*. There are 30–40 cases per year in the UK. The condition develops when a wound is contaminated by the spores of the organism in circumstances that permit germination, specifically in necrotic, anaerobic tissue.

The toxin is called tetanospasmin and is taken up by the terminals of motor neurones and transported to the spinal cord where it inhibits GABAergic and glycinergic descending pathways. As these pathways tend to inhibit motor neurone activity, interference with them produces spasticity (Chapter 85).

Botulism: Botulism is another clostridial toxin disease, this time *Clostridium botulinum*. The toxin blocks the release of acetylcholine by lower motor neurones and causes a flaccid paralysis.

Polio: Polio is caused by a picornavirus. There is serious involvement in only 1–5%. The spread is faecal–oral and dissemination to the target of the lower motor neurones is haematogenous.

Systems pathology

Control of movement

Pyramidal cells in the primary motor cortex

◆ Final output pathway of the brain to the motor neurones in the spinal cord in lateral corticospinal tracts to the anterior horn cells
◆ Receive projections from basal ganglia, cerebellum, higher motor regions and higher regions
◆ Also known as upper motor neurones
◆ Much of their basal activity is inhibitory and serves to suppress primitive reflexes that operate at a subcortical and spinal level and are unwanted in the presence of higher motor skills
◆ Disease states are characterised by paralysis of voluntary movement, increased tone, increased reflexes and upgoing plantars E.g. stroke
◆ Motor neurone disease is characterised by both upper and lower motor neurone defects

Basal ganglia

◆ Receive projections from various sensory pathways and brain regions and assist with the development of motor functions
◆ Project to the primary motor cortex to influence the output of this region
◆ Precise functions remain to be elucidated
◆ Disease states are characterised by increased tone (rigidity), abnormal movements (e.g. tremor, chorea, athetosis) and bradykinesia, but not paralysis of voluntary movement E.g. Wilson's disease, Huntingdon's chorea, Parkinson's disease

Cerebellum

◇ Receives sensory information from proprioreceptors and other somatosensory fibres. Also receives input from vestibular system
◇ Sends fibres to and receives them from the primary motor cortex
◇ Integrates data from these various sources to co-ordinate movement and modify the activity of the primary motor cortex
◇ Disease states are characterised by impaired co-ordination, either of basic motor functions such as balance and eye movements and/or complex skilled movements (including speech) E.g. multiple sclerosis, stroke, Wernicke's encephalopathy

Input from other sensory fibres

◆ Assorted somatosensory fibres such as pressure, pain, fine touch and crude touch, project to the cerebral cortex and the cerebellum and are integrated to assist in the development of optimal motor output signals

Muscle spindle

◆ Measures the degree of stretch in a muscle and tendon Serves to help to maintain the resting state of tone of the muscle and is essential to the spinal stretch reflex Provides crucial proprioreceptive information for co-ordination

Skeletal muscle fibre

Gamma motor neurone

◇ Innervates the muscle spindle and serves to modify the size of the stretch reflex
◇ It is a form of lower motor neurone Increased motor neurone activity stretches the muscle spindle, increasing its sensitivity and therefore increasing the size of any reflex caused by stretching of the muscle spindle

Alpha motor neurone

◆ Final common output pathway from the nervous system to muscle fibres
◆ All higher motor information converges on the α-motor neurone to be relayed to the skeletal muscle fibre to produce movement
◆ Also known as a lower motor neurone
◆ Disease states are characterised by paralysis of movement, wasting, decreased tone, fasiculations and decreased reflexes E.g. Guillain–Barré syndrome

General principles
Upper and lower motor neurone lesions

One of the central principles of the neurology of movement disorders is the division of the motor system into the upper motor neurones and lower motor neurones. Upper motor neurones are the final common output pathway from the brain for the complex pathways that generate and fine tune a motor sequence. They connect to the lower motor neurones, which innervate the skeletal muscles. Lesions confined to upper or lower motor neurones produce specific patterns of features (Table 85.1). Understanding of these features is made easier by the realisation that much of the basal activity in the upper motor neurones is inhibitory and damps down the resting activity of the lower motor neurones and spinal reflex arcs. Furthermore, lower motor neurones are the final pathway for any process, including the reflex arc, to stimulate the muscle.

Fasciculations are believed to arise as part of a failed attempt to reinnervate muscle fibres that have lost their lower motor neurones. The terminals of surviving axons sprout collaterals to denervated muscle fibres. However, once the size of a motor unit supplied by an axon reaches a critical level, it becomes unstable and spontaneous contractions of individual fibres and groups of fibres results.

Table 85.1 Features of upper and lower motor neurone lesions.

	Upper motor neurone	Lower motor neurone
Inspection	Limited or no wasting	Wasting and fasciculations
Posture	Spastic – flexor movements dominate in upper limb and extensor in the lower	No specific features, contractures in late disease
Tone	Increased	Decreased
Power	Decreased	Decreased
Reflexes	Increased	Decreased or absent
Plantars	Upgoing	Downgoing

Nerve root versus peripheral nerve lesion

Different processes damage nerve roots and peripheral nerves and imply different anatomical sites for the pathology. Therefore, for any motor action, or any sensory distribution, it is necessary to know which spinal nerve root innervates the territory and which peripheral nerve supplies it. For example, all of the small muscles of the hand are supplied by C8 and T1, but the median nerve is restricted to the muscles of the thenar eminence. Therefore, paralysis and wasting of the thenar eminence, but sparing of the remainder of the hand, indicates a median nerve palsy, rather than a C8/T1 lesion, in which the entire hand would be affected.

Motor neurone disease

Motor neurone disease is a neurodegenerative disorder of unknown cause. The incidence is 1–3 per 100 000 and the prevalence is 4–6 per 100 000. The disease is rare before 50 years and is more common in males. The condition occurs worldwide, with peaks in Guam and the Japanese Kii Peninsula.

Approximately 5% of cases are inherited as an autosomal dominant condition. This form has an earlier onset and more protracted course. The defect is in the superoxide dismutase gene.

Pathology

There is a loss of upper motor neurone Betz cells in the primary motor cortex, the anterior horn cells of the spinal cord and the motor neurones of the cranial nerve nuclei. This loss of neurones results in thinning of the anterior spinal nerve roots, as well as the lateral corticospinal tracts.

Different patterns of disease are described:
- Amyotrophic lateral sclerosis predominantly affects the lateral corticospinal tracts.
- Progressive muscular atrophy mainly involves the anterior horn cells.
- Bulbar palsy is due to loss of cranial nerve nuclei motor neurones.
- Pseudobulbar palsy is caused by damage to the primary motor cortex neurones that innervate the cranial nerve motor nuclei.

One of the most useful diagnostic features of motor neurone disease is the combination of upper and lower motor neurone features in the same muscle group.

Parkinson's disease

Parkinson's disease is an extrapyramidal neurodegenerative disease that affects the substantia nigra and is characterised by the triad of bradykinesia, rigidity and tremor. The prevalence is one per 100 000 of the general population, but rises to one per 200 in the elderly. Presentation is typically between 40 and 70 years. The disease is more common in whites.

Pathology

There is a loss of pigmented dopaminergic neurones in the pars compacta of the substantia nigra. As a result, the substantia nigra becomes pale (the substantia nigra is not pigmented in children; pigmentation is normally only achieved by the teenage years). Other less well known brainstem pigmented nuclei such as the locus coeruleus and dorsal motor neurone of the vagus also degenerate. As well as a loss of the neurones, the surviving cells display eosinophilic inclusions known as Lewy bodies.

Due to the reserve capacity of the substantia nigra, the condition does not present until around 60% of the neurones have already been lost.

Parkinsonism

Parkinsonism is the term applied to the set of clinical features that are seen in Parkinson's disease. However, as well as being caused by Parkinson's disease, it can also be caused by Wilson's disease, antidopamingeric drugs, MPTP, ischaemia, carbon monoxide poisoning, multiple systems atrophy and progressive supranuclear palsy.

Huntington's chorea

Huntington's chorea is an autosomal dominant disease in which there is an extrapyramidal movement disorder and dementia. The incidence is four per 1 000 000 per year and the prevalence is 7–10 per 100 000. The onset is usually in the fourth and fifth decades and therefore tends to be after an affected individual has already reproduced.

The gene (*Huntingtin*) is situated on the short arm of chromosome 4p16.3 and the mutation involves CAG trinucleotide repeats.

Pathology

The changes are most marked in the caudate nucleus and putamen, which show wasting. This results in enlargement of the lateral ventricles. The usual bulge of the caudate into the lateral ventricle is lost. Generalised cortical atrophy is also present. The disease progresses relentlessly over 10–20 years.

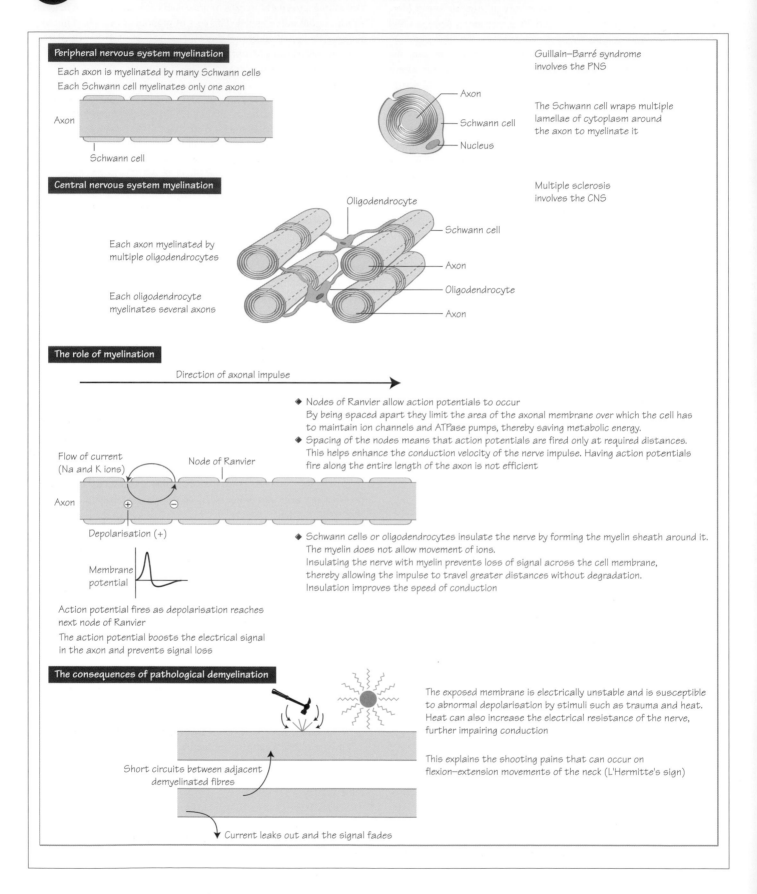

Peripheral nervous system myelination

Each axon is myelinated by many Schwann cells
Each Schwann cell myelinates only one axon

Axon

Schwann cell

Axon

Schwann cell

Nucleus

Guillain–Barré syndrome
involves the PNS

The Schwann cell wraps multiple
lamellae of cytoplasm around
the axon to myelinate it

Central nervous system myelination

Each axon myelinated by
multiple oligodendrocytes

Each oligodendrocyte
myelinates several axons

Oligodendrocyte

Schwann cell

Axon

Oligodendrocyte

Axon

Multiple sclerosis
involves the CNS

The role of myelination

Direction of axonal impulse

Flow of current
(Na and K ions)

Node of Ranvier

Axon

Depolarisation (+)

Membrane
potential

Action potential fires as depolarisation reaches
next node of Ranvier
The action potential boosts the electrical signal
in the axon and prevents signal loss

◆ Nodes of Ranvier allow action potentials to occur
By being spaced apart they limit the area of the axonal membrane over which the cell has
to maintain ion channels and ATPase pumps, thereby saving metabolic energy.
◆ Spacing of the nodes means that action potentials are fired only at required distances.
This helps enhance the conduction velocity of the nerve impulse. Having action potentials
fire along the entire length of the axon is not efficient

◆ Schwann cells or oligodendrocytes insulate the nerve by forming the myelin sheath around it.
The myelin does not allow movement of ions.
Insulating the nerve with myelin prevents loss of signal across the cell membrane,
thereby allowing the impulse to travel greater distances without degradation.
Insulation improves the speed of conduction

The consequences of pathological demyelination

Short circuits between adjacent
demyelinated fibres

Current leaks out and the signal fades

The exposed membrane is electrically unstable and is susceptible
to abnormal depolarisation by stimuli such as trauma and heat.
Heat can also increase the electrical resistance of the nerve,
further impairing conduction

This explains the shooting pains that can occur on
flexion–extension movements of the neck (L'Hermitte's sign)

Systems pathology

Multiple sclerosis

Definition

Multiple sclerosis is a condition in which there are lesions of demyelination within the central nervous system (CNS) that are disseminated in time and space, in the absence of other causes.

Epidemiology

Multiple sclerosis tends to present between the ages of 20 and 40 years. The male : female ratio is 3 : 2. There is a marked geographical variation in the incidence such that the incidence increases with distance from the equator. In equatorial regions, it is one per 100 000 per year, in southern Europe it is 6–14 per 100 000 per year, rising to 30–80 per 100 000 per year in Northern Europe and 250 per 100 000 per year in the Orkneys. This geographical risk is established by the age of 15 years. If a person moves before that age, they acquire the risk of their destination; if they move after 15 years, they take their risk with them. Interestingly, 15 years is approximately the age at which the process of myelination finishes in the brain.

Familial factors are involved in the disease. The risk of developing multiple sclerosis is one in 50 for offspring of a patient, one in 20 for a sibling and one in three for an identical twin.

Pathology

The basic process is demyelination. Macroscopically, this is seen as multiple grey regions within the white matter of the brain and spinal cord that range in size from a couple of millimetres to several centimetres. Any part of the CNS white matter can be affected, but common sites are the optic nerves, long tracts of the spinal cord and the periventricular white matter.

Microscopically, the first changes are perivenular cuffing and permeation of tissue by chronic inflammatory cells, mainly T cells and macrophages. The myelin lamellae of oligodendrocytes vacuolate, split and fragment. The debris is removed by microglia and macrophages. Astrocytes proliferate. Ultimately, the oligodendrocytes are lost. The axons are undamaged.

The cause of the demyelination is uncertain. Defects in the blood–brain barrier and T cell-mediated immunity have been proposed and the variation in incidence with latitude suggests an environmental component.

Pathophysiology

Demyelination of the axons slows axonal conduction. There can be complete conduction block, or a partial block at high frequencies. The demyelinated axons become unstable and can discharge spontaneously, hence some of the paraesthesias that may be encountered in multiple sclerosis. Discharge may also be precipitated by mechanical stress, hence L'Hermitte's sign. An increased temperature slows axonal conduction and this can produce noticeable effects in multiple sclerosis. In addition, demyelinated axons can communicate inappropriately (or short circuit) with each other.

Multiple sclerosis encompasses both motor and sensory features. The former includes complex movement disorders, but the basic paralysis is that of an upper motor neurone lesion as the disease is one of CNS myelin.

Other forms of CNS demyelination

Acute disseminated encephalomyelitis

This acute disease is rare. It can develop after an infection or after a vaccination. The vaccines primarily associated with the disease are smallpox and rabies, neither of which is in routine use. The post-infectious type follows childhood viral infections and can complicate approximately one in 1000 cases of measles.

Numerous foci of demyelination are scattered throughout the brain and spinal cord. The death rate is high and many of the survivors have persistent deficits.

Acute necrotising haemorrhage encephalomyelitis

This tends to affect children and young adults. The name encapsulates the pathological changes, although it should be emphasised that a high volume of white matter is destroyed.

Central pontine myelinolysis

This is a disorder in which there is destruction of the myelin within the pons. It is usually associated with rapid correction of hyponatraemia. The degree of damage can vary from being symptomless to coma or the locked-in syndrome.

Guillain–Barré syndrome

Definition

Guillain–Barré syndrome is an autoimmune condition in which there is acute demyelination of the peripheral nerves.

Epidemiology

The incidence is 1–2 per 100 000 per year and does not show the geographical variation of multiple sclerosis. All ages can be affected and the male to female ratio is equal.

Pathology

The majority of cases of Guillain–Barré syndrome occur 1–3 weeks after a respiratory or gastrointestinal infection. *Campylobacter gastroenteritis* is the most common organism, but a variety of other agents may lead to the condition. Non-infectious causes include lymphoma.

There is an autoimmune reaction against the myelin of the peripheral nervous system. Lymphocytes and macrophages infiltrate the nerve fibre and there is destruction of the myelin. In infectious causes, some form of cross-reactivity may be postulated.

As with multiple sclerosis, the axons are relatively spared. The pathophysiological behaviour is the same. The demyelinated axons have impaired conduction, both in terms of conduction velocity and the magnitude of the total impulse that reaches the synaptic terminal. However, whereas remyelination is unusual in multiple sclerosis, good resolution occurs in Guillain–Barré syndrome, provided that the patient can be supported through the acute paralysis. The process of remyelination is time consuming and recovery can be delayed for up to 18 months if axonal degeneration has recurred as axonal regrowth is a slow process (approximately 1–2 mm per day). There is complete recovery in 85%.

Both motor and sensory nerves are affected. Being a condition of peripheral nervous system myelin, the motor features are those of lower motor neurone lesions. Paralysis of the respiratory muscles occurs in severe disease.

Chronic inflammatory demyelinating polyradiculoneuropathy

This is a rare condition of peripheral nervous system myelin that progresses over months to years. Both motor and sensory neurones are involved.

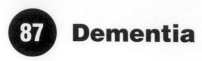 **Dementia**

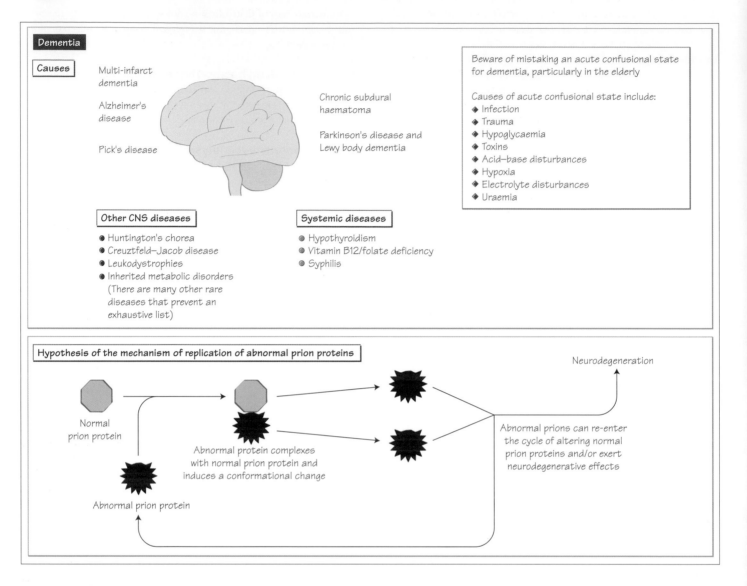

Dementia

Causes

Multi-infarct dementia

Alzheimer's disease

Pick's disease

Chronic subdural haematoma

Parkinson's disease and Lewy body dementia

Beware of mistaking an acute confusional state for dementia, particularly in the elderly

Causes of acute confusional state include:
◆ Infection
◆ Trauma
◆ Hypoglycaemia
◆ Toxins
◆ Acid–base disturbances
◆ Hypoxia
◆ Electrolyte disturbances
◆ Uraemia

Other CNS diseases
● Huntington's chorea
● Creuztfeld–Jacob disease
● Leukodystrophies
● Inherited metabolic disorders (There are many other rare diseases that prevent an exhaustive list)

Systemic diseases
● Hypothyroidism
● Vitamin B12/folate deficiency
● Syphilis

Hypothesis of the mechanism of replication of abnormal prion proteins

Normal prion protein

Abnormal prion protein

Abnormal protein complexes with normal prion protein and induces a conformational change

Neurodegeneration

Abnormal prions can re-enter the cycle of altering normal prion proteins and/or exert neurodegenerative effects

Systems pathology

Alzheimer's disease

Along with multi-infarct dementia, this is the most common form of dementia. The incidence rises with age, such that the prevalence is three per 1000 between 60 and 69 years, 30 per 1000 between 70 and 79 years, and 110 per 1000 between 80 and 89 years. However, the disease has been described at every stage of adult life.

The aetiology is uncertain, but familial forms of the disease exist and centre around presenilin 1 and 2, or the amyloid precursor protein found on chromosome 21. People with Down's syndrome (trisomy 21) develop Alzheimer's disease by 40 years. Possession of the apo eta4 apolipoprotein E polymorphism also predisposes to Alzheimer's disease.

Pathology

There is diffuse atrophy of the brain, with widening of the sulci and thinning of the cerebral cortex and symmetrical enlargement of the lateral ventricles. The involvement of the frontal, parietal and temporal lobes is uniform. In the simplest sense, there is neuronal loss in the affected regions of the brain, although the changes are more complex. The key features are neurofibrillary tangles, plaques and amyloid.

• Neurofibrillary tangles: these are found within neurones and consist of a twisted mass of abnormal tubules. They stain with tau protein.
• Amyloid: amyloid deposition is characteristic of Alzheimer's disease. The form of amyloid encountered is a protein 42 to 43 amino acids in length, that is the result of abnormal cleavage of the amyloid precursor protein encoded on chromosome 21.
• Plaques: amyloid is found in the cores of the extracellular Alzheimer plaques that are scattered throughout the cerebral cortex in which it is admixed with granules and filamentous material. The plaques may be surrounded by degenerated nerve terminals.

There can also be amyloid deposition within the walls of blood vessels.

Although the plaques and tangles are encountered throughout the cerebral cortex, they are particularly common in the hippocampus and entorhinal cortex. The distribution of the tangles and plaques in a postmortem examination of the brain is important in making a postmortem diagnosis of Alzheimer's disease.

Pick's disease

This is a neurodegenerative disease of unknown cause that is much rarer than Alzheimer's disease. The onset tends to be after 65 years and the disease is more common in women.

Pathology

Unlike Alzheimer's disease, Pick's disease tends to affect only the frontal and temporal lobes, while sparing the parietal. This zonation can be very striking, with normal gyri being juxtaposed against atrophied ones. The affected gyri can become paper thin and the involved part of the brain resembles a dry walnut. As with Alzheimer's disease, the lateral ventricles are enlarged.

Microscopically, there is neuronal loss, which is most marked in the first three layers of the cerebral cortex. The remaining neurones are swollen and feature Pick bodies, which can be stained with α-synuclein and are composed of straight fibrils.

Creuztfeld–Jakob disease

Creuztfeld–Jakob disease (CJD) is a prion disorder that is also known as subacute spongiform encephalopathy. The incidence is 1–2 per 1 000 000 per year. The incidence is increased in Libya, North Africa and Slovakia. The disease is familial and autosomal dominant in 5–15%. The onset is in late middle age, although new variant CJD tends to affect younger patients.

Pathology

Prions are proteins that behave as transmissible agents. The prion protein of CJD is naturally occurring within the brain but the wild type form differs from the pathological form in its structural configuration. The pathological form has the ability to alter the configuration of the wild type form to the pathological. The abnormal prion protein is remarkably resistant to most forms of sterilisation and requires autoclaving at 405K and increased pressure for 1 hour to be denatured.

The disease affects the cerebral and cerebellar cortices, either diffusely or predominating in the occipitoparietal region. There is neuronal loss and proliferation of astrocytes. The affected areas show vacuolation, hence the spongiform designation. The cerebellar involvement correlates with the ataxia that is often found in the presentation.

Other prion diseases

CJD dominates the discussion of prion diseases, but there are two other human prion diseases, Gerstmann–Straussler–Schenker syndrome and fatal familial insomnia.

Vascular dementia

This is a common form of dementia and is due to repeated infarction of the cerebral hemispheres, hence the alternative name of multi-infarct dementia. As such, the disease tends to display a stepwise progression, rather than a continuous decline, as each new infarct increases the degree of neuronal loss in a sudden burst.

General considerations

The above diseases share the unfortunate characteristic of being largely untreatable and irreversible. However, there are other conditions that can produce dementia that may be amenable to therapy, provided that the diagnosis is considered and made. These include:
• Vitamin B12 deficiency.
• Coeliac disease.
• Hypothyroidism.
• Hyperviscosity.
• Chronic subdural haematoma.
• Neuronal syphilis.
• Depression.
• Vasculitis.
• Uncontrolled epilepsy.
• Normal pressure hydrocephalus.

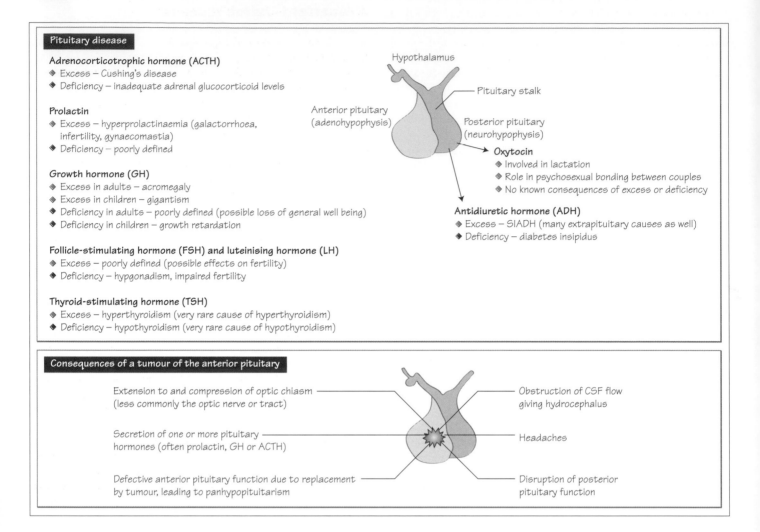

Pituitary disease

Adrenocorticotrophic hormone (ACTH)
◆ Excess – Cushing's disease
◆ Deficiency – inadequate adrenal glucocorticoid levels

Prolactin
◆ Excess – hyperprolactinaemia (galactorrhoea, infertility, gynaecomastia)
◆ Deficiency – poorly defined

Growth hormone (GH)
◆ Excess in adults – acromegaly
◆ Excess in children – gigantism
◆ Deficiency in adults – poorly defined (possible loss of general well being)
◆ Deficiency in children – growth retardation

Follicle-stimulating hormone (FSH) and luteinising hormone (LH)
◆ Excess – poorly defined (possible effects on fertility)
◆ Deficiency – hypgonadism, impaired fertility

Thyroid-stimulating hormone (TSH)
◆ Excess – hyperthyroidism (very rare cause of hyperthyroidism)
◆ Deficiency – hypothyroidism (very rare cause of hypothyroidism)

Hypothalamus

Pituitary stalk

Anterior pituitary (adenohypophysis)

Posterior pituitary (neurohypophysis)

Oxytocin
◆ Involved in lactation
◆ Role in psychosexual bonding between couples
◆ No known consequences of excess or deficiency

Antidiuretic hormone (ADH)
◆ Excess – SIADH (many extrapituitary causes as well)
◆ Deficiency – diabetes insipidus

Consequences of a tumour of the anterior pituitary

Extension to and compression of optic chiasm (less commonly the optic nerve or tract)

Secretion of one or more pituitary hormones (often prolactin, GH or ACTH)

Defective anterior pituitary function due to replacement by tumour, leading to panhypopituitarism

Obstruction of CSF flow giving hydrocephalus

Headaches

Disruption of posterior pituitary function

Syndrome of inappropriate ADH secretion

The syndrome of inappropriate antidiuretic hormone (ADH) secretion (SIADH) is a condition in which the secretion of ADH by the posterior pituitary gland is disregulated, increased and disproportionate to the serum osmolarity.

Causes

In general terms, SIADH can be caused by pathology in the head or the chest, plus a few drugs and miscellaneous entities. A more enumerated list is as follows:
• Cerebral abscess.
• Encephalitis.
• Intracranial haemorrhage.
• Intracranial tumour.
• Meningitis.
• Skull fracture.
• Bronchial cancer.
• Empyema.
• Lung abscess.
• Pneumonia.

• Tuberculosis.
• Hodgkin's lymphoma.
• Pancreatic cancer.
• Prostatic cancer.
• Thymoma.
• Acute intermittent porphyria.
• Guillain–Barré syndrome.
• Hypothyroidism.
• Systemic lupus erythematosus.
• Carbamazepine.
• Chlorpromazine.
• Chlorpropamide.
• Cyclophosphamide.
• Vinca alkaloids.
• Tricyclic antidepressants.

Pathology

The excess ADH causes the kidney to conserve water. This dilutes the plasma and reduces its osmolarity. Oedema tends not to occur because there is no concurrent sodium retention. The reduction in serum osmolarity is mainly through hyponatraemia, which presents as headache, lethargy and weakness, through confusion, cramps and weakness to convulsions, coma and death. Hasty correction of the hyponatraemia may precipitate central pontine myelinolysis.

Diabetes insipidus

Diabetes insipidus is the production of large volumes of dilute urine and is due to either a failure of the posterior pituitary to produce ADH (cranial) or a failure of the kidney to respond to it (nephrogenic).

Causes

Both forms can be familial. Cranial diabetes insipidus tends to be due to trauma, surgical resection of pituitary tumours, infiltration of the posterior pituitary by primary or secondary tumours, infections and diseases such as sarcoidosis, Langerhan's cell histiocytosis and amyloidosis. Nephrogenic causes include obstructive uropathy, hypokalaemia or hypercalcaemia, sickle cell anaemia and amyloidosis.

Pathology

Diabetes insipidus has the opposite biochemical manifestations to SIADH. There is water wasting by the kidney, resulting in an increase in serum osmolarity and hypernatraemia.

Hypopituitarism

Hypopituitarism is a failure of the pituitary gland to secrete adequate levels of its various hormones.

Causes

- Meningitis.
- Encephalitis.
- Syphilis.
- Intracranial tumour including craniopharyngioma.
- Metastases.
- Surgery.
- Skull fracture.
- Infarction.
- Sarcoidosis.
- Langerhan's cell histiocytosis.
- Haemochromatosis.
- Radiation.
- Chemotherapy.
- Anorexia nervosa.

Hypothalamic dysfunction can produce secondary hypopituitarism.

Pathology

The changes within the pituitary will reflect those of the underlying cause. Infarction can either be due to hypertension, when it may be referred to as apoplexy, or secondary to hypotension, most commonly in the postpartum period (Sheehan's syndrome).

The systemic pathophysiology will reflect the degree of hypopituitarism, the pituitary hormones that are affected and the age of the patient. For example, the effects of growth hormone deficiency are poorly described in adults, but are considerable in a child.

Pituitary tumours

Pituitary tumours generally arise in the anterior pituitary and are adenomas. Their classification reflects the size of the tumour and the hormones it secretes.

Microadenomas are under 1 cm in maximum dimension whereas macroadenomas are larger than 1 cm. The tumours form nodules and are soft. The cells are arranged as glandular structures and there is usually little stroma. Adenocarcinomas can also occur and are characterised by the common features of adenocarcinomas in general.

Previously, pituitary adenomas were divided into chromophobe and chromophil (acidophil or basophil) categories. This has been superseded by a classification based on the hormone(s) secreted by the tumour. Macroadenomas are often non-secretory. A secretory tumour can produce more than one hormone. The most common hormones released by the tumour are prolactin, growth hormone and adrenocorticotrophic hormone. Thyroid-stimulating hormone (TSH) secreting tumours are especially rare.

Hormone production by the tumour can be the mechanism of presentation, but the tumour may also declare its presence by mass effects. These can include the non-specific feature of headache, but also the far more specific bitemporal hemianopia. The hemianopia is due to extension of the tumour out of the pituitary fossa to exert pressure on the optic chiasm. Less commonly disseminated is the fact that the tumour may extend in such a way as to impinge upon one of the optic nerves or optic tracts, yielding the corresponding visual field defects.

Rarely, the tumour may not come to medical attention until more extensive local spread has occurred. Other structures that can be involved by local spread include the temporal lobe, cavernous sinus, third ventricle, hypothalamus and skull base (yielding cerebrospinal fluid (CSF) rhinorrhoea).

Craniopharyngioma

A craniopharyngioma is a congenital abnormality that is derived from remnants of Rathke's pouch. The tumour is usually located above the pituitary fossa/sella turcica, but occasionally is positioned within it. The tumour is partially cystic and is often calcified. It is ovoid, lobulated and possesses a smooth surface. The tumour is composed of epithelial cells that can show squamoid differentiation and may have a variety of patterns of growth. The background stroma is formed of loosely arranged stellate cells.

Craniopharyngiomas present with mass effects, usually visual field disturbances, headache, pituitary dysfunction and obstruction to the flow of CSF.

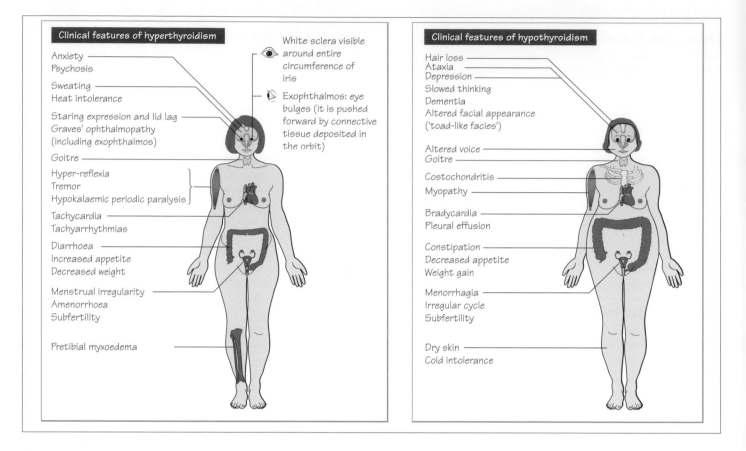

Clinical features of hyperthyroidism

Anxiety
Psychosis

Sweating
Heat intolerance

Staring expression and lid lag
Graves' ophthalmopathy
(including exophthalmos)

Goitre

Hyper-reflexia
Tremor
Hypokalaemic periodic paralysis

Tachycardia
Tachyarrhythmias

Diarrhoea
Increased appetite
Decreased weight

Menstrual irregularity
Amenorrhoea
Subfertility

Pretibial myxoedema

White sclera visible around entire circumference of iris

Exophthalmos: eye bulges (it is pushed forward by connective tissue deposited in the orbit)

Clinical features of hypothyroidism

Hair loss
Ataxia
Depression
Slowed thinking
Dementia
Altered facial appearance
('toad-like facies')

Altered voice
Goitre

Costochondritis

Myopathy

Bradycardia
Pleural effusion

Constipation
Decreased appetite
Weight gain

Menorrhagia
Irregular cycle
Subfertility

Dry skin
Cold intolerance

Hyperthyroidism, e.g. Graves' disease

Definition

Graves' disease is an autoimmune disorder in which there are circulating autoantibodies that cross-react with the thyroid-stimulating hormone (TSH) receptors on thyroid epithelium, causing aberrant stimulation.

Epidemiology

Graves' disease accounts for 75% of cases of hyperthyroidism. It tends to present between 20 and 40 years of age. The male : female ratio is 1 : 5.

Risk factors

There is a strong familial predisposition. In Caucasians, Graves' disease is associated with HLA-A1, -B8 and -DR3, whereas the association is with HLA-B36 in the Japanese and HLA-B46 in the Chinese.

Pathology

The definition given above summarises the basic pathogenetic mechanism. This causes a uniform enlargement of the thyroid, which may reach several times its normal size. The follicular epithelium is hyperplastic and may show papillary infoldings. The high activity of the epithelium means that there is little stored colloid and that which is present often has a scalloped border to it. A lymphocytic infiltrate can be present and may show germinal centre formation.

Many of the features of Graves' ophthalmopathy are specific to the disease and reflect an inflammatory process in the extraocular orbital tissues that shows chronic inflammation and oedema. Ultimately, this can progress to muscle fibre loss and fibrosis. Lid retraction is due to sympathetic overactivation and is found in hyperthyroidism in general. The lid retraction may give the impression of exophthalmos, but genuine exophthalmos is encountered only in Graves' disease and reflects the inflammatory swelling of the orbital soft tissues.

Hypothyroidism, e.g. Hashimoto's thyroiditis

Definition

Hashimoto's thyroiditis is an autoimmune disease in which autoantibodies are directed against the thyroid, leading to loss of thyroid epithelial tissue.

Epidemiology

The disease tends to develop between 30 and 50 years and is considerably more common in women (up to 20 times). There is an association with HLA-DR3 and -DR5.

Pathology

The thyroid shows a widespread infiltrate of chronic inflammatory cells that include lymphocytes, plasma cells and macrophages. There are numerous lymphoid follicles in which germinal centres are present. The infiltrate replaces the normal thyroid tissue.

The follicles are small and atrophic. The follicular cells can exhibit Hürthle cell changes in which they become enlarged and have abundant eosinophilic cytoplasm due to the accumulation of mitochondria. These cells are also known as Ashkenazy cells. It should be noted that Hürthle cells can be also be found in a variety of thyroid tumours and while the term Hürthle cell tumour may be employed, this is not a specific entity in itself but a morphological variant of the other thyroid tumours that are discussed elsewhere.

The autoantibodies are antimicrosomal in most cases and there are antibodies to thyroglobulin in 50%.

Hashimoto's thyroiditis is a risk factor for lymphoma of the thyroid. Hashimoto's thyroiditis generally causes hypothyroidism but in the initial stages of the chronic inflammatory cell infiltrate there may be hyperthyroidism.

DeQuervain's thyroiditis

Definition

DeQuervain's thyroiditis is a granulomatous disease of the thyroid that is due to viral infection. Assorted viruses have been implicated.

Epidemiology

The presentation is usually between 20 and 50 years of age. The male : female ratio is 1 : 3.

Pathology

Initially, the thyroid gland displays an acute inflammatory cell infiltrate. This is followed by an infiltrate of lymphocytes and macrophages, which are accompanied by a granulomatous reaction that includes giant cells. Fibrosis may develop.

At first, there is destruction of follicles. The resulting release of colloid causes transient hyperthyroidism. Once this surge of thyroxine release is over, hypothyroidism ensues while the gland recovers from the inflammatory process. During the process, the gland is enlarged, sometimes asymmetrically.

Riedel's thyroiditis

This is a very rare condition in which there is replacement of the thyroid gland by dense fibrous tissue. This process can extend into the soft tissues of the neck. There is an association with retroperitoneal and mediastinal fibrosis.

Goitre

A goitre is an enlargement of the thyroid gland. The term is generally reserved for non-neoplastic processes. Globally, the most common cause is iodine deficiency. In the UK, goitres are usually multinodular goitres. Rarely, inherited defects in the synthesis of thyroid hormones (dyshormogenesis) are the cause.

A goitre due to iodine deficiency will demonstrate diffuse enlargement in response to persistent stimulation by TSH, which is in turn due to inadequate levels of circulating thyroxine due to a lack of the iodine required for the production of the thyroxine.

The aetiology of multinodular goitres is uncertain but the disorder may represent an abnormal hyperplasia. Like most thyroid conditions, it is more common in women. The thyroid is composed of multiple nodules that are separated by fibrous bands. The nodules contain thyroid follicles which range in size from very small to very large. The large follicles contain abundant colloid. The degree of enlargement can be marked, reaching 500 g (N = 130 g) or more, and is usually asymmetrical. Significant enlargement can compress the trachea. There may also be retrosternal extension of the goitre.

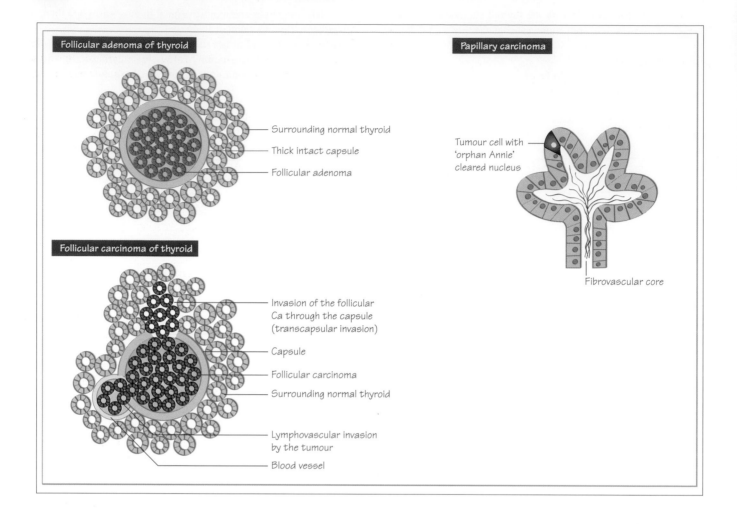

Follicular adenoma

Definition

Follicular adenoma is a benign glandular tumour of the follicular epithelium of the thyroid.

Pathology

Follicular adenomas are typically solitary lesions and are composed of thyroid follicles. The follicles may be similar in size to those of the adjacent gland, or smaller (microfollicular) or larger (macrofollicular). The adenoma is always surrounded by a well-defined capsule and the adenoma does not invade through the capsule.

Clinical correlations

Follicular adenomas are one cause of a solitary nodule in the thyroid gland. The nodule is 'cold' on radionucleotide scanning in 90% of cases, requiring that distinction from a malignant tumour be made by other means. The adenoma is hormonally active ('hot') in 10% and can therefore be a cause of hyperthyroidism.

Follicular carcinoma

Definition

Follicular carcinoma is a malignant tumour that is derived from the follicular epithelium of the thyroid gland.

Epidemiology

The tumour tends to present around 50 years of age and accounts for 5% of thyroid cancers, with an incidence of about one per 1 000 000 per year. It is more common in women.

Pathology

Most of the architectural and cytological features of a follicular carcinoma resemble those of an adenoma, although a wider variety of growth patterns may be seen. However, follicular carcinomas display invasion through their capsule and into the adjacent thyroid gland. There is also invasion of lymphovascular channels outside the capsule. These two features define the lesion as a follicular carcinoma rather than an adenoma. Some tumours show only focal invasion and are termed microinvasive. Others exhibit widespread invasion and are designated widely invasive.

Pattern of spread
Minimally invasive carcinomas are very seldom associated with distant metastases. Widely invasive tumours frequently demonstrate distant metastases. These are haematogenous and are frequently to the bone.

Papillary carcinoma
Definition
Papillary carcinoma is a malignant tumour of the epithelium of the thyroid that exhibits characteristic nuclear features.

Epidemiology
Papillary carcinoma has an incidence of 15 per 1 000 000 per year and constitutes 80% of thyroid cancers. The average age at presentation is 40 years and the tumour is more common in females.

Pathology
There is a considerable variation in the size of tumours at the time of presentation. Some are found incidentally as microscopic foci, while others are large. The tumours are generally white and firm and only 10% have a macroscopically apparent capsule. Many tumours are single but intrathyroid deposits may be found, giving a multifocal lesion.

Papillary carcinoma is defined by a set of microscopic features that are present in the nuclei of the constituent cells. The cells are crowded and overlapping. They possess grooves in their nuclei. An exaggerated version of the nuclear groove is the cytoplasmic nuclear pseudoinclusion in which the fold that produces the groove effect is so marked as to give the impression of a blob of cytoplasm within the nucleus. The nuclei are also optically clear. These are referred to as 'orphan Annie' nuclei, named after a cartoon character of rapidly decreasing familiarity to newer generations of medical students. A single nucleus does not show all of the features, but they are widespread throughout the tumour as a whole.

Many papillary carcinomas have a papillary architecture in which the cells line delicate fibrovascular papillae that have a complex arrangement. However, other variants exist, the most problematic of which is the follicular variant. This type possesses a follicular architecture but the tumour cells display the typical nuclear characteristics of a papillary carcinoma. The importance of recognising papillary carcinoma is that this tumour is often multifocal and requires total thyroidectomy, whereas others, e.g. follicular carcinoma, can be treated by local (partial) resection. Other variants also exist but are rare.

Papillary thyroid carcinomas often include psammoma bodies.

Pattern of spread
Direct extension beyond the thyroid gland is encountered in around 25% of cases. Local cervical lymph node metastases are common and may be the mass that causes the tumour to be recognised. Distant metastases are less common than in other types of thyroid cancer, but the lung is the principal site if they do occur.

Medullary carcinoma
Definition
Medullary carcinoma is a thyroid malignancy that is derived from the calcitonin-secreting interfollicular C cells.

Epidemiology
The tumour is familial in 20%, either as part of the multiple endocrine neoplasia 2 (MEN2) syndrome or as an isolated inherited condition; the rest are sporadic. Familial cases present 10 years earlier at 35 years.

Pathology
The tumour is circumscribed but non-encapsulated, firm and grey and tends to be found in the upper part of the thyroid.

The cells are ovoid to polyhedral and have granular, eosinophilic cytoplasm. The cells can be arranged in nests, trabeculae, papillae or glandular formations in a highly vascular stroma that may be sclerotic and often includes amyloid. The cells express calcitonin.

Pattern of spread
There is local invasion. Lymph node metastases are cervical and mediastinal. Distant metastases are to the lungs, liver and bone.

Prognosis
The best prognosis is in young females with the familial form.

Anaplastic carcinoma
Definition
Anaplastic carcinoma is a highly malignant tumour of the thyroid epithelium that does not show differentiation into any other subtype.

Epidemiology
Anaplastic carcinoma is a disease of the elderly. The female predominance of the lower grade lesions is lost.

Pathology
This carcinoma is a rapidly growing mass that invades widely through the tissues of the neck where it can compress structures such as the trachea or oesophagus. Haemorrhage and necrosis are frequent.

Various cell morphologies are seen, all of which share the characteristic of being markedly atypical.

General staging
All thyroid tumours are staged using the TNM system (see Chapter 28). Size and extrathyroid extension are the main defining variables.

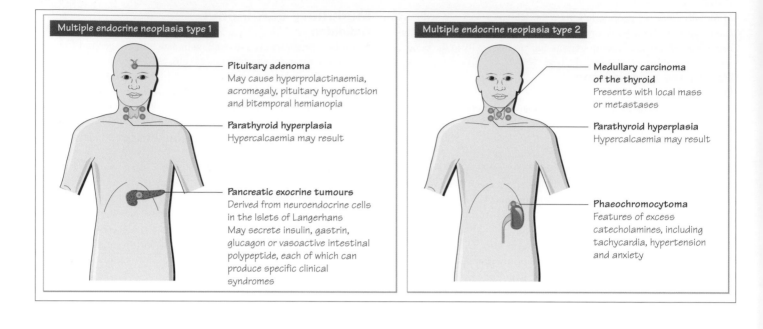

Multiple endocrine neoplasia type 1

Pituitary adenoma
May cause hyperprolactinaemia, acromegaly, pituitary hypofunction and bitemporal hemianopia

Parathyroid hyperplasia
Hypercalcaemia may result

Pancreatic exocrine tumours
Derived from neuroendocrine cells in the Islets of Langerhans
May secrete insulin, gastrin, glucagon or vasoactive intestinal polypeptide, each of which can produce specific clinical syndromes

Multiple endocrine neoplasia type 2

Medullary carcinoma of the thyroid
Presents with local mass or metastases

Parathyroid hyperplasia
Hypercalcaemia may result

Phaeochromocytoma
Features of excess catecholamines, including tachycardia, hypertension and anxiety

Table 91.1 Clinical features of hyper- and hypoparathyroidism.

Hyperparathyroidism
(due to Ca2+ liberation from bone)
- Hypercalcaemia-related
  - Nausea, vomiting, anorexia
  - Thirst and polyuria
  - Lethargy, coma, convulsions
- Osteopenia-related
  - Bone pain, pathological fracture
- Calcium deposition-related
  - Renal stones, nephrocalcinosis
- Other
  - Peptic ulcer, MEN, pancreatitis

Hypoparathyroidism
(reflect hypocalcaemia)
- Sensory nerve impairment
  - Tingling and numbness
- Muscle spasm
  - Cramps (especially laryngeal muscles, causing stridor), hyper-reflexia, tetany (+ve Chvostek's Trousseau's signs)
- Agitation and convulsions (especially in children)

Systems pathology

The parathyroids are small glands that are located in the neck. They produce parathyroid hormone (PTH), which is involved in regulating calcium metabolism. PTH causes an increase in blood calcium, a fall in blood phosphate and increased bone resorption.

The anatomy of the parathyroid glands is variable. The normal arrangement is two glands, superior and inferior, on each side, deep to the thyroid. However, the number can vary and the glands may be situated within the thyroid, the thymus or pericardium or be positioned behind the oesophagus.

Hyperparathryoidism
Primary
In primary hyperparathyroidism, there is an inappropriate, excessive elevation of PTH secretion. It is due either to parathyroid hyperplasia (15–20%), a parathyroid adenoma (80%) or parathyroid carcinoma (2–3%) and is the joint commonest cause of hypercalcaemia along with malignancy. Primary hyperparathyroidism tends to present from 20 to 50 years and is slightly more common in women.

Hyperplasia affects more than one gland, whereas adenomas and carcinomas usually occur in only one gland. In hyperplasia the changes are diffuse within the affected glands, whereas in an adenoma or carcinoma there is a compressed rim of normal parathyroid around the edge of the tumour. In addition, tumours lose the admixed fat that is seen within a non-neoplastic parathyroid gland.

As with the adrenal tumours, the separation of a parathyroid adenoma from a carcinoma on histological grounds is problematic. The definitive criterion, the presence of distant metastases, is clinically unhelpful as the aim is to predict dissemination and prevent it. However, parathyroid carcinomas tend to be larger, associated with greater degrees of hypercalcaemia and feature fibrous bands.

Secondary
Secondary hyperparathyroidism is a response to hypocalcaemia. The usual setting is chronic renal failure.

Tertiary
Tertiary hyperparathyroidism follows long-term secondary hyperparathyroidism and is due to the development of autonomous parathyroid hyperplasia that does not respond to the usual homeostatic mechanisms.

Bone changes
The usual action of PTH is to increase the activity of osteoclasts to elevate levels of bone resorption. This mobilises calcium from the skeleton into the blood as well as promoting bone turnover and remodelling. This is seen histologically as a greater number of osteoclasts on the surface of the bone and within the trabeculae. There is an accompanying increase in the number of osteoblasts as part of the remodelling process.

In hyperparathyroidism, there is a net loss of bone. There is inadequate replacement of the resorbed bone by irregular trabeculae of woven bone. Fibrosis develops around the sites of reabsorption and also within the marrow spaces. Cystic change may occur in the fibrotic regions, hence the term osteitis fibrosa cystica. Some regions of fibrosis contain abundant haemosiderin and numerous osteoclasts and are referred to as brown tumours.

Howship's lacunae are scalloped zones on the surface of the bone that contain giant multinucleated osteoclasts.

Hypoparathyroidism
This is a deficiency of PTH and results in hypocalcaemia and hyperphosphataemia. The causes include inadvertent removal of parathyroid tissue at thyroidectomy, autoimmune causes, neck irradiation, haemochromatosis, di George syndrome, inherited genetic defects and a deficiency of magnesium (which is required for PTH metabolism).

Pseudohypoparathyroidism
Pseudohypoparathyroidism comprises three conditions in which the metabolic features of a deficiency of PTH are present, but in which PTH levels are elevated. The basic process is a failure of the body to respond to PTH. In most cases, this is due to a defect in the α-subunit of the G protein involved in the PTH receptor.

Most patients manifest Albright's hereditary osteodystrophy in which there is a short stature, round face, brachydactyly and heterotopic calcification.

Pseudopseudohypoparathyroidism
Remarkably, *pseudo*pseudohypoparathyroidism exists and is so-called because it seems to be pseudohyoparathyroidism but is not. Calcium and PTH levels are normal, but the appearances of Albright's hereditary osteodystrophy are present and thus the condition may be a mild form of type 1a pseudohypoparathyroidism.

Multiple endocrine neoplasia
The multiple endocrine neoplasia (MEN) syndromes are inherited conditions in which there is a tendency to form tumours within specific endocrine organs. The prevalence is one in 10 000 to one in 30 000.

MEN1
MEN1 is the association of parathyroid hyperplasia, pituitary adenomas and pancreatic endocrine tumours and is sometimes referred to as Werner's syndrome. The condition is autosomal dominant with the gene responsible, *menin*, located on chromosome 11q13. Menin is believed to be a tumour suppressor gene. The genetic behaviour of the disease is considered to be an example of Knudson's two hit hypothesis.

The pancreatic tumours can secrete a variety of hormones, with gastrin and insulin accounting for the majority. The pancreatic tumours tend to be responsible for mortality in MEN1.

MEN2a
MEN2a is also known as Sipple's syndrome and features medullary carcinoma of the thyroid, parathyroid hyperplasia and phaeochromocytoma. It is autosomal dominant and is due to mutations in the *RET* proto-oncogene, which is located on chromosome 10q11.2 and is a tyrosine kinase. In MEN2, mutations in *RET* result in an abnormally elevated level of signalling.

MEN2b
MEN2b has the same cause and pattern of tumours as MEN2a but differs in that sufferers have an additional tendency to develop submucosal fibromas and possess a physique reminiscent of that seen in Marfan's disease.

Familial medullary thyroid carcinoma
This is sometimes grouped with MEN2 as it is also due to a mutation in the *RET* proto-oncogene. While the incidence of parathyroid hyperplasia and phaeochromocytoma in MEN2 is around 70–80% for each, medullary carcinoma is encountered in almost 100% of cases.

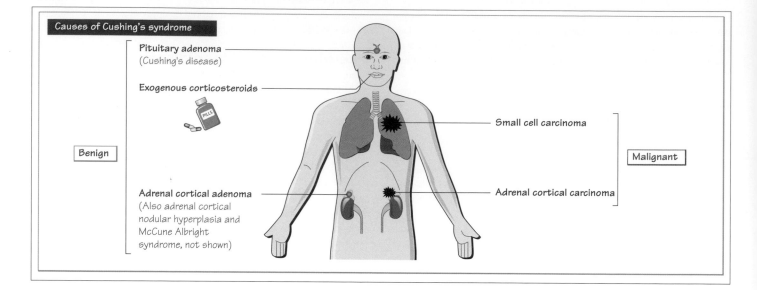

Causes of Cushing's syndrome

Pituitary adenoma
(Cushing's disease)

Exogenous corticosteroids

Benign

Adrenal cortical adenoma
(Also adrenal cortical
nodular hyperplasia and
McCune Albright
syndrome, not shown)

Small cell carcinoma

Malignant

Adrenal cortical carcinoma

Phaeochromocytoma

Definition
Phaeochromocytoma is a cathecholamine-producing tumour of the adrenal medulla that may also arise from sympathetic ganglia.

Epidemiology
Phaeochromocytoma is a rare tumour that accounts for one in 1000 cases of hypertension. The tumour tends to present in young to middle-aged adults. In 10% of cases the tumour is familial, often as part of multiple endocrine neoplasia 2 (MEN2).

Pathology
Phaeochromocytoma is bilateral in 10% of cases and malignant in 10%; the tumour has an extra-adrenal location in 10%. The tumour arises in the adrenal medulla and forms an orange-brown mass.

A phaeochromocytoma is formed of nests of cells that are divided by a delicate fibrovascular stroma. Sustentacular cells are specialised supporting cells that are found at the edges of the nests.

The distinction between benign and malignant phaeochromocytomas can be difficult in the absence of metastases. Malignant tumours tend to be larger, but conventional histological parameters such as lymphovascular invasion lose their usual utility.

Addison's disease

Definition
Addison's disease is primary adrenocortical deficiency.

Epidemiology
The incidence is approximately eight per 100 000 per year with an equal male to female ratio and a wide age range.

Causes
• Autoimmune causes.
• Tuberculosis.
• Metastatic tumour.
• Lymphoma.
• Amyloidosis.
• Haemochromatosis.
• Intra-adrenal haemorrhage.
• Adrenoleukodystrophy.
• Hereditary unresponsiveness to adrenocorticotrophic hormone (ACTH).
• Polyglandular deficiency type I.
• Polyglandular deficiency type II.
• Bilateral adrenalectomy.

Pathology
• Autoimmune adrenalitis accounts for 70% of cases. The adrenal glands are atrophied due to loss of the cortical cells. Almost all patients have autoantibodies to the 21-hydroxylase enzyme.
• Polyglandular deficiency type I is an autosomal recessive condition that encompasses Addison's disease, chronic mucocutaneous candidiasis, hypoparathyroidism, dental enamel hypoplasia, alopecia and primary gonadal failure.
• Polyglandular deficiency type II is autosomal dominant, associated with HLA-DR3 and features Addison's disease, hypothyroidism, type 1 diabetes mellitus, hypogonadism, pernicious anaemia and vitiligo.

Clinical correlations
Many of the features of Addison's disease can be predicted from a knowledge of the role of adrenal corticosteroids but are outside the size constraints of this book. However, attention is drawn to the frequent coexistence of hypothyroidism and hypoadrenalism in the elderly. Rapid correction of hypothyroidism in these patients places an overwhelming stress demand on the adrenal gland and precipitates an Addisonian crisis. This can be averted by giving exogenous corticosteroids with the thyroid replacement. Dexamethasone has the advantage of not interfering with the synacthen tests that will be required.

Secondary hypoadrenalism
This is typically due to an abrupt cessation of exogenous corticosteroids

Systems pathology

in situations where the duration and dose of the exogenous steroids has led to the suppression of endogenous ACTH release and reversible atrophy of the adrenal cortex. The other rare causes are pituitary surgery, hypopituitarism and hypothalamic disease.

Cushing's syndrome

Cushing's syndrome is the condition that results from prolonged exposure to inappropriately increased levels of glucocorticoids.

Causes

- ACTH-secreting pituitary tumour (Cushing's disease).
- Other ACTH-secreting tumour (e.g. small cell carcinoma of the lung).
- Exogenous steroids.
- Adrenal adenoma.
- Adrenal carcinoma.
- McCune–Albright syndrome.
- Macroscopic nodular adrenal hyperplasia.
- Alcohol.

Pathology

- Cushing's disease causes 70–80% of cases of Cushing's syndrome (after exogenous steroids are excluded). The presentation is usually in the third or fourth decade and the male : female ratio is 1 : 3. Cushing's disease is produced by a pituitary adenoma that secretes ACTH. The adenoma is normally a microadenoma. The persistently elevated ACTH causes bilateral hyperplasia of the adrenal cortex.
- Ectopic secretion of ACTH contributes 15–20% of cases and in half of these the source is a small cell carcinoma of the lung. Other sources include carcinoid tumours, phaeochromocytoma and thyroid medullary carcinoma. Cushing's disease due to ectopic ACTH secretion by a malignant tumour often lacks some of the typical Cushingoid appearances due to superimposed tumour cachexia. In addition, hyperkalaemia tends to be more prominent than in other causes of Cushing's syndrome.
- Adrenal adenomas and carcinomas account for around 10% of cases. Both form masses centred on the adrenal cortex that are composed of cells which resemble those of the normal adrenal cortex. As with parathyroid tumours and phaeochromocytomas, reliable distinction between benign and malignant tumours on histological grounds may not be straightforward as the usual parameters that are employed

elsewhere are of less value. However, carcinomas tend to be larger and may feature regions of necrosis.

Incidental adrenal adenomas that are non-functioning are much more common than those that cause Cushing's syndrome. Their main clinical significance is that they can be discovered on abdominal CT scans that have been performed for other reasons. This can lead to further investigations to confirm the innocuous nature of the lesion.

- McCune–Albright syndrome is a G protein disease in which a mutation in the α-subunit leads to aberrant activation of adenyl cyclase. There is fibrous dysplasia, cutaneous pigmentation and hyperfunction of the pituitary, thyroid and adrenal glands and the gonads.
- Excessive consumption of alcohol can yield a pseudo-Cushing's syndrome.

Mineralocorticoid excess

Causes

- Conn's syndrome.
- Adrenal carcinoma.
- Glucocorticoid suppressible hyperaldosteronism.
- Congenital adrenal hyperplasia.
- Syndrome of apparent mineralocorticoid excess (SAME).
- Excess ACTH.

Pathology

- Conn's syndrome is an aldosterone-producing adrenal adenoma that tends to occur between 30 and 50 years with a male : female ratio of 1 : 2. It is around 20–30 times more common than an aldosterone-secreting adrenal carcinoma.
- Glucocorticoid suppressible hyperaldosteronism is an autosomal dominant condition located on chromosome 8 in which the regulatory region for 11β-hydroxylase is fused with the coding sequence for aldosterone synthetase. This aberrantly renders aldosterone synthesis under the control of ACTH.
- SAME is a consequence of the response of the kidney to aldosterone and cortisol. The renal aldosterone receptor actually has an equal affinity for aldosterone and cortisol. However, the enzyme 11β-hydroxysteroid dehydrogenase converts cortisol to cortisone, thereby shielding the kidney from cortisol. In SAME, this enzyme is either congenitally defective, or becomes inhibited by agents such as liquorice and carbenoxolone.

Systems pathology

Diabetes mellitus

Vascular problems are at the root of most diabetic complications and include:
- **Accelerated atherosclerosis** due to increased lipolysis, liberating FFA and cholesterol
- Diabetic **smokers** are particularly at risk of ischaemic necrosis and **gangrene** of extremities, **strokes** and **myocardial infarction**
- **Impaired wound healing** due to a combination of factors: atheroma of large and medium sized vessels and glycation of basement membrane proteins and wound-site collagen by AGEPs
- The classic '**diabetic foot**' is either cold, due to ischaemic problems, or warm and ulcerated due to peripheral neuropathy. In a 'Charcot's foot' the foot is warm and the joints are damaged

Diabetic neuropathies of several types, due to hyperglycaemic damage and damage to small nutrient vessels to nerves:
- Autonomic neuropathy: postural hypotension, atonic bladder, impotence, diarrhoea
- Distal sensory neuropathy: typical 'glove and stocking' distribution
- Distal motor neuropathy: wasting of muscles of hand and foot
- Diabetic amyotrophy: wasted quadriceps muscles, painful skin
- Mononeuritis multiplex favours 3rd cranial nerve, thus affects eye movements, but usually spares pupillary reflex

AGEP = advanced glycosylation end products

Ocular problems: occur 10-15 years earlier than the general population, affect 1/3 diabetic patients and cause blindness within 30 years in 5%
- Cataract formation: angiogenic factors cause new vessel formation over the lens, rendering it opaque Possibly glycation of proteins in lens matrix as well
- Retinopathies: stiffened capillaries due to glycated basement membranes leak, causing 'blot' haemorrhages, 'hard' exudates of plasma proteins and 'dot' microaneurysms. 'Cotton wool spots' occur when there is axonal ischaemic damage. Capillary proliferation causes proliferative retinopathy, scarring and related traction can cause retinal detachment
- The macula is often spared – its involvement is implied by impaired visual acuity

Renal disease
Occurs in 35-45% of type I DM, <20% type II DM, about 15–25 years after diagnosis
Stiffening of collagen due to cross-linkage of AGEPs, causing vascular rigidity and hypertension, retinopathy and renal vascular damage with glomerulosclerosis

Infection
- Skin infections, due to increased glucose in sweat
- Fungal infections, e.g. Candidiasis ('thrush') affecting vagina or pharynx
- Urinary tract infections (UTI), due to glycosuria, providing an energy source for pathogenic bacteria. Diabetics with UTI are at increased risk of acute papillary necrosis
- Sinusoidal colonisation by Aspergillus or Mucormycosis species

Comparison of hyper and hypoglycaemic symptoms

Hyperglycaemia
- Polydipsia
- Polyuria
- Fatigue
- Slow wound healing
- Impaired vision
- Ketone breath
- Coma

Hypoglycaemia
- Increased appetite
- Headache
- Weakness
- Loss of concentration
- Nausea
- Vomiting
- Blurred vision
- Coma

Causes of hypoglycaemia, other than excess insulin treatment in diabetes:
- Alcohol excess
- Renal or hepatic failure
- Tumour: Insulin-secreting tumour, e.g. neuroendocrine tumour of pancreas or duodenum, or tumours secreting insulin-like growth factor receptor II (IGF-II), e.g. pleural fibromas or sarcomas
- Adrenocortical failure
- Hypopituitarism

The urine in diabetes mellitus (DM) is sweet (*mellitus* = honey), due to failure of the pancreatic hormone, insulin, to clear glucose from the blood into the cells. It is characterised by 'starvation in the midst of plenty' since glucose is available in the blood, but cannot be utilised by the cells. This is in contrast to diabetes insipidus, due to failure of antidiuretic hormone (ADH) secretion by the pituitary, where the urine is very dilute.

The pancreatic islets of Langerhans make glucagon in α-cells, insulin in β-cells, pancreatic polypeptide in γ-cells and somatostatin in δ-cells. The islets have an independent blood supply and secrete hormones directly into the blood, with effects throughout the body.

Insulin is secreted in response to high plasma glucose. Glucose is converted to adenosine triphosphate (ATP) and, via several paths, stimulates an influx of Ca^{2+} into the cell, which causes insulin in granules within the β-cell to be secreted into the blood. Insulin stimulates insulin receptors on all other body cells to move their glucose transporter molecules to their surface membranes so that they can take in glucose to meet their energy needs.

Glucagon has the reverse action, and is released in response to low blood glucose levels. It mediates the catabolism of starch and other energy reserves to form glucose.

Epidemiology
• **Type I DM**: the incidence is 25 per 100 000, usually in white northern Europeans; prevalence is 0.5% of the UK population.
• **Type II DM**: the incidence is rising rapidly in the developed world, with a prevalence of 3–5% of the UK population. Subtypes of type II DM are:
  • **Maturity onset diabetes of the young**: the prevalence is 1–2% of diabetic patients, and so is rare.
  • **Gestational diabetes**: this occurs in about 4% of pregnancies, usually in the third trimester.

Aetiology and pathogenesis
• **Type I DM**: molecular mimicry following viral infection of the pancreas (e.g. mumps) is thought to lead to an autoimmune destruction of β-cells. There is a strong association with other autoimmune diseases.
• **Type II DM**: several possible points in the insulin–glucose pathway are affected; insulin receptor insensitivity is implicated by the fact that some patients have higher than normal insulin levels. Insulin receptor insensitivity may be related to adiponectin levels in the obese.
  • **Maturity onset diabetes of the young**: several gene defects have been identified affecting β-cell function, e.g. *MODY* 2 in which there is a glucokinase defect.
  • **Gestational diabetes**: the aetiology is unclear, but low adiponectin (which sensitises insulin receptors) levels may play a part. Thirty to 50% develop type II DM in the next 10 years.

Clinical features
Type I diabetes mellitus
Type I DM usually presents in under 25-year-olds (average age 13 years) who are normally thin. The symptoms can be insidious, with a gradual onset of malaise, weight loss and weakness, often with poor wound healing or skin infections. The classic symptoms are polydipsia, polyuria and nocturia, all of which are explained by the high urine output dictated by a high excretion of glucose, which is accompanied by excessive water loss due to osmotic diuresis.

Hyperglycaemia causes fat cells to undergo lipolysis, liberating fatty acids for energy production. In the process, ketone bodies accumulate, causing a metabolic acidosis. Ketone bodies, excreted in the breath, impart a characteristic 'acid-drop' smell. Ketone bodies impair brain function. Patients may be tachypnoeic (as the body attempts to correct the metabolic acidosis by excreting CO_2) and present with nausea or vomiting.

If the disease is not recognised at this stage, a calamitous presentation with ketoacidosis and hyperglycaemic coma may be the presenting feature, progressing to coma and death if untreated.

Treatment is with insulin and great caution as excessive amounts of insulin can cause such a profound drop in blood glucose that a hypoglycaemic coma with an even quicker onset of death may occur (the brain requires glucose for energy).

Type II diabetes mellitus
Type II DM is typically a disease of adulthood, often occurring in the elderly as an unsuspected phenomenon (identified on routine urine testing at a check up or when the patient presents with another complaint), or there may be mild symptoms of thirst and increased urine production, including nocturia. Increasingly it is presenting in younger, obese people as part of the metabolic syndrome. There is evidence for a genetic predisposition for type II DM.

Treatment is with drugs that stimulate insulin release from β-cells. Some patients respond at first to drugs, but may eventually require insulin.

Clinical diagnosis
Fasting hyperglycaemia and glycosuria are present in untreated diabetes. A glucose tolerance test shows elevated levels of blood glucose 2 hours after a 75 g glucose meal.

Gross features
On gross examination the pancreas appears unremarkable. However, there may be features such as atherosclerosis at unusual sites, e.g. the renal or pulmonary arteries, which should raise suspicion of DM.

Microscopic features
In type I DM there may be lymphocytic infiltration of the islets of Langerhans. More obvious in many patients is the typical diabetic glomerulosclerosis (Chapter 67).

Complications
These are summarised in the figure opposite. Complications involve all parts of the body, in particular the eye, blood vessels, nerves and kidney and relate to the presence of:
• Increased glucose, which dehydrates cells by drawing water from them by osmosis, which is then lost in the urine by osmotic diuresis.
• The generation of free radicals in pancreatic β-cells by oxidative phosphorylation of the excessive quantities of glucose, which accumulate within the cell, and the production of reactive oxygen species (ROS), which damage the β-cells and impair their ability to form and secrete insulin.
• Glycation of proteins throughout the body, including plasma albumin and tissue collagen, which form advanced glycation end-products that cross-link proteins such as collagens.

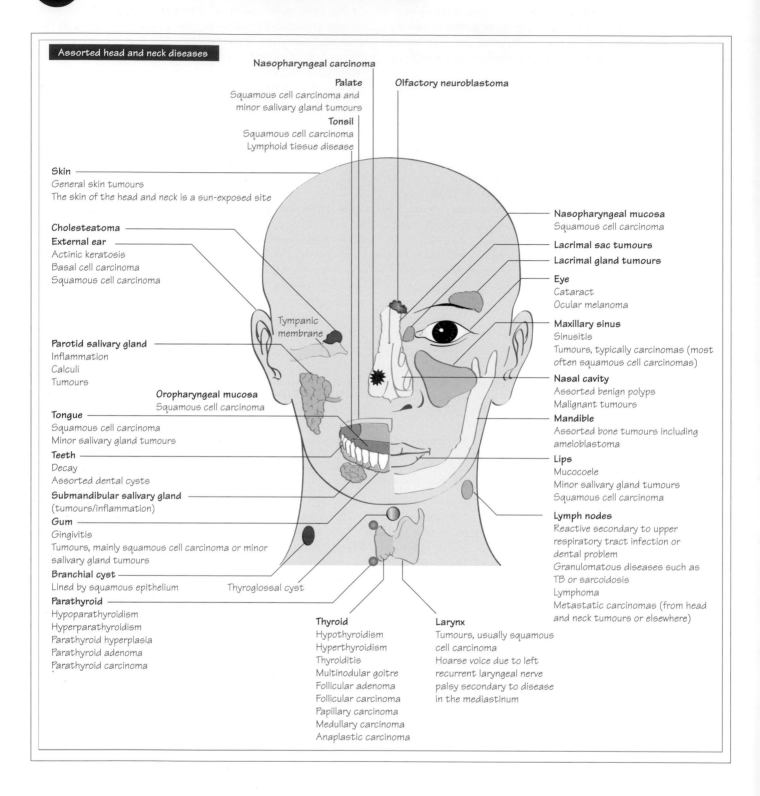

Assorted head and neck diseases

Nasopharyngeal carcinoma

Palate
Squamous cell carcinoma and minor salivary gland tumours

Tonsil
Squamous cell carcinoma
Lymphoid tissue disease

Olfactory neuroblastoma

Skin
General skin tumours
The skin of the head and neck is a sun-exposed site

Cholesteatoma
External ear
Actinic keratosis
Basal cell carcinoma
Squamous cell carcinoma

Tympanic membrane

Parotid salivary gland
Inflammation
Calculi
Tumours

Oropharyngeal mucosa
Squamous cell carcinoma

Tongue
Squamous cell carcinoma
Minor salivary gland tumours

Teeth
Decay
Assorted dental cysts

Submandibular salivary gland
(tumours/inflammation)

Gum
Gingivitis
Tumours, mainly squamous cell carcinoma or minor salivary gland tumours

Branchial cyst
Lined by squamous epithelium

Thyroglossal cyst

Parathyroid
Hypoparathyroidism
Hyperparathyroidism
Parathyroid hyperplasia
Parathyroid adenoma
Parathyroid carcinoma

Thyroid
Hypothyroidism
Hyperthyroidism
Thyroiditis
Multinodular goitre
Follicular adenoma
Follicular carcinoma
Papillary carcinoma
Medullary carcinoma
Anaplastic carcinoma

Larynx
Tumours, usually squamous cell carcinoma
Hoarse voice due to left recurrent laryngeal nerve palsy secondary to disease in the mediastinum

Nasopharyngeal mucosa
Squamous cell carcinoma

Lacrimal sac tumours
Lacrimal gland tumours

Eye
Cataract
Ocular melanoma

Maxillary sinus
Sinusitis
Tumours, typically carcinomas (most often squamous cell carcinomas)

Nasal cavity
Assorted benign polyps
Malignant tumours

Mandible
Assorted bone tumours including ameloblastoma

Lips
Mucocoele
Minor salivary gland tumours
Squamous cell carcinoma

Lymph nodes
Reactive secondary to upper respiratory tract infection or dental problem
Granulomatous diseases such as TB or sarcoidosis
Lymphoma
Metastatic carcinomas (from head and neck tumours or elsewhere)

Systems pathology

Head and neck pathology encompasses the diseases that are encountered in ENT surgery and maxillofacial surgery. Thyroid disease can also fall within the remit of head and neck surgeons.

The head and neck territory includes a variety of complex structures and organs, each of which can have numerous disorders. Within the space constraints of this book, it is possible only to give a very brief overview of a few of these.

Cholesteatoma

Cholesteatoma is a rather bizarre entity that occurs in the middle ear. It is an expansile cystic mass that is formed by cytologically innocuous, keratinising stratified squamous epithelium. Although not a malignant tumour, it nevertheless has the capacity to be locally destructive, possibly wrecking the middle and inner ear and even invading through the skull into the temporal lobe of the brain. The origin of cholesteatomas is uncertain, but theories revolve around retraction pockets of epithelium that arise from the tympanic membrane.

Salivary glands

Like most organs, the salivary glands can be affected by acute or chronic inflammation, the pathological changes of which reproduce the common elements of these two processes. Sjögren's syndrome is a specific, autoimmune disease in which the chronic inflammatory response is directed against salivary (and lacrimal gland) tissue. Sjögren's syndrome can be associated with other organ-specific autoimmune diseases.

Also in common with other secretory, duct-based organs, the salivary glands can develop calculi.

Tumours

Despite their small size in relation to total body mass, the salivary glands can generate a wide variety of tumours. It is important to remember that as well as the three major salivary glands, salivary gland tissue is also distributed in the lips, oral mucosa, tongue and larynx – all of which may manifest salivary gland tumours. The lung as well is also a rare site of salivary-type tumours.

The pleomorphic adenoma is the commonest primary salivary gland tumour and the parotid gland is frequently affected. Although benign, a pleomorphic adenoma can recur with considerable tenacity if not completely excised. As the name implies, a pleomorphic adenoma can adopt a variety of guises, but common to them all is the biphasic composition of an epithelial–myoepithelial element and a stromal component. The former can adopt numerous configurations, while the latter is characteristically myxochondroid and particularly striking on fine needle aspiration (FNA) slides.

Warthin's tumour is a benign neoplasm of the parotid gland in which complex papillary structures are lined by an outer layer of cuboidal cells and an inner layer of columnar cells that have granular, eosinophilic (oncocytic) cytoplasm. The stroma of the papillae contains a dense lymphoid infiltrate. The histological appearance is very characteristic.

Adenoid cystic carcinoma is a relatively low grade malignancy that nevertheless has an avidity for invading nerves, which enables it to recur with considerable facility. Microscopically, the tumour is formed by numerous arcades and cords and pseudoglandular and cribriform structures.

Other tumours include basal cell adenoma, canalicular adenoma, acinic cell carcinoma, mucoepidermoid carcinoma and salivary duct carcinoma, but these do not exhaust the list.

Nasal polyps

The commonest form of nasal polyps, the inflammatory or allergic type, are benign lesions that consist of polypoid, oedematous nasal mucosa (ciliated columnar glandular mucosa) in which there is a heavy, chronic, inflammatory cell infiltrate that features abundant eosinophils.

Various other morphological types of nasal polyps exist, including the inverted type in which stratified squamous mucosa grows inwards into the core of the polyp, such that the basal layer is on the outside rather than the inside. These have a tendency to local recurrence.

Unilateral nasal polyps are more likely to be of a problematic subtype than bilateral ones.

Tumours

Even allowing for the salivary gland neoplasms mentioned above, there are many head and neck tumours due to the diversity of tissue types that are normally present in this territory.

Squamous cell carcinoma

Squamous cell carcinoma is the commonest head and neck malignant tumour, due to the wide distribution of squamous epithelium in the head and neck mucosa. The lips, oral cavity, tongue, tonsils, larynx and sinuses can all generate squamous cell carcinomas. The principal risk factor is smoking. Alcohol has a lesser role. In the oral cavity, chewing betel nuts is a specific and characteristic risk factor, although in the UK the majority of cases of oral and glossal squamous cell carcinoma will arise in the absence of betel nut exposure.

Head and neck carcinomas spread to the cervical lymph nodes. The chain of lymph nodes that is associated with head and neck tumours runs along the vicinity of the sternocleidomastoid muscle and is divided into five anatomical levels. Carcinomas tend to spread down this chain in sequence. Clearance of the chain by a neck dissection is part of the surgical management of many head and neck cancers.

Nasopharyngeal carcinoma

Nasopharyngeal carcinoma is a malignant neoplasm that is closely linked to the Epstein–Barr virus. The incidence is very high in the Far East. The tumour tends to occur between 15 and 25 years of and in the seventh decade.

The malignant cells grow diffusely or as sheets and are accompanied by a very dense, chronic, inflammatory cell background. The majority of the tumours are non-keratinising.

Olfactory neuroblastoma

Olfactory neuroblastoma is a malignant neuroectodermal tumour that arises from the olfactory tissue in the roof of the nasal cavity. The tumour can demonstrate a variety of microscopic patterns, but is composed of ovoid cells in a fibrillary background.

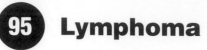

Classification of lymphoma

Lymphoma

- Hodgkin lymphoma
  - Classical Hodgkin lymphoma (95%)
    - Lymphocyte rich
    - Nodular sclerosing
    - Mixed cellularity
    - Lymphocyte depleted
  - Nodular lymphocyte predominant Hodgkin lymphoma (5%)
- Non-Hodgkin lymphoma
  - B cell (>90%)
    - **Low grade**
      - Follicular lymphoma
      - Mantle cell lymphoma
      - Nodal marginal zone lymphoma
      - Extranodal marginal zone lymphoma of MALT type
      - Splenic marginal zone lymphoma
      - Lymphoplasmacytoid lymphoma
      - Plasma cell neoplasms
      - Small lymphocytic lymphoma/chronic lymphocytic leukaemia
      - Hairy cell leukaemia
    - **High grade**
      - Diffuse large B cell lymphoma
      - Mediastinal (diffuse) large B cell lymphoma
      - Burkitt lymphoma and Burkitt-like lymphoma
      - Primary effusion lymphoma
      - Intravascular B cell lymphoma
      - (Grade 3b follicular lymphoma)
  - T cell (<10%)
    - Peripheral T cell lymphoma not otherwise specified (50%)
    - Anaplastic large cell lymphoma
    - Precursor T lymphocytic leukaemia
    - T cell large granular lymphocytic leukaemia
    - Aggressive NK cell leukaemia
    - Adult T cell lymphoma/leukaemia
    - Extranodal NK-T cell lymphoma, nasal type
    - Enteropathy associated T cell lymphoma
    - Hepatic gamma-delta T cell lymphoma
    - Subcutaneous panniculitis-like T cell lymphoma
    - Mycosis fungoides and Sézary syndrome
    - Angioimmunoblastic T cell lymphoma

Ann Arbor staging system for lymphoma

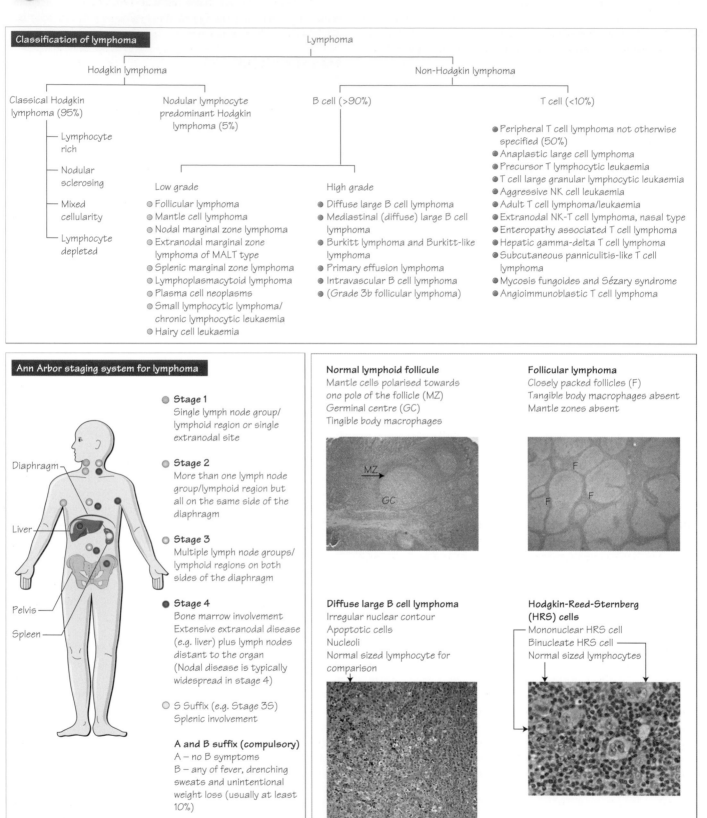

Diaphragm
Liver
Pelvis
Spleen

- **Stage 1**
  Single lymph node group/lymphoid region or single extranodal site

- **Stage 2**
  More than one lymph node group/lymphoid region but all on the same side of the diaphragm

- **Stage 3**
  Multiple lymph node groups/lymphoid regions on both sides of the diaphragm

- **Stage 4**
  Bone marrow involvement Extensive extranodal disease (e.g. liver) plus lymph nodes distant to the organ (Nodal disease is typically widespread in stage 4)

- **S Suffix** (e.g. Stage 3S)
  Splenic involvement

A and B suffix (compulsory)
A – no B symptoms
B – any of fever, drenching sweats and unintentional weight loss (usually at least 10%)

Normal lymphoid follicule
Mantle cells polarised towards one pole of the follicle (MZ)
Germinal centre (GC)
Tingible body macrophages

Follicular lymphoma
Closely packed follicles (F)
Tangible body macrophages absent
Mantle zones absent

Diffuse large B cell lymphoma
Irregular nuclear contour
Apoptotic cells
Nucleoli
Normal sized lymphocyte for comparison

Hodgkin-Reed-Sternberg (HRS) cells
Mononuclear HRS cell
Binucleate HRS cell
Normal sized lymphocytes

Hodgkin lymphoma

Hodgkin lymphoma is a malignant condition of lymphocytes that is characterised by the presence of Hodgkin–Reed–Sternberg cells (HRSCs).

Epidemiology and risk factors

The incidence is 2–3 per 100 000 per year with a male : female ratio of 2–3 : 1. Two age peaks exist, at 15–40 years and over 60 years. The disease is less common in Afro-Caribbeans. An identical twin has a 99-fold increased risk if the twin has the condition. Epstein–Barr virus (EBV) infection may be implicated in Hodgkin lymphoma.

Pathology

The affected lymph nodes are enlarged and show diffuse replacement of their architecture by a population of lymphoid cells and other leucocytes in which HRSCs are scattered. HRSCs are the crucial diagnostic element of Hodgkin lymphoma, although they account for only a small minority of the total cells. Emphasis is usually placed on the classic variant of HRSCs, but others exist and are often more abundant.

All HRSCs share the property of being considerably enlarged relative to normal lymphocytes. The classic form has a bilobed nucleus, each lobe of which possesses a large, prominent, eosinophilic nucleolus. The nucleolus is often surrounded by a region of clearing.

The mononuclear variant is similar to the classic form but has only one nuclear lobe. Multilobated HRSCs exist. Lacunar cells exhibit artefactual shrinkage of the cytoplasm away from the cell borders. Mummified cells represent dead cells. The lymphocytic and histiocytic, or popcorn, cell tends to be encountered only in the nodular lymphocyte predominant variant; its nucleus is large and convoluted, but the nucleoli are absent.

Most HRSCs are believed to be derived from B cells that have suffered a series of mutations which remove their ability either to produce immunoglobulins or to complete their differentiation.

Classification

The subclassification of Hodgkin lymphoma has recently been revised. The four traditional variants are designated classic Hodgkin lymphoma and constitute the considerable majority. The newcomer is nodular lymphocyte predominant Hodgkin lymphoma (NLPHL).

Classic Hodgkin lymphoma is divided on the basis of the background in which the HRSCs are found into lymphocyte rich, nodular sclerosing, mixed cellularity and lymphocyte depleted. Advances in treatment have rendered this classification of little to no significant prognostic value.

• Lymphocyte-rich Hodgkin lymphoma features sheets of lymphocytes, with other leucocytes being sparse.

• Mixed cellularity Hodgkin lymphoma has a mixture of lymphocytes, plasma cells, histiocytes and eosinophils.

• Lymphocyte-depleted usually occurs in people in poor general health, has a paucity of lymphocytes but is rich in histiocytes and granulocytes.

• The nodular sclerosing form is the commonest (75%). Bands of fibrous tissue divide the node into nodules of lymphoid tissue that tend to be dominated by lymphocytes, although eosinophils and macrophages are often well represented. The capsule of the lymph node is usually thickened. Sometimes the fibrous bands are poorly developed. Two grades are distinguished by the density of the HRSC population.

NLPHL contributes 5% of cases. The lymph node has an abnormal nodular architecture that is rich in lymphocytes. Popcorn cells are scattered in this background, often between the nodules.

Distribution

Hodgkin lymphoma tends to present in lymph nodes, particularly the cervical, mediastinal, inguinal and axillary. Spread is usually in a contiguous fashion, reaching neighbouring nodal groups sequentially. Involvement of the liver, spleen and bone marrow can occur, but usually late. Sites outside the haematoreticular system may be affected, but are unusual and primary Hodgkin lymphoma in these locations is rare.

Non-Hodgkin lymphoma (NHL)

Non-Hodgkin's lymphoma is a malignant tumour of lymphoid cells. The incidence is 13 per 100 000 per year. The age range is wide.

Pathology

The classification of NHL is complex. The current system is that of the World Health Organisation. Common features are the presence of an architecturally abnormal proliferation of atypical lymphocytes within the affected lymphoid tissue that replaces the normal architecture. The lymph nodes are enlarged. NHL is more likely to arise in sites outside the haematoreticular system than Hodgkin lymphoma. The classification may be simplified into three groups: low grade B cell lymphomas, high grade B cell lymphomas and T cell lymphomas.

T cell lymphomas: These constitute the minority of NHLs (10%) and include lymphomas with natural killer (NK) cell differentiation. They are frequently aggressive and difficult to treat.

Low grade B cell lymphomas: These encompass the greatest number of entities. Many are relatively indolent, so patients may survive for considerable periods with the disease. However, cure is difficult because the proliferative rate is relatively low targeting with chemotherapy is problematic.

• The commonest low grade B cell NHL is follicular lymphoma. This tends to occur in the elderly and has a characteristic t(14;18)(q32;q21) translocation that rearranges the *bcl-2* gene.

• Extranodal marginal zone B cell lymphoma of the MALT type arises in mucosal lymphoid tissue, e.g. the gastrointestinal tract, lung and skin. Some cases develop in the salivary glands and elsewhere. The gastric type is driven by infection with *H. pylori*, to the extent that in early disease eradication of the infection can control the lymphoma.

• Mantle cell lymphoma tends to present with stage 4 disease, so its prognosis is poor, belying its low grade categorisation. There is a characteristic t(11;14)(q13;q32) translocation.

High grade B cell lymphomas: These are dominated by the diffuse large B cell lymphoma. This is an aggressive disease, but its high proliferation rate renders it more chemosensitive.

• Burkitt's lymphoma is a specific high grade B cell NHL of which endemic and non-endemic forms exist. The endemic variant occurs in African children and is strongly associated with EBV infection. It typically involves the jaw, with the breasts and ovaries being other characteristic sites. The non-endemic type has a weaker link with EBV.

Staging

Both Hodgkin lymphoma and NHL are staged using the Ann Arbor system.

Prognosis

The prognosis in Hodgkin lymphoma is excellent in stage 1 with a 5-year survival of over 90%. This falls to 50–70% by stage 4, which is still very good compared with most other stage 4 malignancies.

The diverse composition of NHL prevents general comments on the prognosis other than those above, with the addition that many untreated TB or cell NHLs have a prognosis of weeks to months.

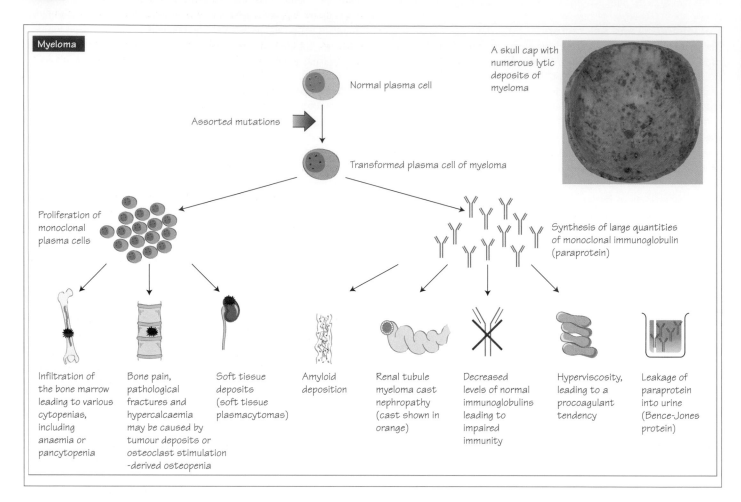

Myeloma

Normal plasma cell

A skull cap with numerous lytic deposits of myeloma

Assorted mutations

Transformed plasma cell of myeloma

Proliferation of monoclonal plasma cells

Synthesis of large quantities of monoclonal immunoglobulin (paraprotein)

Infiltration of the bone marrow leading to various cytopenias, including anaemia or pancytopenia

Bone pain, pathological fractures and hypercalcaemia may be caused by tumour deposits or osteoclast stimulation -derived osteopenia

Soft tissue deposits (soft tissue plasmacytomas)

Amyloid deposition

Renal tubule myeloma cast nephropathy (cast shown in orange)

Decreased levels of normal immunoglobulins leading to impaired immunity

Hyperviscosity, leading to a procoagulant tendency

Leakage of paraprotein into urine (Bence-Jones protein)

208 *Pathology at a Glance.* By C.J. Finlayson and B.A.T. Newell. Published 2009 by Blackwell Publishing. ISBN: 978-1-4051-3650-1

Systems pathology

Definition

Myeloma is a systemic, clonal, malignant, neoplastic disease of plasma cells.

Epidemiology

The incidence is 4–5 per 100 000 per year, with a male : female ratio of 5 : 3. The disease tends to present in the seventh and eighth decades, and is more common in Afro-Caribbeans.

Pathology

Immunoglobulin synthesis

Myeloma is a tumour of plasma cells. The plasma cells are clonal and therefore all produce the same immunoglobulin composed of the same heavy and light chains; occasionally, only the light chain is produced and, rarely, the plasma cells do not secrete their synthesised immunoglobulin.

Normally, two-thirds of circulating immunoglobulins have a kappa light chain. However, in myeloma, this ratio is reversed such that two-thirds of myelomas bear lambda light chains.

IgG is the most common immunoglobulin made by myelomas, being found in 70%. A further 20% synthesise IgA. Light chain-only variants encompass 5–10%. IgM, IgD and IgE forms are rare, but IgM paraprotein production is encountered in another haematoreticular neoplasm, lymphoplasmacytoid lymphoma (Waldenstrom's macroglobulinaemia).

The monoclonal immunoglobulin can be detected as a paraprotein in the blood. On plasma electrophoresis, this is seen as a very narrow, intense band. The band is narrow because it is produced by a single type of immunoglobulin molecule, which has an identical mass in all copies. The usual peaks for the immunoglobulin classes in serum are broader due to their heterogenous composition and masses.

The light chain component can pass into the urine, where it may be detected as Bence-Jones protein.

Osteopenia

Myeloma cells often secrete osteoclast-stimulating factors which liberate calcium from bones, causing osteopenia. This can cause bone pain and may lead to pathological fracture.

Histopathology

The microscopic features of myeloma are relatively straightforward. The tumour consists of aggregates of plasma cells. These are primarily located in the bone marrow, which can show various patterns and degrees of infiltration. The morphology of the plasma cells may not differ significantly from that of normal plasma cells, or the neoplastic plasma cells may exhibit nuclear atypia such as enlargement, prominent nucleoli or bilobation.

Myeloma also affects the skeleton in general and yields lytic deposits. The skull is frequently involved and shows multiple small lesions.

Extraskeletal plasma cell tumours can also develop. The microscopic features are the same but the term plasmacytoma is employed, particularly when dealing with an isolated, extramedullary lesion that is not associated with an underlying myeloma.

In rare cases, the neoplastic plasma cells circulate in large numbers in the blood and the term plasma cell leukaemia is employed.

Clinical diagnosis

Myeloma is also referred to as multiple myeloma and this designation highlights an aspect of the disease that is necessary to distinguish it from a solitary plasmacytoma. The diagnostic criteria are as follows:

1 Major criteria:
- Elevated blood immunoglobulin levels above subtype-specific thresholds (IgG >30 g/L, IgA >20 g/L) or urine Bence-Jones proteins above specified thresholds.
- Plasmacytoma proven by biopsy.
- Bone marrow infiltration by plasma cells of at least 30%.

2 Minor criteria:
- Lesser degrees of paraproteinaemia.
- Bone marrow infiltration of 10–30%.
- Multiple skeletal lesions detected radiologically.
- Immunoparesis.

The diagnosis requires one major and one minor criterion in a symptomatic patient, or three minor criteria in a symptomatic patient.

Monoclonal gammopathy of uncertain significance (MGUS) is a disorder in which a paraprotein is present, but at a lower level than myeloma and without skeletal abnormalities. There is progression to myeloma in 10–30%.

Complications

- The excessive production of a clonally derived immunoglobulin can lead to a lack of normal immunoglobulins (immunoparesis). This impairs the immune response.
- Infiltration of the bone marrow by the plasma cells can overwhelm and replace the normal haematopoietic tissue, leading to bone marrow failure. This may exacerbate the immunocompromisation.
- Hyperviscosity can arise due to the increased protein content of the blood. This induces a procoagulant tendency, with cerebrovascular accidents being one of the most serious consequences.
- Pathological fractures may occur due to destruction of bone by deposits of myeloma.
- Hypercalcaemia can develop in 25% and is related to stimulation of osteoclasts by the myeloma or osteopenia.
- The synthesis of large quantities of immunoglobulin light chains by the myeloma can lead to amyloidosis (AL type).
- Renal failure is encountered in approximately 30% of patients and reflects a variety of causes. Light chains are toxic to the renal tubules, where they can precipitate as casts within the tubules. Hypercalcaemia may cause renal failure. Amyloidosis can be complicated by renal failure. The immunocompromised state that may result from myeloma can lead to repeated urinary tract infections and chronic pyelonephritis. The proliferative activity of the myeloma, specifically the nucleic acid metabolism, can elevate serum urate levels, leading to urate nephropathy. The myeloma may infiltrate the kidney (rare). Chemotherapy treatment can be nephrotoxic.

Prognosis

The average survival in treated patients is 3–5 years. The prognosis is better in younger individuals and those who can tolerate the more aggressive therapies. Poor prognostic features include anaemia and renal failure.

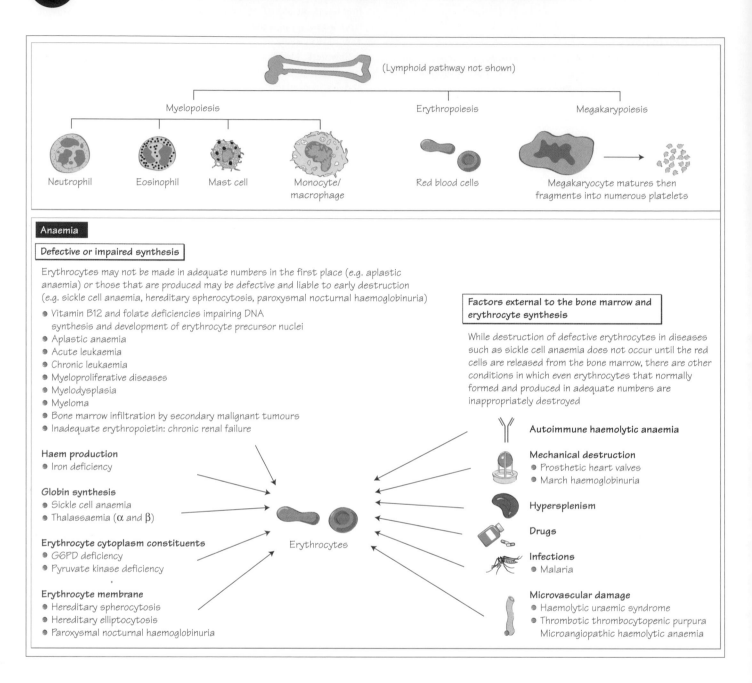

Constraints of space mean that only a very brief overview can be given of a few selected topics in haematology.

Leukaemia

The leukaemias are malignant clonal populations derived from bone marrow stem cells. Myeloid leukaemias arise from myeloid precursors and lymphoblastic/lymphocytic leukaemias are of lymphoid origin.

Leukaemias are acute or chronic. In acute lymphoblastic leukaemia (ALL), there is an unregulated proliferation of lymphoid blasts which fail to undergo differentiation. By contrast, chronic lymphocytic leukaemia

(CLL) is a proliferation of mature small lymphocytes. Similarly, acute myeloblastic leukaemia (AML) is a proliferation of early myeloid precursors which do not differentiate, whereas chronic myeloid leukaemia (CML) is also due to unregulated stem cell proli-feration, but with subsequent differentiation of the offspring to mature myeloid forms.

ALL and CLL may be of either B or T cell lineage. The T cell forms are rarer and more aggressive.

AML is divided into eight subclasses. Groups M0–M3 are from early myeloid cells, M0 being the most primitive. M4 is myelomonocytic, M5 is monocytic, M6 is erythroid and M7 is megakaryoblastic.

Genetics

Numerous genetic abnormalities have been described in the various leukaemias and are of use in some subclassifications of AML. However, the most well known genetic abnormality is the Philadelphia chromosome of CML. This is due to the t(9;22)(q34;q11) translocation that creates the bcr-abl fusion protein. The normal abl protein is a tyrosine kinase and the chimeric protein has a markedly increased tyrosine kinase activity.

Pathology

The nuances of the pathology are diverse, as to be expected from a varied group of entities, but the common theme is that the neoplastic proliferation occurs in the bone marrow and is associated with the presence of neoplastic cells in the blood. In ALL and AML the neoplasm overruns the bone marrow and overwhelms the normal haematopoietic tissue. Thus, there is anaemia and thrombocytopenia. While the overall white count is elevated by the neoplastic population, the production of functional leucocytes is also decimated, so the patients are profoundly neutropenic.

In CML and CLL, there is typically adequate bone marrow reserve as the neoplastic cells coexist with normal haematopoietic elements.

Both CML and CLL can undergo transformation to higher grade lesions. CML may convert to AML (two-thirds) or ALL (one-third). CLL may transform to diffuse large B cell lymphoma.

Clinical correlations

Both ALL and AML present quickly with bone marrow failure and are rapidly fatal if untreated. Treatment is with high dose chemotherapy and is attended by its own significant mortality. Patients with CML and CLL can be quite well and may live for years with limited intervention. The monoclonal antibody imatinib (Glivec) targets the mutated tyrosine kinase receptor in CML and has provided effective new treatment.

Myelodysplasia

Myelodysplasia tends to occur in older people and is a disease in which there is defective haematopoiesis that produces peripheral blood cytopenias. Some cases will have a pancytopenia and marrow failure.

Five subclasses are described: refractory anaemia, refractory anaemia with ring sideroblasts, refractory anaemia with excess blasts, chronic myelomonocytic leukaemia and 5q- isolated syndrome.

As well as the problems caused by defective haematopoiesis, myelodysplasia may be complicated by transformation into AML.

Myeloproliferative disorders

Myeloproliferative disorders are clonal bone marrow stem cell proliferation diseases in which there is overproduction of one or more mature haematopoietic cells. As the definition implies, there is overlap with CML, such that CML is classed as one of the myeloproliferative disorders. The others are polycythaemia rubra vera (PRV) (erythrocytes), essential thrombocythaemia (platelets) and myelofibrosis (fibrosis of the bone marrow and extramedullary haematopoiesis in the liver and spleen).

In PRV, the clinical manifestations relate to the elevated haematocrit, elevated blood viscosity and increased tendency to thrombosis. A hypercoagulable state is also the main problem in essential thrombocythaemia, although, paradoxically, clotting may be impaired as the platelets produced by the megakaryocytes are functionally defective.

Precise criteria exist for diagnosing the various myeloproliferative disorders. The Philadelphia chromosome trumps the other criteria such that its presence excludes PRV, essential thrombocythaemia and myelofibrosis. Recently, the JAK-2 mutation has become a useful diagnostic tool.

Both PRV and essential thrombocythaemia can progress to myelofibrosis. Like CML, the other myeloproliferative diseases can also transform to AML.

Anaemia

Anaemia is a diverse group of conditions in which there is a low blood concentration of haemoglobin. Parallel classification systems exist and are clinically useful in narrowing down the cause when confronted by a low haemoglobin result.

Anaemia is considered in terms of the size of the red cells (microcytic, normocytic or macrocytic) as indicated by the mean corpuscular volume (MCV) and the amount of haemoglobin in the erythrocyte (hypochromic or normochromic). Different conditions cause different patterns of these parameters.

• **Macrocytic anaemia**: this is encountered in deficiencies of folate or vitamin B12. The pathogenesis centres round the role of these two substances in DNA synthesis. Macrocytic anaemia also occurs in diseases in which the bone marrow prematurely releases late red cell precursors into the peripheral blood before they have completed maturation to an erythrocyte. This is seen in aplastic anaemia, myelodysplasia and some haemolytic anaemias. The late precursors (e.g. reticulocytes) are larger than normal erythrocytes, but are measured as erythrocytes by the automated haematology analysers and thereby skew the MCV.

• **Hypochromic, microcytic anaemia**: this occurs in iron deficiency and thalassaemia (defective synthesis of the α- or β-chains or haemoglobin).

• **Normochromic, normocytic anaemia**: this includes the anaemia of chronic disease, sometimes sickle cell anaemia and many haemolytic anaemias.

Alongside this classification is the division into haemolytic anaemias (hereditary spherocytosis, glucose-6-phosphate dehydrogenase (G6PD) deficiency, sickle cell anaemia, thalassaemia, autoimmune and paroxysmal nocturnal haemoglobinuria) and non-haemolytic anaemias (iron deficiency, vitamin B12 and folate deficiency, anaemia of chronic disease, anaemia of chronic renal failure). Also intersecting the two previous classifications are the hereditary (sickle cell anaemia, G6PD deficiency, thalassaemia) versus acquired (vitamin deficiencies, autoimmune haemolytic anaemia) division and subtyping into defective haemoglobin synthesis (sickle cell anaemia, thalassaemia, iron deficiency) versus defective red cell membranes (hereditary spherocytosis) versus others (autoimmune haemolytic anaemia, chronic renal failure, aplastic anaemia).

Thrombocytopenia

Thrombocytopenia is a low platelet count. It may be seen as part of a more generalised bone marrow failure, or be isolated. Other than drug-induced thrombocytopenia, the commonest cause is idiopathic thrombocytopenic purpura – an autoimmune disease.

Neutropenia

Neutropenia is a low blood neutrophil count. It usually occurs as part of generalised bone marrow failure, but isolated forms can arise (drugs, various syndromes). Severe neutropenia places the patient at serious risk of overwhelming bacterial and fungal infection and should be taken very seriously.

The neuromuscular junction

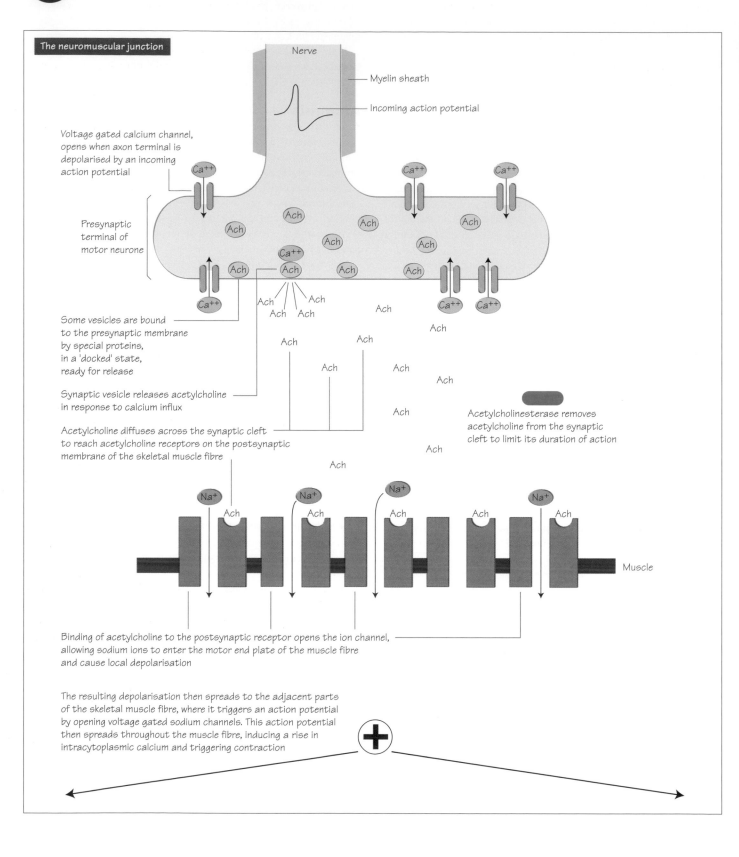

Nerve

Myelin sheath

Incoming action potential

Voltage gated calcium channel, opens when axon terminal is depolarised by an incoming action potential

Presynaptic terminal of motor neurone

Some vesicles are bound to the presynaptic membrane by special proteins, in a 'docked' state, ready for release

Synaptic vesicle releases acetylcholine in response to calcium influx

Acetylcholine diffuses across the synaptic cleft to reach acetylcholine receptors on the postsynaptic membrane of the skeletal muscle fibre

Acetylcholinesterase removes acetylcholine from the synaptic cleft to limit its duration of action

Muscle

Binding of acetylcholine to the postsynaptic receptor opens the ion channel, allowing sodium ions to enter the motor end plate of the muscle fibre and cause local depolarisation

The resulting depolarisation then spreads to the adjacent parts of the skeletal muscle fibre, where it triggers an action potential by opening voltage gated sodium channels. This action potential then spreads throughout the muscle fibre, inducing a rise in intracytoplasmic calcium and triggering contraction

Systems pathology

Myasthenia gravis

Definition

Myasthenia gravis is an autoimmune condition in which there are circulating autoantibodies that are directed against the neuromuscular junctions of skeletal muscle.

Epidemiology

The incidence is four per 1 000 000 per year and the prevalence is four per 100 000 per year. The male : female ratio is 2 : 3. The disease presents in the third and fourth decades in females and the sixth and seventh decade in males.

Pathology

In 85% of cases, the autoantibodies are IgG directed against the acetylcholine receptors of the neuromuscular junction. Some of the remaining 15% of cases feature IgM autoantibodies that target sodium ion channels. The action of the autoantibodies on the acetylcholine receptor impairs transmission of the signal from the synaptic terminal of the motor neurone to the muscle. This decreases the stimulus to the muscle, which is perceived by the patient as weakness. Repeated or prolonged activity places a stress on the motor neurone to maintain a supply of synaptic vesicles. If the receptors on the muscle are depleted, this stress becomes critical – hence the exacerbation of myasthenia gravis towards the end of the day, or with repeated activity.

Microscopic changes at the neuromuscular junction are subtle and include widening of the synaptic cleft.

Many patients (approximately 60%) have thymic hyperplasia. In 10%, there is a thymoma (one of the primary neoplasms of the thymus). Patients without thymic disease show an association with HLA-B8 and -DR3. The latter is commonly found in organ-specific autoimmune disease.

Clinical correlations

As the underlying pathophysiology is analogous to the jamming of a radio signal, boosting the signal can overcome the problem. Hence, inhibitors of acetylcholinesterase are used in the treatment of myasthenia gravis as they increase the quantity and duration of availability of acetylcholine at the neuromuscular junctions.

Eaton–Lambert syndrome

This is a rare autoimmune condition that can affect a wide age range and has a male : female ratio of 5 : 1. In 50% of cases it occurs as a paraneoplastic phenomenon and under these circumstances is typically associated with bronchial small cell carcinoma.

As with myasthenia gravis, neurotransmission at the neuromuscular junction is impaired. However, in contrast to myasthenia gravis, the problem lies on the presynaptic part of the junction, in the form of autoantibodies that are directed against presynaptic calcium channels. Interference with these channels prevents the influx of calcium that is essential to cause the release of synaptic vesicles. Thus, muscle weakness occurs.

Whereas in myasthenia gravis repeated use of a muscle worsens the weakness, rapid repeated contractions in Eaton–Lambert syndrome may provide some relief. This is because such rapid stimulation elevates the intracytoplasmic levels of calcium in the presynaptic terminal, partially overcoming the reduction in the size of the calcium influx.

Polymyositis

Polymyositis is an autoimmune condition that targets skeletal muscle. It may be combined with dermatological manifestations, when it is referred to as dermatomyositis.

The disease is rare and tends to present between 30 and 60 years and is more common in women. As well as arising in isolation, polymyositis/dermatomyositis may be encountered in association with a connective tissue disorder or malignancy.

Pathology

Affected muscles show destruction of fibres by an infiltrate of lymphocytes and macrophages. The disease tends to involve the proximal muscles and spares the distal muscles in 75%.

The underlying process in the skin follows a lichenoid pattern, but more critical to remember is the presence of periorbital oedema and a periorbital lilac rash that is named after a flower of a similar hue, the heliotrope.

Myotonic dystrophy

Myotonic dystrophy is an autosomal dominant condition that has an incidence of 14 per 100 000 live births and tends to manifest between 20 and 30 years. The gene is located on chromosome 19q13.3 and the mutated form shows the CTG trinucleotide repeat phenomenon.

The disease primarily affects the muscles of the face, neck (including the larynx) and distal extremities. There is muscle wasting, which can give a characteristic facial appearance. Myotonia itself is delayed relaxation of a muscle after voluntary contraction or prolonged contraction after brief percussion.

The majority of patients have cardiac abnormalities, usually conducting system defects. Cataracts are present in 90%. Progression is slow over 15–20 years.

Duchenne muscular dystrophy

This is an X-linked recessive disease that occurs in 30 per 1 000 000 live male births. The onset is between 3 and 15 years. The gene responsible is at Xp21. This usually codes for the protein dystrophin, which is normally located on the inner surface of the sarcolemma of skeletal muscle fibres.

The disease shows muscle wasting and the affected muscles exhibit replacement by fat and connective tissue. This can give the confusing appearance of pseudohypertrophy in the earlier stages, although most muscles do eventually decrease in size. A muscle biopsy will demonstrate variation in the size of the muscle fibres with necrosis of fibres. Fatty and fibrous replacement is seen. Dystrophin is absent.

Dilated cardiomyopathy is common. Three-quarters of patients die before 25 years of age.

Becker muscular dystrophy is also produced by a mutation in the dystrophin gene but has milder features. Patients remain able to walk until 25–30 years of age.

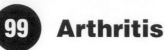

Rheumatoid arthritis: chronic inflammation due to autoimmune disease

◆ The initiating antigenic stimulus for rheumatoid arthritis is not clear, though recent suggestions include Mycobacterial infection

◆ In 50–70% of patients, Rheumatoid factor (RhF), an anti-self antibody directed against Fc IgG is produced – IgM isotype is the most commonly tested anti-RF antibody

◆ Recently described is anti-cyclic citrullinated peptide (anti-CCP), an IgG antibody which is more sensitive than RhF in the diagnosis of rheumatoid arthritis, positive in nearly 90–95% of patients. Patients positive for both anti CCP and RhF have severe erosive joint destruction. Anti-CCP testing is very expensive so anti-RF is used for screening

◆ Antibody–antigen complexes circulate in the blood

◆ The complexes are arrested in capillaries in joint linings or connective tissue. Th cells in this disease appear to react against collagen components, (e.g. collagen 2), which may explain the disease localisation

◆ Lymphoid tissue develops in the synovium: there are large follicles with germinal centres and abundant plasma cells and Th cells. There is generalised upregulation of class II MHC molecules, including synovial epithelium. Capillary endothelial cells upregulate adhesion molecules. The inflammatory focus expands, and bony destruction occurs, together with an inflammatory layer on the joint surface: 'pannus'

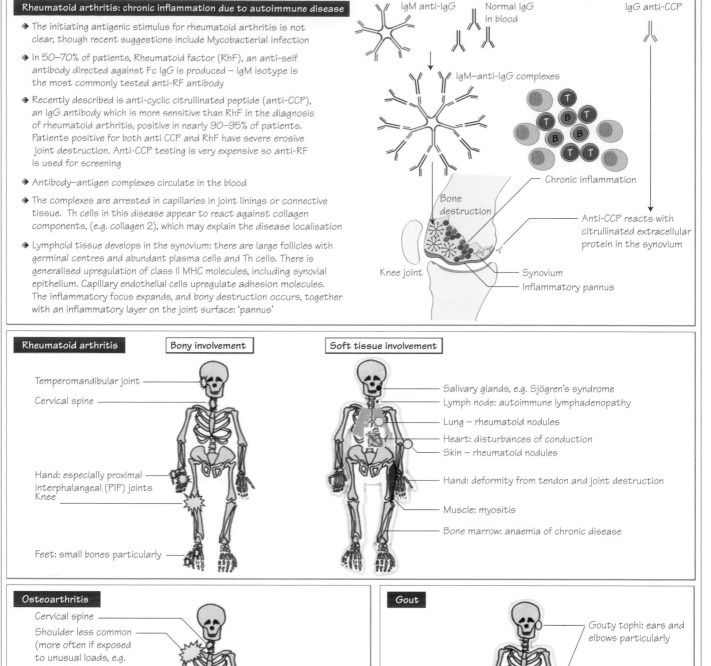

Systems pathology

Rheumatoid arthritis

Rheumatoid arthritis (RA) is a chronic, inflammatory, multisystem disorder that typically involves the joints.

Epidemiology and pathology

The prevalence is 1% worldwide. The disease usually presents in the fourth and fifth decades but the age range is wide. The overall male : female ratio is 1 : 3, but varies with age, being 1 : 10 at 30 years and equal at 65 years.

The disease is autoimmune. HLA-DR4 is present in 70% of sufferers, compared with 20% of the general population.

Affected joints show an inflammatory response and associated cytokine and cellular cascades. There is proliferation of the synovium which forms villous folds. There is severe chronic inflammation, typically with lymphoid follicles. Fibrin is present.

The changes described are reversible, but if granulation tissue affects the articular cartilage, irreversible damage can develop. The granulation tissue is referred to as pannus and interferes with the nutrition of the cartilage, as well as causing its degradation. The pannus can extend into the underlying bone, or across the joint to form adhesions. Fibrosis of the granulation tissue can worsen the adhesions.

Approximately three-quarters of patients have circulating rheumatoid factor (RF), as somewhat confusingly do 5% of the unaffected population. RF is a circulating antibody, usually IgM, that is directed against the Fc portion of altered IgG. Its presence opens up the possibilities of immune complex-related phenomena. Recently IgG anti-cyclic citrullinated peptide (anti-CCP) has been found to be present in 90–95% of RA patients. Though too expensive for screening purposes, it is useful both for confirming the diagnosis and in predicting the severity of RA, which is worst if both anti-RF and anti-CCP are present.

Rheumatoid nodules are a feature in 20–30% of patients. Numerous sites can be affected but they are typically found in the skin. They consist of a central region of fibrinoid necrosis that is surrounded by fibrous tissue and macrophages. Rheumatoid nodules are usually associated with the presence of rheumatoid factor.

Clinical correlations

• Characteristic deformities of the hands occur. Many of these have as their basis damage to the articular cartilage, which leads to subluxation of the joint – the direction of which is determined by the balance of tone in the long flexors, extensors and small muscles of the hand.
• The spine is affected in 80% and the cervical spine is the most susceptible. Atlantoaxial subluxation can occur. Cervical spine involvement can lead to nerve and cord compression.
• Rheumatoid nodules can be responsible for features in a variety of organs. Of particular note are conduction disturbances in the heart and pulmonary nodules.
• Felty's syndrome is often seized upon by students and comprises the interesting combination of lymphadenopathy, splenomegaly, anaemia, thrombocytopenia and neutropenia. However, it occurs in only 1% of patients and usually after at least 10 years of the disease.

Osteoarthritis

Osteoarthritis is a degenerative condition of synovial joints. The disease is more common with increasing age, particularly over the age of 60. The male : female ratio is 1 : 2.

Most cases of osteoarthritis are primary, but various secondary conditions exist. These secondary conditions tend to share the properties of predisposing the joint to increased damage and include the following:

• Obesity.
• Hypermobility syndromes.
• Recurrent dislocation.
• Recurrent haemarthrosis.
• Intra-articular fracture.
• Septic arthritis.
• Inflammatory arthropathy.
• Osteochondritis (such as Perthe's disease).
• Congenital dysplasias.
• Neuropathies yielding Charcot's joints (such as syringomyelia).
• Haemochromatosis.
• Sickle cell disease.
• Gout.
• Pseudogout.
• Corticosteroids.

The joints most commonly affected are the load bearing joints of the hips and knees, or the joints of the phalanges.

There is degeneration of the articular cartilage, which becomes irregular and has a fibrillated surface. The underlying bone can show cyst formation. There is loss of width of the joint space. New bone formation can occur on the edges of the joints to yield osteophytes.

Gout

Gout is a form of abnormal metabolism that results in the deposition of crystals of uric acid in the tissues, primarily the joints.

Epidemiology and pathology

Gout is primarily a disease of affluent societies. It is generally rare below 30 years of age in both genders and also before the menopause in women.

The basic pathological process is hyperuricaemia. The elevated concentration of uric acid increases the likelihood of precipitation of urate crystals from solution. This may be induced by a reduction in temperature and this has been invoked as an explanation for why exposed sites such as the big toe and the ear are characteristic sites of involvement .

General factors that can contribute to hyperuricaemia include alcohol, dehydration, obesity and stress. Impaired excretion of urate is encountered in chronic renal failure and primary hyperparathyroidism and with thiazide and loop diuretics. Excess production is found in the Lesch–Nyhan syndrome, myeloproliferative disorders and carcinomas. Chemotherapy may release large volumes of uric acid into the circulation by liberating it from killed cancer cells.

In acute gouty arthritis, crystals of uric acid are present in the fluid within the joint and these can be discerned by polarised light microscopy. The gout crystals provoke acute inflammation. Neutrophils try to phagocytose the gout crystals, but are unsuccessful and release the destructive contents of their granules in this failed process.

Tophi are chronic accumulations of urate crystals that have a chalky appearance. The ear is the classic site, but cartilage elsewhere can be involved as well as the skin and, rarely, deeper organs. The urate crystals induce a fibrotic and macrophage response. Urate can precipitate in the urine to form stones.

Other forms of arthritis

Inflammatory arthritis can be encountered in various other conditions, including systemic lupus erythematosus, psoriatic arthropathy and Reiter's syndrome. The histopathological changes alone are often those of a chronic inflammatory process without specific nuances.

Systems pathology

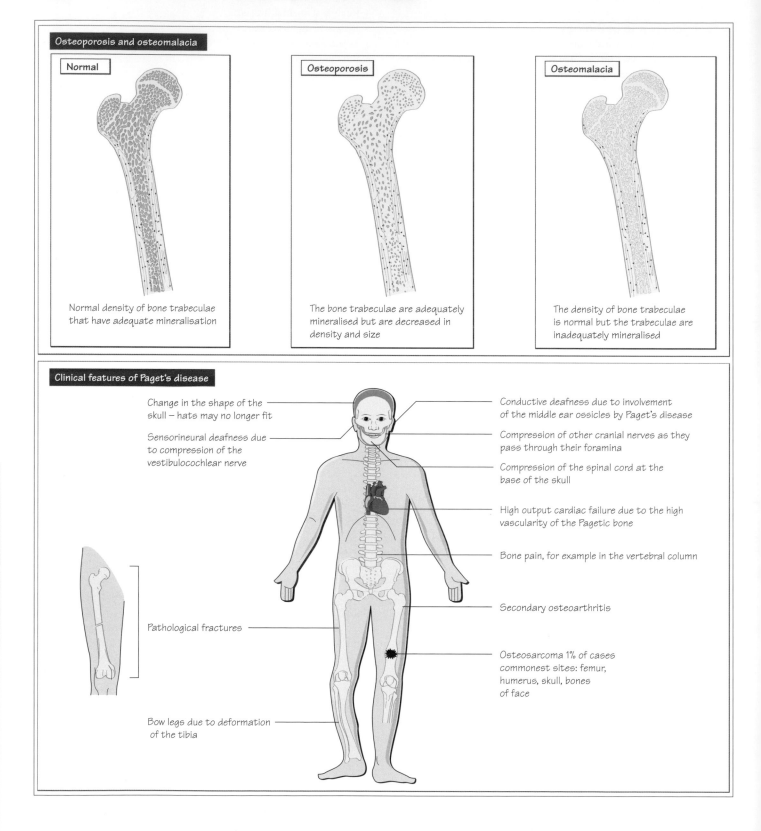

Osteoporosis and osteomalacia

Normal

Normal density of bone trabeculae that have adequate mineralisation

Osteoporosis

The bone trabeculae are adequately mineralised but are decreased in density and size

Osteomalacia

The density of bone trabeculae is normal but the trabeculae are inadequately mineralised

Clinical features of Paget's disease

Change in the shape of the skull – hats may no longer fit

Sensorineural deafness due to compression of the vestibulocochlear nerve

Conductive deafness due to involvement of the middle ear ossicles by Paget's disease

Compression of other cranial nerves as they pass through their foramina

Compression of the spinal cord at the base of the skull

High output cardiac failure due to the high vascularity of the Pagetic bone

Bone pain, for example in the vertebral column

Secondary osteoarthritis

Osteosarcoma 1% of cases commonest sites: femur, humerus, skull, bones of face

Pathological fractures

Bow legs due to deformation of the tibia

Osteoporosis

Osteoporosis is a reduction in the mass of bone per unit volume. The remaining bone has a normal composition and mineralisation. The condition is considerably more common in women, especially in the post-menopausal period. Other risk factors include:

- Being Caucasian.
- Being thin.
- Family history.
- Reduced physical activity.
- Smoking.
- Alcohol abuse.
- Cushing's syndrome.
- Hyperthyroidism.
- Acromegaly.
- Hypogonadism.

The rate of bone loss varies between bones and between regions of the same bone. The spine and femur are particularly susceptible, especially the femoral head. The bone loss is seen as thinning of the cortex and the trabeculae. The disease is better assessed by radiological means rather than conventional histopathology.

Osteomalacia

Osteomalacia is inadequate mineralisation of the osteoid framework of bone and is known as rickets in children. The causes include: vitamin D deficiency, vitamin D-dependent rickets types 1 and 2, chronic renal failure, renal tubular disorders, malabsorption and phosphate depletion.

Paget's disease

Paget's disease is a disorder in which there is excessive bone turnover and resulting disorganisation of the architecture of the bone. The disease is common in those of Anglo-Saxon descent and is rare in Japan and Scandinavia. As with osteoarthritis, the prevalence rises with age, reaching 10% in those over 80 years.

Pathology

Paget's disease may affect one, several or many bones, and part or the whole of a bone. The skull and tibia are particularly common sites.

In the initial stage of the disease there is intense activity of the bone resorbing osteoclasts, which become larger than usual. This provokes increased activity in the osteoblasts with the rapid laying down of new bone. This new bone is structurally deficient. The bone marrow develops highly vascular fibrous tissue. Later in the disease the osteoclast activity subsides, leaving a legacy of hard dense bone that is less vascular. The previous frantic activity can be seen as an irregular, disordered pattern of cement lines within the bone. The bones remain weak.

Clinical consequences

Affected bones are susceptible to pathological fractures. The weakened nature of the bone can deform under repeated mechanical loading (typically tibial bowing). Furthermore, secondary osteoarthritis may arise. The high bone turnover yields an elevated alkaline phosphatase. The other complications are shown in the figure.

Osteomyelitis

Definition and epidemiology

Osteomyelitis is an infection of the bone and bone marrow. The condition usually affects children and the incidence has fallen considerably in developed countries.

Microbiology

Three-quarters of cases are due to *Staphylococcus aureus*. Special mentions are required for *Salmonella* species in sickle cell disease and *Pseudomonas aeruginosa* in intravenous drug abusers. Other organisms include *Streptococcus pneumoniae*, *S. pyogenes*, *Haemophilus influenzae* and *Escherichia coli*, *Mycobacterium tuberculosis* and *Brucella*.

Pathology

The infection usually spreads haematogenously from another focus. Fractures, surgery and metallic implants are predisposing factors. Direct spread is perhaps surprisingly uncommon as a cause.

No bone is invulnerable, but the metaphyses of long bones are at most risk, especially the distal femur, proximal tibia and humerus. This distribution has the advantage of being similar to that of osteosarcoma, thereby reducing efforts at memorisation. The vertebral column is also a common site. The metaphyses may be susceptible due to the sluggish blood flow in their dilated sinusoids.

As is expected for a bacterial infection, the result is acute inflammation. The exudate raises the pressure within the bone, potentially resulting in first venous, then arterial, infarction. With no barriers to its spread within the marrow cavity, the infection extends rapidly throughout this compartment of the bone such that the marrow fills with pus. The pus enters the Haversian system and accumulates beneath the periosteum to form an abscess which elevates the periosteum and yields a useful radiological feature.

If the abscess surrounds much of the diaphysis, the penetrating arteries may thrombose, exacerbating any infarction. The resulting volume of dead bone is known as a sequestrum. A shell of new subperiosteal bone, the involucrum, forms around the sequestrum. The involucrum is typically irregular and perforated, permitting pus to track into the neighbouring soft tissues, or reach the surface of the skin as a sinus.

Clinical correlations

- Extension of the process into a joint yields septic arthritis, particularly in joints such as the hip and shoulder where the metaphysis is within the capsule.
- In children, the infection can damage the growth plate, leading to altered growth.
- Metastatic abscesses or septicaemia can occur.
- Chronic osteomyelitis may develop and be accompanied by amyloidosis.

Septic arthritis

Septic arthritis is infection of a joint. Unlike osteomyelitis, the age distribution is not biased towards the young. Infection of a joint can be due to spread from an infected bone, a penetrating wound, surgery or haematogenous spread. Predisposing factors include the following:

- Arthritic joint damage.
- Prosthetic joint.
- Chronic disease such as diabetes mellitus, systemic lupus erythematosus or chronic renal failure.
- Immunosuppression.
- Alcoholism.
- Intravenous drug abuse.

The causative agents are similar to osteomyelitis, although viral infection must also be considered.

The pathological process is that of acute inflammation. Particular nuances that relate to septic arthritis are the destruction of cartilage by the proteolytic enzymes released by neutrophils and fibrosis in the healing phase. If untreated, the infection can cause serious damage to the joint and therefore permanent functional impairment.

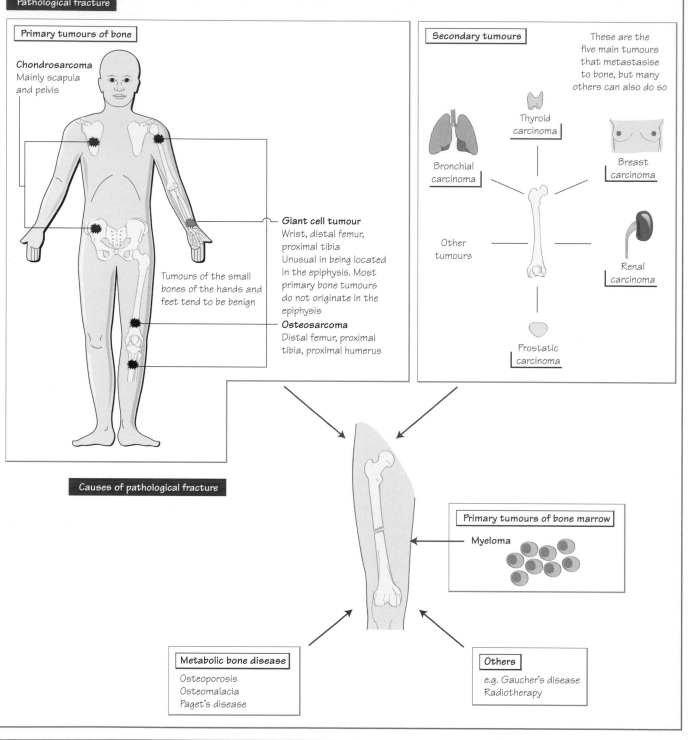

Pathological fracture

Primary tumours of bone

Chondrosarcoma
Mainly scapula and pelvis

Tumours of the small bones of the hands and feet tend to be benign

Giant cell tumour
Wrist, distal femur, proximal tibia
Unusual in being located in the epiphysis. Most primary bone tumours do not originate in the epiphysis

Osteosarcoma
Distal femur, proximal tibia, proximal humerus

Secondary tumours

These are the five main tumours that metastasise to bone, but many others can also do so

Bronchial carcinoma

Thyroid carcinoma

Breast carcinoma

Other tumours

Renal carcinoma

Prostatic carcinoma

Causes of pathological fracture

Primary tumours of bone marrow

Myeloma

Metabolic bone disease

Osteoporosis
Osteomalacia
Paget's disease

Others

e.g. Gaucher's disease
Radiotherapy

Systems pathology

218 *Pathology at a Glance.* By C.J. Finlayson and B.A.T. Newell. Published 2009 by Blackwell Publishing. ISBN: 978-1-4051-3650-1

Secondary tumours

Traditionally, discussion of secondary tumours in a chapter on neoplasms of a particular organ is left until the end of the section. However, secondary tumours of the bone are considerably more common than primary bone tumours and therefore are mentioned first.

There are five primary malignancies that are particularly likely to metastasise to bone. These are thyroid, bronchial, breast, renal and prostatic carcinomas. All but the last of these are osteolytic; prostatic adenocarcinoma is osteosclerotic. Attention is drawn to the usefulness of this quintet for multiple choice questions. Note that other malignant tumours are not precluded from displaying bone metastases.

Osteosarcoma

Definition
Osteosarcoma is a malignant connective tissue tumour that produces osteoid.

Epidemiology
The incidence is three per 1 000 000 per year. Three-quarters of cases occur between the ages of 10 and 25 years. Over half of those patients aged more than 40 years have Paget's disease. The tumour is more common in males.

Pathology
Most osteosarcomas affect the metaphysis of a long bone. The distal femur, proximal tibia and proximal humerus are the usual sites.

The tumour is an irregular, destructive mass, which may appear sclerotic, fleshy or telangiectatic. The tumour spreads along the marrow cavity, as well as destroying the cortex to invade into and through the periosteum into the adjacent soft tissue. Raising of the periosteum by the tumour results in new spicules of bone being formed perpendicular to the cortical surface of the bone. On X-ray, this is seen as sunray spiculation. The other key radiological term is Codman's triangle, the boundaries of which are formed by the new, raised periosteum on two sides and the old periosteum as the base of the triangle, while the centre of the triangle is new reactive bone.

The cells of origin are primitive bone-forming cells. The quantity of bone and osteoid produced by the tumour can range from considerable to limited, but the presence of osteoid is the defining characteristic of the neoplasm. The cells may be plump to spindle shaped and are cytologically atypical. Cartilage formation can be encountered.

Direct spread along the bone can be temporarily slowed by the epiphyseal cartilage plate in children, but haematogenous dissemination occurs early and the lungs are the principal location.

The 5-year survival is approximately 30%.

Paraosteal osteosarcoma is a less aggressive variant that is found between the ages of 30 and 60 years. The key feature is that the tumour is situated on the outside of the bone and is a well defined, lobulated mass.

Ewing's sarcoma

Ewing's sarcoma should be considered with the entity of primitive neuroectodermal tumour (PNET). The neoplasms effectively have the same histological properties but are distinguished by their primary site. Ewing's sarcoma affects bone whereas a PNET affects other sites, including the brain.

Ewing's sarcoma and PNET are highly aggressive tumours that tend to develop in young people aged between 5 and 20 years.

Pathology
Ewing's sarcoma variant can arise anywhere along the diaphysis or metaphysis of a long bone. In contrast to osteosarcoma, Ewing's sarcoma mainly involves the pelvis, scapulae and ribs.

The tumour is composed of closely packed, relatively small, hyperchromatic cells that have a high nuclear : cytoplasmic ratio. Such tumours are referred to as small round blue cell tumours. The differential diagnosis includes Ewing's sarcoma/PNET, nephroblastoma, lymphoma/leukaemia, retinoblastoma and rhabomyosarcoma. Determining the nature of the tumour requires complex immunohistochemical panels supplemented by cytogenetic analysis. In the case of Ewing's sarcoma/PNET, there is a characteristic t(11;22)(q24;q12) translocation that involves the c-myc oncogene (CD99).

The 5-year survival is approximately 25%.

Chondrosarcoma

Chondrosarcoma is a malignant tumour that forms cartilage. Unlike osteosarcoma and Ewing's sarcoma, it is a tumour of the middle-aged and elderly. Also unlike osteosarcoma, it is primarily a tumour of the axial skeleton, with the pelvis and shoulder being the main sites. The majority of tumours arise without a precursor lesion, but in 10% there is a pre-existing benign cartilage tumour.

The tumour is either central, developing within the medullary cavity, or peripheral, growing on the surface of the bone.

Microscopically, the tumour produces lobules of cartilage and permeates the marrow spaces. Low grade lesions typically lack the usual cytological features of malignancy and diagnosis requires integration of the clinical, radiological, macroscopic and microscopic features.

The tumour tends to be slow growing and causes morbidity by local recurrence rather than metastases.

Giant cell tumour

This lesion is also known as an osteoclastoma. It is benign but locally aggressive. The age range is 20 to 40 years. The anatomical locations are the distal femur, proximal tibia and wrist. In contrast to osteosarcoma, the tumour usually arises in the end of the bone rather than the metaphysis.

Osteoclastomas are osteolytic and cause expansion of the end of the affected bone, leaving a soft, reddish, haemorrhagic tumour surrounded by a thin shell of bone. The tumour is composed of numerous ovoid and spindle-shaped cells with a minority of multinucleate giant cells.

Osteoid osteoma

This is a benign tumour of the long bones of adolescents and young adults. It has a central nidus of irregular trabeculae or woven bone and osteoid, set in a highly vascular stroma surrounded by a mass of sclerotic bone.

An osteoblastoma is microscopically indistinguishable. It differs from osteoid osteoma only in size (it is larger, with the cut off being 1 cm) and by a tendency to be found in the spine.

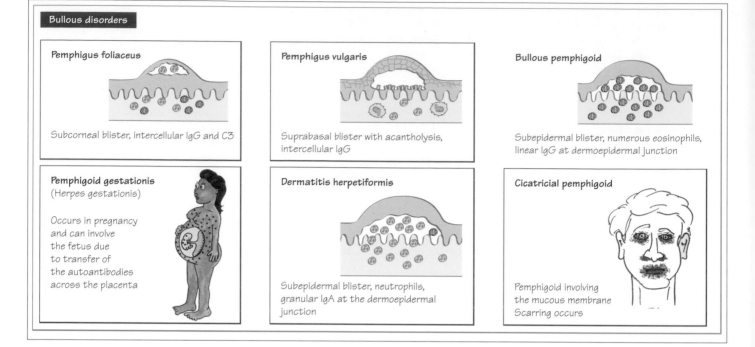

Bullous disorders

Pemphigus foliaceus
Subcorneal blister, intercellular IgG and C3

Pemphigus vulgaris
Suprabasal blister with acantholysis, intercellular IgG

Bullous pemphigoid
Subepidermal blister, numerous eosinophils, linear IgG at dermoepidermal junction

Pemphigoid gestationis (Herpes gestationis)
Occurs in pregnancy and can involve the fetus due to transfer of the autoantibodies across the placenta

Dermatitis herpetiformis
Subepidermal blister, neutrophils, granular IgA at the dermoepidermal junction

Cicatricial pemphigoid
Pemphigoid involving the mucous membrane Scarring occurs

The inflammatory dermatoses comprise a diverse range of conditions, such that textbooks of dermatopathology are typically comfortably in excess of 1000 pages. Therefore, an exploration of even the commonest conditions is difficult within the format of this book, but an introduction to the basic patterns of inflammation is possible.

Terminology
There are many specific terms in dermatopathology that are used to describe changes within the skin. Some of the most common are:
• **Acantholysis**: splitting of the attachment between epidermal cells, often giving a microscopic appearance of the epidermis falling apart.
• **Acanthosis**: thickening of the epidermis.
• **Bulla**: a blister over 5 mm.
• **Erythematous**: red.
• **Hyperkeratosis**: an increase in the thickness of the keratin layer. The normal thickness of the keratin layer varies between different sites. For example, palmar and plantar skin have abundant keratin.
• **Macule**: a small, flat spot.
• **Nodule**: a big lump (bigger than 5 mm).
• **Papule**: a small lump (under 5 mm).
• **Parakeratosis**: persistence of basophilic nuclear material within the keratin layer.
• **Plaque**: flat lesion over 20 mm in width but shallow.
• **Spongiosis**: oedema within the epidermis.
• **Vesicle**: a blister under 5 mm.

Basic categories
Spongiotic diseases
The spongiotic group of disorders includes eczema. The hallmark is oedema within the epidermis. The accumulation of fluid in the intercellular spaces causes the keratinocytes to appear to be further apart from each other, often with accentuation of the intercellular bridges. The oedema is typically accompanied by an inflammatory infiltrate within the dermis, in conjunction with movement of inflammatory cells, usually lymphocytes, into the epidermis – a process referred to as exocytosis.

Lichenoid diseases
The most well known lichenoid disorder is lichen planus. Erythema multiforme also falls into this category, as do the lupus erythematosus spectrum and cutaneous graft versus host disease. The pathology here is centred on the dermoepidermal junction. There is a chronic inflammatory cell infiltrate in the upper dermis that has a band-like configuration and is usually rich in lymphocytes. The inflammation produces degeneration of the basal layer of the epidermis such that it can become irregular and poorly defined. The keratinocytes may become swollen (vacuolar degeneration), and necrotic keratinocytes can form eosinophilic bodies that are known as Civatte bodies.

Psoriasiform diseases
As the name implies, the model for psoriasiform disorders is psoriasis. The pathological process is increased turnover of the epidermis. This is seen as elongation of the rete ridges in a fairly regular pattern. This acanthosis is usually accompanied by hyperkeratosis and often parakeratosis. Chronic inflammation is present in the dermis.

In psoriasis, parakeratosis is usual and is associated with loss of the underlying granular layer. There is thinning of the epidermis where it overlies the projections of the papillary dermis (suprapapillary thinning).

Systems pathology

Table 102.1 Types and properties of bullous disorders.

Disease	Location of blister	Target protein	Immunofluorescence	Inflammatory cells	Other
Pemphigus foliaceus	Intracorneal or subcorneal	Desmoglein 1	IgG and C3 Throughout epidermis, but sparing basal layer	Few neutrophils in blister Neutrophils and eosinophils in dermis	
Pemphigus vulgaris	Suprabasal	Desmoglein 3	IgG Intercellular regions of epidermis, sparing upper part	Few cells in blister Mild mixed infiltrate in the dermis	Tombstone appearances of surviving basal keratinocytes A few acantholytic cells in the blister
Bullous pemphigoid	Subepidermal	Bullous pemphigoid antigens 1 and 2	IgG and C3 Basement membrane, uniform, linear staining	Eosinophils in blister Eosinophils in dermis	
Pemphigoid gestationis (herpes gestationis)	Subepidermal	Bullous pemphigoid antigen 2	C3, sometimes IgG Basement membrane, uniform and linear staining	Eosinophils, lymphocytes and histiocytes in blister and dermis	Occurs only in pregnancy Can affect the fetus
Dermatitis herpetiformis	Subepidermal	Uncertain	IgA Granular pattern in dermal papillae	Neutrophils predominant over eosinophils initially Neutrophils in oedematous dermal papillae is characteristic	Associated with coeliac disease Very itchy so blisters often rupture due to scratching
Cicatricial pemphigoid	Subepidermal	Bullous pemphigoid antigen 2 Epiligrin	Similar to bullous pemphigoid	Neutrophils at first, eosinophils and lymphocytes later	Scarring Affects mucous membranes, notably eye and oral

Bullous diseases

Bullous diseases are those that form blisters. Examples include bullous pemphigoid, dermatitis herpetiformis and pemphigus vulgaris (and its other variants). The blisters are caused by defective intercellular adhesions at different levels of the epidermis and the dermoepidermal junction, which in turn are usually secondary to an autoimmune response directed against the relevant proteins. Different conditions are due to defects in particular parts of this network and therefore produce different patterns of disease. This is most readily manifest by the level of the epidermis at which the blister is formed. Table 102.1 gives the location of the blister in a few different bullous disorders and also the protein that is targeted and the pattern of immunofluorescence. Superficially placed blisters tend to be more prone to rupture than deeper located bullae.

Categorisation of bullous disorders is based upon the location of the blister, the accompanying inflammatory cell infiltrate and the pattern of immunofluorescence. Immunofluorescence studies the deposition of the various immunoglobulins, complement and fibrinogen in the epidermis in terms of the location of the deposition and its pattern.

Granulomatous diseases

As well as systemic diseases such as sarcoidosis, and infections like tuberculosis, leprosy and leishmaniasis, there are also specific dermatological conditions that feature cutaneous granulomas. These include necrobiosis lipoidica and granuloma annulare, although the granulomas in the latter are often extremely poorly formed.

Vasculopathic diseases

Disorders of blood vessels can yield skin conditions. The cause may either be a systemic vasculitis or be of another vascular aetiology, such as urticaria.

Clinical correlations

Dermatological conditions that involve a large area of skin, such as erythema multiforme/toxic epidermonecrolysis and severe psoriasis, can produce systemic complications due to disruption of the normal function of the skin. Burns can also be considered in this respect.

- Thermoregulation is impaired as the insulating effect of the skin is lost.
- Fluid balance is compromised. The skin is waterproof and is resistant to the passive loss of fluid on exposure to the air. However, the underlying tissues are not resilient to passive fluid loss on exposure to the air. Thus, in conditions in which large areas of skin are lost, there are substantial increases in the volume of water lost through the cutaneous surface of the body.
- The skin is part of the innate immune system in its capacity as a barrier. Widespread disruption of this barrier provides easier access for infectious organisms.

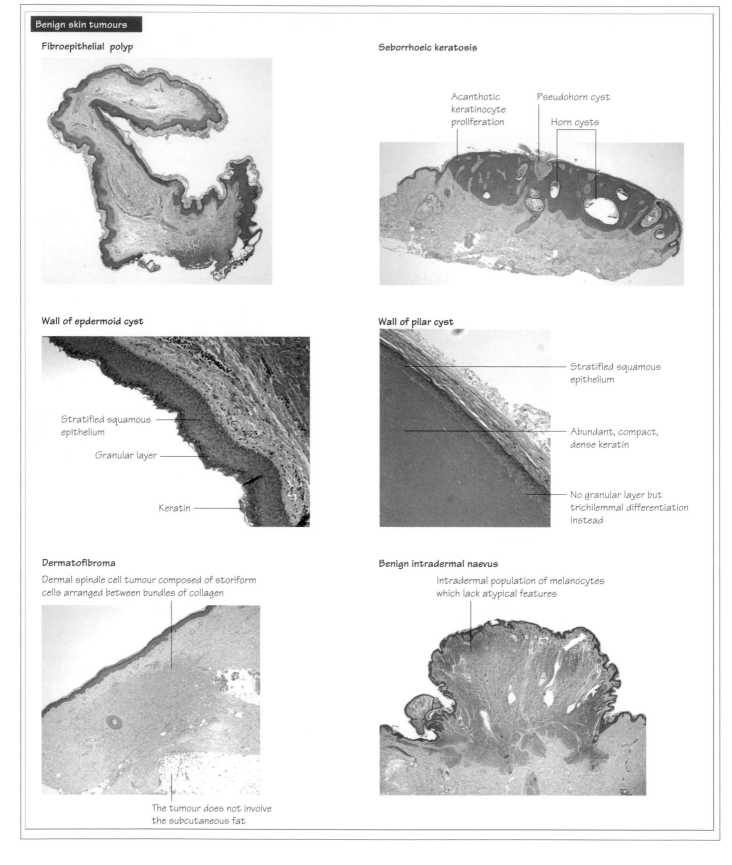

Benign skin tumours

Fibroepithelial polyp

Seborrhoeic keratosis

Acanthotic keratinocyte proliferation

Pseudohorn cyst

Horn cysts

Wall of epdermoid cyst

Stratified squamous epithelium

Granular layer

Keratin

Wall of pilar cyst

Stratified squamous epithelium

Abundant, compact, dense keratin

No granular layer but trichilemmal differentiation instead

Dermatofibroma

Dermal spindle cell tumour composed of storiform cells arranged between bundles of collagen

The tumour does not involve the subcutaneous fat

Benign intradermal naevus

Intradermal population of melanocytes which lack atypical features

A wide range of benign tumours can develop in the skin and their number can support, in specialist textbooks, chapters that themselves exceed the size of this book. Therefore, only a small proportion of the entities will be discussed here, but they are the lesions that are likely to be encountered in everyday practice.

Fibroepithelial polyp

These are small, common entities also known as skin tags. They have simple microscopic features and consist of a polyp of skin with a fibrous core.

Seborrhoeic keratosis

The seborrhoeic keratosis, also known as the seborrhoeic wart or basal cell papilloma, is a benign tumour of the epidermal keratinocytes. It may arise anywhere on the body and tends to be more common in late middle age and the elderly.

Seborrhoeic keratoses are typically brown, well defined, relatively small and appear warty. They are said to look as if there are 'stuck on'. The tumour is composed of keratinocytes, usually arranged as acanthotic, papillomatous projections with overlying hyperkeratosis, or as a more endophytic nodule without papillomatous projections. Infoldings of the tumour yield horn cysts and pseudohorn cysts.

Epidermoid cyst

Contrary to popular belief, the term sebaceous cyst is not a correct alternative designation for this entity. Epidermoid cysts can arise in a variety of places and are believed to develop due to entrapment of a small quantity of epidermis in the dermis. This forms a cyst that is lined by epidermal stratified squamous epithelium, which has the usual granular layer of skin and makes keratin. Hence the contents are often soft and creamy.

Pilar cyst

Pilar cysts are typically located on the scalp. They are frequently multiple and individuals who develop them often have a tendency to develop further pilar cysts. They are similar to epidermoid cysts except that their stratified squamous epithelium shows pilar (hair follicle) type differentiation such that it does not have a granular layer and produces very dense and compact keratin in an abrupt transition from the squamous cells.

Dermatofibroma

Dermatofibromas are dermal tumours that may be found in many locations, although the limbs are among the more common sites. The precise cell of origin is uncertain, although an older synonym that indicates some of the lines of thought is fibrous histiocytoma.

Dermatofibromas are fairly small and can produce a nodule. They consist of spindle-shaped cells with bland nuclei arranged between thickened bundles of collagen. The tumour is separated from the epidermis by a thin zone of uninvolved dermis and the overlying epidermis is usually acanthotic. Unlike dermatofibrosarcoma protuberans, they do not infiltrate the subcutaneous fat.

Melanocytic naevi

Melanocytic naevi are colloquially known as moles. While the term naevus implies that the tumour is present at birth, this is often not the case and is reflected in the specific variant, congenital naevus.

Melanocytic naevus NOS

These naevi are the junctional, compound and intradermal naevi. The distinctions are of little to no clinical relevance, other than that the junctional naevus is more likely to be flat, whereas the other two will be nodular. In all three cases, the naevi are small, with regular edges and are pigmented.

The three terms reflect the location of the melanocytes, either at the dermoepidermal junction, at the dermoepidermal junction and in the dermis, or in the dermis alone. The hypothesis is that after arising from the neural crest, cutaneous melanocytes normally migrate to the dermoepidermal junction. In the case of the melanocytic naevus, as some of the melanocytes mature, they descend into the dermis. As more time elapses, the junctional component descends, leaving only the intradermal melanocytes. This phenomenon is of relevance to histopathologists as the permissible extent and nature of a junctional melanocytic population in a melanocytic tumour can vary with the age of the patient.

Blue naevus

Blue naevi are dermal melanocytic naevi in which the melanocytes are generally spindle cell shaped and produce large amounts of pigment. However, due to the deep nature of the pigment and the differential refraction of different wavelengths of light, the naevi appear blue (the Tindall effect).

Halo naevus

The halo naevus possesses an area of pallor around it. This is due to a lymphocytic response to the naevus, which causes regression of the lesion. The microscopic features of the melanocytic component itself are similar to usual naevi but are accompanied by a very dense infiltrate of lymphocytes.

Congenital naevus

These naevi are present at birth. Many of their basic features are similar to the standard naevus, although they can show some nuances. Congenital naevi are often hair bearing and can be larger than acquired naevi. In some cases, they may be extremely large and can occupy half or more of the trunk. This can be problematic because large congenital naevi are at an increased risk of undergoing malignant transformation, but excising the affected area of skin is difficult.

Spitz naevus

The old name for a Spitz naevus is juvenile melanoma. The term is unfortunate as the lesion is not malignant (although malignant variants do exist). It occurs mainly in children and young adults and is normally a red nodule. Recognition of the lesion microscopically is outside the scope of this book, although it should be noted that the appearances can be confused with a genuine melanoma.

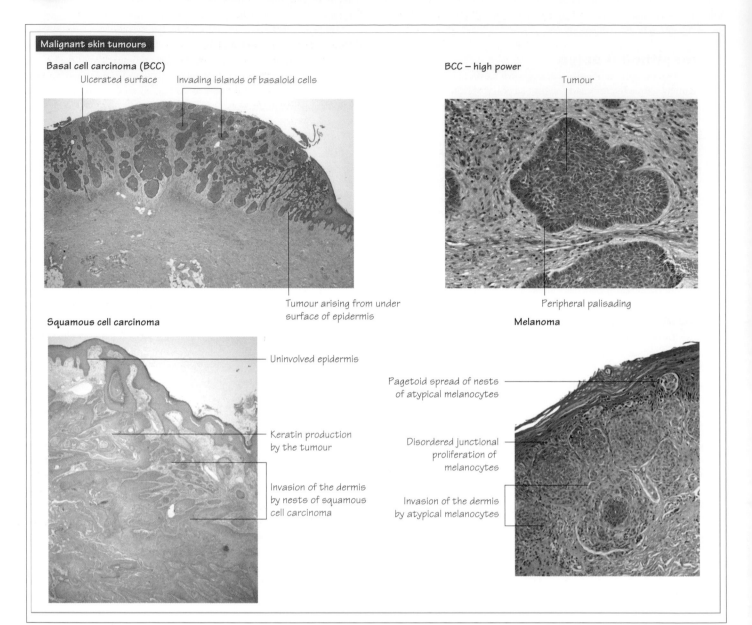

Malignant skin tumours

Basal cell carcinoma (BCC)
- Ulcerated surface
- Invading islands of basaloid cells
- Tumour arising from under surface of epidermis

BCC – high power
- Tumour
- Peripheral palisading

Squamous cell carcinoma
- Uninvolved epidermis
- Keratin production by the tumour
- Invasion of the dermis by nests of squamous cell carcinoma

Melanoma
- Pagetoid spread of nests of atypical melanocytes
- Disordered junctional proliferation of melanocytes
- Invasion of the dermis by atypical melanocytes

Basal cell carcinoma (BBC)

Epidemiology

Basal cell carcinoma is the commonest skin malignancy. The incidence increases with age, with late middle age and the elderly most affected.

Risk factors

The ultraviolet light component of sunlight is the main aetiological component. Other less significant factors are X-rays, arsenic and immunosuppression. Basal cell carcinomas are also a feature of Gorlin's syndrome and xeroderma pigmentosa, where they develop at an early age.

Pathology

The majority (80%) of BCCs arise on the head and face, with most of the remainder being located on the shoulders, back and chest. Basal cell carcinomas generally form a nodule, with the traditional description alluding to raised edges and a pearly appearance. The tumour may be ulcerated. The superficial subtype may have a more plaque-like appearance with poorly defined edges.

Although several different histological subtypes of BCC exist, they all share the feature of being composed of relatively uniform basaloid cells that resemble those of the basal layer of the epidermis. The cells tend to form islands, at least some of which will be

Systems pathology

connected to the underside of the epidermis. The cells line up around the edges of the island to form a palisade. Separation of the islands from the dermis is a frequently found artefact and is of diagnostic utility.

Most of the histological subclassification is of little clinical relevance, but the superficial, morpheic (infiltrative) and micronodular forms have a greater tendency to local recurrence.

Pattern of spread

Despite its designation as a carcinoma, a BCC is remarkably inept at metastasising, with distant spread occurring in only one in 2000 cases and then only usually to local lymph nodes. However, the tumour is relentlessly locally aggressive and before modern treatment could literally destroy huge parts of the face.

Squamous cell carcinoma (SCC)
Epidemiology
Like BCCs, SCCs are derived from keratinocytes and share a similar age distribution.

Risk factors
Sun exposure is again the main risk factor. Infection with human papilloma virus may also have a role. Immunosuppression is of greater significance than in BCC in that most immunosuppressed patients, particularly transplant patients, who develop skin tumours tend to have SCCs rather than BCCs. Chronic ulcers may also be complicated by SCCs.

Pathology
Cutaneous SCC have similar features to SCC that are found at other sites.

Pattern of spread
Spread is usually to regional lymph nodes, although the frequency with which this occurs varies with the location of the primary tumour. Perineal and penile SCC region spreads to lymph nodes in 30–80% of cases. Those arising in chronic ulcers metastasise in 10–30%, while SCC that develop in sun-exposed regions spread in only 1–5% of cases.

Melanoma
Definition
Melanoma is a malignant tumour that is derived from melanocytes.

Epidemiology
Melanoma has a less slanted age distribution than basal cell carcinoma, with an incidence of around 12 per 100 000 per year.

Risk factors
Sun exposure is the key agent. Unlike basal cell and squamous cell carcinoma, in which the sun exposure tends to be chronic, in melanoma it is intermittent and, in particular, associated with burning. Other factors include dysplastic naevi, xeroderma pigmentosa and family history.

Pathology
A wide variety of sites can be affected and melanoma can arise in numerous other organs. Melanomas are typically pigmented brown but the rarer amelanotic form lacks melanin. Melanomas tend to be larger than naevi, irregular in pigmentation, outline and contours, may itch or bleed and change in size. The microscopic features are summarised in the figure.

If the atypical melanocytes are confined to the epidermis, the tumour is an *in situ* lesion. However, if atypical melanocytes invade the dermis, the melanoma is invasive. Two patterns of invasive melanoma exist:
- In radial growth phase, the tumour is considered to still be spreading primarily in a horizontal fashion.
- In the vertical growth phase the emphasis is on invasion down into the dermis. The prognosis is worse as access to the deeper lymphovascular structure that permits dissemination is more likely.

The criteria for distinguishing the two phases are beyond the remit of this book.

Both radial and vertical growth phase melanomas are characterised by the Breslow thickness. This is a very important prognostic parameter and is the distance from the granular layer to the deepest invasive melanocyte. Related to the Breslow thickness is Clarke's level, although this is more qualitative and relates the melanoma to one of five structural layers of the skin.

Assorted melanoma subtypes exist. The commonest is the superficial spreading type. Nodular melanomas are in the vertical growth phase and tend to be thick. Lentigo maligna melanoma develops on the face of elderly people. Acral lentigenous melanoma is found on the palms and soles and is the only melanoma to occur with any frequency in Afro-Caribbeans.

Pattern of spread
Melanoma can metastasise to local and distant lymph nodes, other sites in the skin and numerous internal organs. Melanoma is one of the tumours that is most likely to spread to the kidney and heart.

Prognosis
The prognosis is intimately related to the Breslow thickness, with melanomas less than 0.75 mm thick having a 98% 5-year survival and those more than 1.5 mm thick showing a 5-year survival of around 40–60%. Complete excision of the primary is also vital. Melanomas can recur many years after the primary.

Actinic keratosis and Bowen's disease
These are two precursor lesions to keratinocyte malignancies and share the common property of dysplasia within the epidermis without invasion of the dermis.
- Actinic keratoses tend to occur on the head and neck as small, crusted lesions. They can have a variable degree of disordered epidermal maturation but are associated with hyperkeratosis and parakeratosis.
- Bowen's disease in the more stringent use of the term refers to red scaly patches on the face and legs of the elderly, typically women, in which the patches show full thickness, usually very marked, epidermal dysplasia. The term is sometimes used more liberally for any lesion that has these histopathological features, although some argue it must be reserved for those entities which have both the clinical and histological characteristics. To overcome this problem, the term Bowenoid keratosis is employed, which implies a lesion with full thickness dysplasia.

Benign breast disease

Sclerosing adenosis
Glandular structures infiltrate the breast stromal tissue and may resemble IDC. However these are pinched-off TDLU, which are lined by both epithelium and myoepithelium and are benign. They probably result from previous inflammation followed by scarring around the TDLU.
See chapter 106

Epithelial hyperplasia
Lining intraductal cells proliferate, along with myoepithelial cells, to expand the duct. Often this causes obstruction to the flow of secretions and may cause cystic dilatation of the TDLU. 'Atypical epithelial hyperplasia' is considered to be a precursor to in situ lobular and ductal neoplasia and is discussed in chapter 106

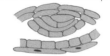

Phyllodes tumour
This exceptionally rare tumour is the malignant counterpart of the benign fibroadenoma and is usually large, 5 cm diameter or more. The glandular element is benign. It is the stromal element whch is cellular and behaves in a malignant fashion, though often this is low-grade and only very slowly progressive locally

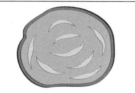

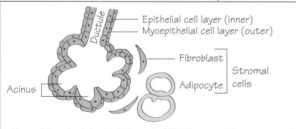

Epithelial cell layer (inner)
Myoepithelial cell layer (outer)
Ductule
Fibroblast
Stromal cells
Acinus
Adipocyte

Normal terminal duct lobular unit (TDLU) comprising an extra-lobular, then intralobular terminal duct, which opens into the multiple acini which form the lobule. Most carcinomas are thought to arise from the TDLU

Fibrocystic change
Cystically dilated lobules and ducts, surrounded by an often dense hyaline stroma, probably represent the end result of repeated episodes of inflammation and repair. The breast is diffusely nodular and firm to palpation, without the crisp, hard-edged lump often palpated in malignant disease

Radial scar
Stellate form of fibrocystic disease which may mimic a cancer (see text)

Nipple
15–20 collecting ducts receive secretions from the entire lobular and ductal system and open onto the surface

Intraduct papilloma
These benign tumours present with a bloodstained nipple discharge. The differential diagnosis is from a papillary intraductal carcinoma. Benign intraduct papillomas have a connective tissue core and are lined by a double cell layer of epithelium and myoepithelium

Myoepithelium
Epithelium

Epithelial and myoepithelial elements
Dense connective tissue stroma with few fibroblasts

Fibroadenoma
This is a very common benign tumour of breast, which is usually smooth and easily palpable and generally 2–3 cm in diameter. It is very well circumscribed and consists of two elements: epithelium and stroma. The epithelium consists of glandular epithelium and myoepithelium from the TDLU and the bland connective tissue is secreted by the stromal cells associated with the breast lobule. Rarely, giant (benign) fibroadenomas, 5–10cm diameter, are encountered, particularly in young Afro-Caribbean women

Hamartoma
A circumscribed mass of haphazardly arranged breast tissue. This may resemble a fibroadenoma

Systems pathology

Fibroadenoma

Definition
Fibroadenoma is a benign tumour of the breast epithelium and stroma.

Epidemiology
Fibroadenomas are common tumours and tend to occur in women under the age of 30 years.

Pathology
Fibroadenomas are usually small (under 3 cm), firm and circumscribed. They are mobile within the breast and grow slowly. The cut surface has a vaguely lobulated pattern and is usually light grey.

Both stromal and epithelial elements are present in the tumour, although admixed mature adipose tissue tends not to be seen. The epithelium is present as elongated duct-like structures, which frequently appear to be compressed by the stroma. The stroma has a modest density of cells and often features regions of myxoid change. The stroma can also display additional characteristics such as hyalinisation, calcification or osteochondroid change.

The epithelium can exhibit hyperplastic or metaplastic changes. While carcinoma in situ may also develop, this is rare.

Hamartoma

Definition
A breast hamartoma is a benign mass that is composed of all components of the normal breast.

Epidemiology
Although hamartomas can be encountered in a wide range of ages, they tend to occur in peri-menopausal women.

Pathology
Hamartomas are well demarcated, usually encapsulated lesions that range in size from 1 to 20 cm. Depending upon the precise composition of the lesion, the cut surface may resemble normal breast or appear like a lipoma or fibroadenoma.

A hamartoma demonstrates the normal constituents of breast in the form of benign breast ducts and lobular units, fibrous stroma and mature adipose tissue. The proportions of each may vary. Distinction from normal breast requires that the lesion is recognised as being discrete and may therefore require additional data from radiological investigations, particularly in the case of a core biopsy.

Fibrocystic/benign breast change

Definition
Fibrocystic and benign breast change encompasses a variety of benign, non-neoplastic processes that affect the breast epithelial structures.

Epidemiology
Fibrocystic change is common and, while affecting women in the reproductive years, tends to involve a slightly older age group than fibroadenoma. It is most frequently seen in women aged from 30 to 50 years.

Pathology
The process can be localised within the breast or be a more diffuse process. Varying degrees of circumscription are encountered. The lesion may be dominated by a cystic component or fibrosis, in the latter case having a firm, grey-white appearance. Several microscopic elements can be found.

- Simple cystic change is due to dilatation of the terminal duct lobular units and yields cysts lined by an inner layer of breast epithelium and an outer layer of myoepithelial cells.
- Apocrine metaplasia is frequently associated with cyst formation. The epithelial cells have abundant granular eosinophilic cytoplasm, larger nuclei and may show decapitation secretion in which blebs of their adluminal cytoplasm are shed into the lumen.
- Sclerosing adenosis is a proliferation of breast acini set within a fibrous stroma. Importantly, the adenosis retains the lobular architecture of normal breast and the normal bilayered epithelium. This distinction is crucial in differentiating the lesion from lower grade carcinomas.
- A radial scar is an important lesion that can mimic carcinoma on imaging due to its stellate shape. The lesion retains this configuration microscopically due to dense fibrosis which imparts the stellate morphology. Adenosis is found within the radial scar but again retains the bilayered epithelial arrangement.
- Particularly in the case of radial scar, benign breast disease can show coexisting changes of hyperplasia, or even rarely carcinoma in situ.

Papilloma
Breast papillomas are benign lesions that tend to be found in the larger ducts and usually present in the fourth and fifth decades. Obstruction of these ducts by the papillomas can lead to a nipple discharge. As with papillomas elsewhere in the body, the breast papilloma has a branching fibrovascular core that is lined by epithelial structures, in this case the normal bilayered epithelial–myoepithelial tissue of the breast. Caution is warranted in the histopathological assessment of biopsies due to the existence of papillary carcinomas. More peripherally located papillomas can also arise.

Epithelial hyperplasia
Hyperplasia is a benign, epithelial proliferation. It is also referred to as hyperplasia of usual type or hyperplasia without atypia. Ductal epithelial hyperplasia is benign but has an increased risk of subsequent carcinoma of approximately 1.5 times.

The affected TDLU contain an increased number of epithelial cells that are admixed with myoepithelial cells. Although the cells may form a solid proliferation that occupies the lumen, they are more commonly arranged to form multiple, small, secondary lumens within the contour of the duct. The cells are haphazardly arranged. Separating hyperplasia from carcinoma in situ is not always straightforward, but a detailed discussion of this diagnostic process is outside the remit of this book and lies in the postgraduate arena.

Others
Various other non-malignant entities can occur within the breast. Proliferations of the myoepithelial cells can occur. Benign mesenchymal tumours such as haemangiomas and lipomas may develop. Abscesses may be seen in lactating women. Awareness of the diversity of breast lesions is useful. Beware 'inflammatory carcinoma' which clinically mimics the redness, induration and heat of acute inflammation.

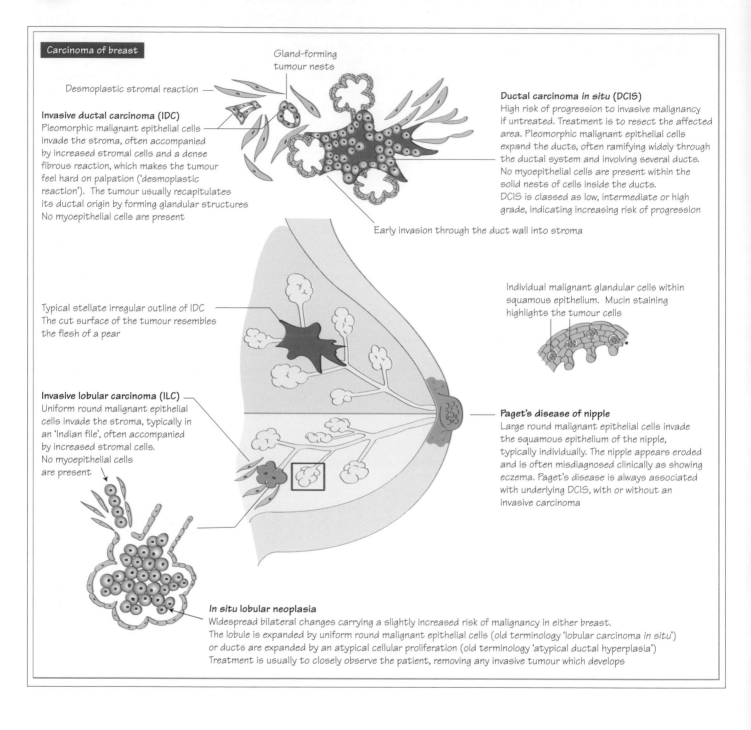

Carcinoma of breast

Gland-forming tumour nests

Desmoplastic stromal reaction

Invasive ductal carcinoma (IDC)
Pleomorphic malignant epithelial cells invade the stroma, often accompanied by increased stromal cells and a dense fibrous reaction, which makes the tumour feel hard on palpation ('desmoplastic reaction'). The tumour usually recapitulates its ductal origin by forming glandular structures
No myoepithelial cells are present

Ductal carcinoma *in situ* (DCIS)
High risk of progression to invasive malignancy if untreated. Treatment is to resect the affected area. Pleomorphic malignant epithelial cells expand the ducts, often ramifying widely through the ductal system and involving several ducts. No myoepithelial cells are present within the solid nests of cells inside the ducts.
DCIS is classed as low, intermediate or high grade, indicating increasing risk of progression

Early invasion through the duct wall into stroma

Typical stellate irregular outline of IDC
The cut surface of the tumour resembles the flesh of a pear

Individual malignant glandular cells within squamous epithelium. Mucin staining highlights the tumour cells

Invasive lobular carcinoma (ILC)
Uniform round malignant epithelial cells invade the stroma, typically in an 'Indian file', often accompanied by increased stromal cells.
No myoepithelial cells are present

Paget's disease of nipple
Large round malignant epithelial cells invade the squamous epithelium of the nipple, typically individually. The nipple appears eroded and is often misdiagnosed clinically as showing eczema. Paget's disease is always associated with underlying DCIS, with or without an invasive carcinoma

***In situ* lobular neoplasia**
Widespread bilateral changes carrying a slightly increased risk of malignancy in either breast.
The lobule is expanded by uniform round malignant epithelial cells (old terminology 'lobular carcinoma *in situ*')
or ducts are expanded by an atypical cellular proliferation (old terminology 'atypical ductal hyperplasia')
Treatment is usually to closely observe the patient, removing any invasive tumour which develops

Systems pathology

Definition

Breast carcinoma is a malignant epithelial tumour of the breast.

Epidemiology

Breast carcinoma is the commonest cancer in women, although in the United Kingdom, lung cancer is closing the gap. The incidence is approximately 110–120 per 100 000 women per year. The disease does occur in males, but male breast cancer accounts for only 1% of cases. The majority of cases present over the age of 50 years, particularly from 50 to 65 years.

Risk factors

Numerous risk factors have been involved, many of which are related to exposure of the breast to endogenous oestrogens. Thus, early menarche, late menopause, nulliparity and later age at first full-term birth all elevate the risk. In relation to this, exogenous hormones in the form of the oral contraceptive pill have also been suggested to increase the risk of developing breast cancer.

Dietary factors have been invoked, such as a westernised diet. Increased weight is also a risk factor and may relate to higher oestrogen levels in heavier women. Alcohol is a mild risk factor. Unlike many other cancers, smoking has not been demonstrated to increase the risk.

Assorted other breast diseases, such as hyperplasia, are associated with a small increase (1.5–2 times) in the risk.

Familial breast cancer accounts for 10% of cases and is linked to the *BRCA1* and *BRCA2* genes.

Pathology

Two separate divisions exist for breast cancer. There is the categorisation into ductal and lobular and the separation into in situ and invasive disease.

The division into ductal and lobular subtypes reflects derivation of these two subtypes from the ductal and lobular components of the **terminal duct lobular unit (TDLU)**. In practice, the distinction has been made on the basis of the different morphologies displayed by the two subtypes. More recent work has uncovered at least one molecular difference in that most cases of ductal carcinoma express e-cadherin, while this cell surface adhesion molecule is lost in 80% of cases of lobular carcinoma.

Ductal carcinoma in situ (DCIS)

Ductal carcinoma in situ is believed to be a precursor lesion for invasive carcinoma, but progression from in situ carcinoma to carcinoma is not obligatory. DCIS has a relative risk factor of 8–11 times for subsequent invasive carcinoma. The process is centred on the ducts, but can spread into the lobules in extensive disease. The affected ducts are expanded by a proliferation of cells that show varying degrees of cytological atypia, which forms the basis for the categorisation into three grades. The cells have a more orderly arrangement than in hyperplasia and admixed myo-epithelial cells are not present. Several grades of DCIS are recognised: low, intermediate and high. The higher the grade, the greater is the risk of progression to invasive ductal carcinoma.

Paget's disease of the nipple: This is a variant of DCIS in which the atypical cells extend up the ductal system to reach the skin of the nipple, where they are scattered within the epithelium.

In-situ lobular neoplasia (ISLN)

This term encompasses lesions previously known as 'atypical lobular hyperplasia' and 'lobular carcinoma in situ'. 'Lobular carcinoma in situ' affects the terminal lobules. These are expanded by a monotonous population of cells that can often look quite bland. In 'atypical ductal hyperplasia' the terminal ducts are expanded by similar cells. While there is an increased risk of developing invasive carcinoma, it is low and is insufficient to justify prophylactic mastectomy, particularly as the side and site of development of the carcinoma cannot be predicted from the location of the ISLN.

Invasive carcinoma

Both ductal and lobular carcinomas are adenocarcinomas and are frequently associated with coexisting in situ disease.

Invasive ductal carcinoma (IDC): IDC comprises around 75% of breast malignancies. There is a wide variation in the macroscopic properties, both in terms of shape and size, although the tumour is usually firm to hard. There is also considerable variation in the microscopic features. Tubule formation is present to a greater or lesser degree, but the cells are also arranged in nests, sheets, cords and islands. The degree of pleomorphism and mitotic activity varies and, with tubule formation, form the basis for the three-tier Nottingham grading system.

Important variants of IDC with a better prognosis are:
• Medullary IDC, in which syncytial sheets of cells are set within a dense lymphoid background, in the absence of DCIS.
• Mucinous IDC, where the tumour elaborates abundant extracellular mucin.
• Tubular IDC, in which there are numerous tubules lined by cells that are only mildly atypical.

Invasive lobular carcinoma: This constitutes 5–15% of breast malignancies. It is poorly defined macroscopically. Tubule formation is rare and the cells are instead arranged in single files or cords that infiltrate through the stroma. Concentration of the cells around pre-existing structures, in a targetoid arrangement, is characteristic. The cells are usually small and show only mild to moderate pleomorphism. Grading is by the Nottingham system.

Pattern of spread

Direct spread is to the skin and chest wall. Local lymphatic extension is to the axillary nodes, but also the internal mammary and supraclavicular lymph nodes. Distant haematogenous metastases can be to numerous sites, but bone, lung and liver are the most common.

Staging

The TNM system is used (see Chapter 28). Tumour size and tethering to the skin are important parameters.

Prognosis

The 5-year survival is approximately 80%, with a 20-year survival of 60%. However, breast cancer is a tumour that can characteristically recur after long intervals. The expression of the c-erb2 protein and oestrogen and progesterone receptors can affect the prognosis and treatment.

Case studies and questions

Case 1: Acute collapse with chest pain

A 63-year-old man presents to accident and emergency with a 30-minute history of severe, central crushing chest pain that radiates to his left arm and is associated with nausea. On examination, he is unwell and clammy. His pulse is 90 beats per minute and his blood pressure is 100/60 mmHg. Bibasal crackles are heard.

1 *What is the most likely diagnosis and what risk factors can easily be ascertained?*

2 *The patient's ECG is given below. What does it show and what is the diagnosis?*

Thrombolytic treatment is instituted, in combination with aspirin and analgesia and the patient is transferred to a cardiac care unit. Two days after admission, he complains of a sudden onset of shortness of breath. On examination, his jugular venous pressure is raised and he has a parasternal heave and a pansystolic murmur, heard best at the lower left sternal edge, that does not radiate to the carotid arteries. Widespread crackles are heard throughout his lung fields. His ECG shows no new acute event.

3 *What is likely to have happened?*

4 *What is the mechanism?*

5 *What treatment may help to reduce the incidence of rupture of the ventricular septum, free ventricular wall or papillary muscles?*

6 *What are the underlying pathological processes that cause myocardial infarction?*

7 *What other organs might be affected by this underlying process?*

8 *What other complications of myocardial infarction can occur?*

Case 2: Recent weakness and malaise

A 31-year-old man consults his general practitioner as he has been troubled by impotence and a reduced libido for the last 3 months. He has also noticed that he is tired, feels lethargic, is unable to exercise as much as usual, is constipated, has remarked a reduction in the quantity of his body hair and generally feels unwell. His previous medical history is unremarkable except for a concussion and a fractured skull that he suffered 6 months previously when he was playing rugby.

On examination he is pale and has a smaller than expected quantity of body hair in the axillary and genital regions. His testes appear to be small. His blood pressure is 95/60 mmHg and he has a postural drop to 80/50 mmHg on standing. The patient mentions feeling dizzy when he stands and requires a few moments to recover. His muscle bulk is disproportionately low for the degree of normal physical activity he indicated in his history.

The GP suspects a diagnosis and requests a series of related blood tests, the results of which are as follows:

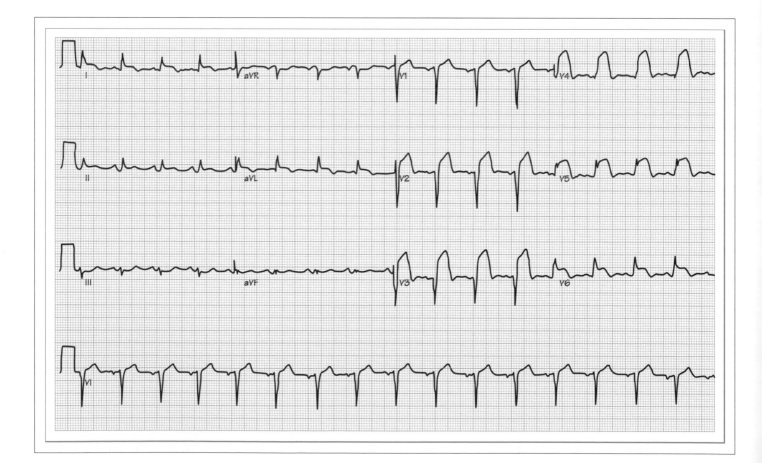

Na$^+$:	131 mmol/L (135–145)
K$^+$:	5.3 mmol/L (3.5–5)
Urea:	6.4 mmol/L (2.5–6.7)
Creatinine:	88 µmol/L (70–170)
Glucose:	3.0 mmol/L (3.5–5 fasting)
Ca^{2+} (corrected):	2.69 mmol/L (2.1–2.65)

1 *What abnormalities are present in the blood tests?*

2 *What condition could explain the electrolyte, renal function, calcium and glucose abnormalities?*

Further test results arrive:

TSH:	0.1 mU/L (0.5–5)
T4:	25 mmol/L (70–140)
FSH:	2 IU/L (5–20)
LH:	2 IU/L (5–20)
Testosterone	1 ng/L (3–10)

3 *What hormonal abnormalities are present and is anything unusual about them?*

4 *What is the overall unifying diagnosis and what are its causes?*

5 *What other hormones could be affected and what specialised tests might be performed to confirm the assorted endocrine abnormalities?*

Case 3: At the breast clinic

In a breast lump outpatient clinic, the first patient is a 28-year-old woman who has a 2 cm mobile lump within her right breast. The lump is well defined. A fine needle aspiration (FNA) is performed in the clinic and the lump is reported as a fibroadenoma. The radiology concords with this.

1 *What is a fibroadenoma?*

The second patient is a 43-year-old woman who had a recent core biopsy to investigate generalised lumpiness in the upper outer quadrant of her right breast. The lumpiness varies with her menstrual cycle. The report from her core biopsy concords with the radiological findings and gives a diagnosis of fibrocystic disease.

2 *What is fibrocystic disease?*

The next patient is a 59-year-old woman who mentions a 3-month history of a lump in her left breast. On examination, the lump is hard and irregular and seems to be fixed within the breast. An FNA is undertaken within the clinic and the lump is reported as carcinoma.

3 *What is a carcinoma?*

In addition to imaging studies, a core biopsy of the lump is performed. It is reported as a grade 2 invasive ductal carcinoma that is positive for oestrogen and progesterone receptors but negative for c-erb-B2.

4 *What is the main division of types of breast carcinoma? What is the significance of the receptor status?*

The patient has a wide local excision of her breast lump in combination with a level one and two axillary node dissection.

5 *What features of the pathology are of particular interest to the surgeon and oncologist?*

Although the patient has clear excision margins, she also has metastases in five axillary lymph nodes. Oncological treatment is instituted. Nine months later she reports shortness of breath when she is seen in the outpatient department. On examination she has bilateral dull percussion notes at both lung bases in conjunction with decreased expansion and decreased breath sounds. A chest X-ray is requested to confirm the clinical diagnosis.

6 *What will the chest X-ray show?*

Cytological aspiration of the pleural fluid reveals carcinoma cells. Further staging investigations are performed and disclose lesions in the liver on CT imaging and in the bone on nuclear imaging. In the clinical context, these lesions are considered to be metastases.

7 *What other tumours commonly metastasise to bone?*

Case 4: Recent onset neurological signs

A 55-year-old right-handed man presents to his general practitioner with a 4-month history of what he describes as 'strange twitches in my left hand'. The twitches occur without warning or any apparent precipitating factor and consist of sharp, involuntary, purposeless jerking movements that last for a few seconds to a few minutes and happen on average twice per day. Once an episode starts, the patient cannot do anything to make it stop. The jerking movements have recently started to involve the forearm and occasionally the elbow. There are no associated sensory symptoms. The patient has not noticed any other movement problems and has no other symptoms. His previous medical history is unremarkable.

The patient states that he initially attributed the problem to the combination of being busy at work and having to use a new computer keyboard and mouse (he works as the deputy manager of the IT department in a large business). However, he had never had any similar sort of problem before and decided that something needed to be done when the problem progressed beyond his hand into his arm.

On examination, the patient's cranial nerves, right upper limb and both lower limbs are normal. However, there is an increase in tone in the forearm and wrist of the left upper limb. The tone is spastic in quality, rather than rigid. Even allowing for the fact that it is the patient's non-dominant arm, the GP thinks that power is reduced to grade 4+/5 in all muscle groups below the elbow. There is also hyperreflexia in the left upper limb. Co-ordination and sensation are normal. The patient's gait is normal.

1 *What sort of pattern of motor features does the patient have in his left upper limb?*

2 *Given that the patient has episodic, abnormal, involuntary movements of a limb, what diagnosis should be considered?*

A few days after seeing his GP, having been referred to the neurology outpatient department, the patient is at home when he suddenly and without warning loses consciousness. This is followed by generalised jerking and shaking of all four limbs and a loss of sphincteral control. The patient is unresponsive and unrousable during this episode, which was witnessed by both his wife and son. The patient's son telephones for an ambulance, which arrives a few minutes after the episode started. The patient's wife and son estimate the duration of the event as a few minutes. The patient is taken to accident and emergency.

3 *What event has the patient just suffered and what diagnosis does the history as a whole suggest?*

A CT scan is performed of the patient's brain and reveals a tumour in the inferior part of the primary motor cortex of the right cerebral hemisphere.

4 *What is the most basic classification of tumours?*

5 *What complications can a brain tumour cause?*

6 *What non-neoplastic lesions can behave as a space-occupying lesion?*

Case 5: Shortness of breath

A 60-year-old man is seen in the outpatient department with a history of exertional dyspnoea. Further questioning reveals that he has also had a cough for the last 3 years. The cough is generally productive, although usually of only small amounts of inoffensive sputum. He is a smoker, having smoked 20 cigarettes a day since the age of 19.

1 *What other information should be sought as part of the respiratory history?*

The patient also mentions that he is feeling slightly more short of breath than usual, and on examination he has scattered wheezes in both lung fields.

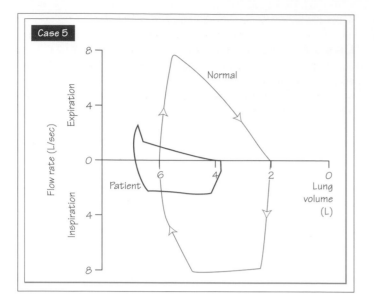

Case 5

Flow volume loop diagram showing Normal and Patient curves, with Flow rate (L/sec) on vertical axis (Expiration above, Inspiration below) and Lung volume (L) on horizontal axis.

2 *What particular diagnosis should be considered and what simple measurement can be performed in the clinic room to pursue this?*

Lung function tests are requested. The patient's flow volume loop is shown in the diagram.

3 *What pattern of change is present?*

The lung function tests also reveal that the patient's defect does not improve with the administration of bronchodilators and a diagnosis of chronic obstructive pulmonary disease (COPD) is made. Appropriate medication and advice are given. Several months later, the patient attends accident and emergency. He is acutely short of breath, has a cough that is productive of large quantities of green sputum and has a low grade pyrexia. Widespread wheeze is present throughout both lung fields.

4 *How can his shortness of breath be assessed at the bedside and what complication has occurred?*

The patient's blood gases (taken while the patient is breathing room air) are as follows:

pH	7.19	(7.35–7.45)
Po_2	7.1 kPa	(11.0–12.6)
Pco_2	7.0 kPa	(4.7–6.0)
HCO_3^-	17 mmol	(19–24)

5 *What is the basic pattern of disease and what is its implication?*

Treatment is begun and the patient recovers over the next week. Over the next 2 years he has four more admissions for infective exacerbations of COPD but manages to stop smoking and his respiratory function remains relatively stable between exacerbations.

6 *What is the basic pathology of COPD?*

7 *What organisms are likely to cause an infective exacerbation and what is the body's typical response to them?*

Two years later, the patient presents to his GP with a 6-week history of weight loss in association with haemoptysis. A chest X-ray reveals a right hilar mass.

8 *What is the most likely diagnosis and how does it relate to his COPD?*

9 *What are the main histological categories for this diagnosis?*

Case 6: Facial rash and joint problems

A 24-year-old woman presents to her general practitioner because she is troubled by aches and pains in her hands, as well as by a rash on her face. The aches and pains in her hands have been present for 3 months and are worse with prolonged use of her hands. She also notices that her finger joints feel stiff if she rests her hands for a long period of time. However, there is no functional impairment.

The rash has been present for 2 months. It occurs over the bridge of her nose and cheeks and seems to be exacerbated by spending time in the sun. The patient has not been using any new soaps, other skin care products, cosmetics or washing powders. She is not taking any medication.

Other than the rash on the patient's face, examination is unremarkable. The GP requests some blood tests and X-rays of the hands and arranges to see the patient with the results.

The patient returns to the GP 3 weeks later and reports a new symptom of swelling of her ankles. At the GP's request she is able to provide a urine sample for dipstick analysis in the surgery. The dipstick shows the presence of protein in the urine but no blood. The patient's blood pressure is normal.

1 *What is the likely unifying diagnosis?*

2 *What blood test in particular will have been especially useful to the GP in reaching a diagnosis?*

3 *What does the coexistence of the proteinuria and peripheral oedema suggest?*

4 *What patterns of renal disease can be encountered in systemic lupus erythematosus (SLE)?*

5 *What complications can occur in nephrotic syndrome?*

The patient is started on treatment and experiences an improvement in her renal function, as well as her joint pains. However, 18 months later she attends the rheumatology outpatient clinic for a follow-up appointment and reports a 3-day onset of weakness in her right arm that is associated with numbness and tingling along the back of the arm, forearm and hand.

On examination, the cranial nerves, left arm and both lower limbs are normal. Tone is not increased in the right upper limb but there is decreased power (grade 4/5) for extension of the right elbow, right wrist and fingers of the right hand. The biceps reflex is normal but the brachioradialis and triceps reflexes are reduced. Sensation is also impaired in the distribution described by the patient.

6 *Are the motor features of upper or lower motor neurone type?*

7 *What nerve root(s) would need to be affected to produce this distribution of features?*

8 *Which peripheral nerve(s) would need to be involved to produce this distribution of features?*

9 *Where is the neurological lesion and does this relate to the patient's previous diagnosis?*

10 *What is the basic pathology of SLE?*

11 *What organs can be affected by SLE?*

Case 7: Longstanding upper GI tract problems

A 53-year-old man attends the gastroenterology outpatient department for the results of his recent upper gastrointestinal endoscopy that was performed during a recent admission for melaena. The patient is aware from the endoscopist's report that he had a gastric ulcer but is anxious to learn the histopathological opinion on the biopsy.

The biopsy report reads: 'The three full thickness pieces of moderately acutely and chronically inflamed non-specialised gastric mucosa are accompanied by ulcer slough. Moderate numbers of *Helicobacter pylori* are observed. No intestinal metaplasia or atropy are seen. No dysplasia or malignancy is identified. Conclusion – gastric biopsy: *H. pylori*-associated ulceration.'

1 *What would you tell the patient if he asks about the biopsy report and asks 'is it cancer, doctor'?*

2 *What is the significance of the H. pylori?*

The patient is prescribed *H. pylori* eradication therapy. The regimen includes metronidazole.

3 *What advice must be given to the patient?*

The patient is also scheduled for a repeat endoscopy in 6 weeks.

4 *Why?*

The patient is well for the next 8 years, over which time his weight has increased a lot. He then presents to his general practitioner with a 4-month history of a burning retrosternal pain. The pain is worse at night when he goes to bed and can be precipitated by bending over. There is no relationship of the pain to exertion and no radiation to the neck or arms.

5 *What is the likely diagnosis and with what abnormality is it likely to be associated?*

In view of the patient's previous history, another upper GI endoscopy is performed. No ulcer or tumour is seen, but there are red tongues of velvety mucosa that extend into the oesophagus from the gastro-oesophageal junction. The photograph illustrates the microscopical appearance of a biopsy from one of these tongues of mucosa.

6 *What is the basic type of mucosa shown below and what is the diagnosis?*

7 *What basic pathological process has occurred in Barrett's oesophagus?*

Thirteen years later the patient is referred to the gastroenterology outpatient clinic with a 2-month history of dysphagia that is worse for solids than liquids and is associated with weight loss of 5 kg and a general feeling of lethargy.

8 *What are the causes of dysphagia?*

9 *In view of the patient's history, which cause of the dysphagia should be particularly considered?*

Case 8: The wisdom of the ancients

In 123 AD a Roman legionary on duty in ancient Britain sustained a javelin wound in the thigh (in what these days would be termed friendly fire), during a battle against the Celts on Hadrian's Wall. The wound became swollen, red and warm and was excruciatingly painful. The chief physician in the fortress valetudinarium (hospital) was familiar with the teachings of Cornelius Celsus and recognised the signs of acute inflammation.

1 *Which of the cardinal features of inflammation described by Celsus in 1 AD were manifested by this patient? Give an explanation for each.*

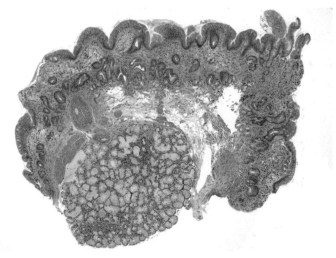

Over the next few days, thick yellow fluid began to discharge from the wound and the soldier became febrile. The physician debrided the wound by scraping the sides and base of the wound site, then covered it with a boiled cloth. His patient settled after drinking an extract of willow bark.

2 *Explain the nature of the thick yellow discharge and how it formed.*

3 *Explain why the patient developed a fever.*

When the physician lifted the cloth a couple of days later, the scab came away with it and there were punctuate red bleeding points in a bed of pink healthy-looking tissue. He cleaned the wound again and replaced the boiled cloth with another.

4 *Why did the wound site show this appearance?*

Gradually the wound healed, leaving a pale, puckered scar which was smaller than the original injury site.

5 *How do scars form?*

Case 9: A small boy with big problems

A 4-year-old boy is seen in the paediatric outpatient department as he is small for his age despite having a good appetite. His parents also report that he tends to have a lot of coughs and colds. The boy's parents wonder if something could be wrong with their son's bowels as he passes large motions.

On examination, the boy is below the 98th centile for height but seems happy and well cared for. No focal lesions are identified. Assorted investigations are carried out.

1 *Given the combined aspects of frequent respiratory tract infections, impaired growth and a possible bowel disorder, what diagnosis should be considered and what test can be used to support it?*

The diagnosis is confirmed.

2 *What is the genetic basis for the condition?*

3 *What sorts of conditions tend to be autosomal recessive?*

4 *What types of diseases tend to be autosomal dominant?*

Treatment is begun and the boy's growth improves. However, as he grows older, he develops more frequent chest infections.

5 *What process is occurring in his lungs and which organism is typically involved?*

At the age of 15, the patient notices twitches of his left hand. These come in bursts that last for several minutes and are associated with weakness. The twitches are sometimes quite marked movements of the whole hand. Over the course of a week, his forearm becomes involved. He also reports headaches. On examination, he has increased tone, increased brachioradialis reflex and decreased power in his left upper limb. Co-ordination and sensation are normal.

6 *What has happened?*

The diagnosis is confirmed.

7 *What other conditions predispose to the lesion?*

The brain abscess is treated and the patient recovers normal neurological function. His bronchiectasis continues to cause problems, but he is adapting to it.

8 *What is the chance that he will pass on the cystic fibrosis gene to any children he may father?*

Case 10: A pregnant woman with viral hepatitis

Maria, a 35-year-old prostitute and intravenous drug user, presents to the consultant hepatologist at her local hospital, after she was found by her general practitioner to have abnormal liver function tests. She is 14 weeks pregnant. Further serological studies reveal that she is positive for hepatitis B and C.

1 *What are the main routes by which adults catch hepatitis A, hepatitis B, hepatitis C and hepatitis D (delta virus)?*

The consultant hepatologist takes serum in order to find out whether replicating virus is present in the blood, i.e. whether there is evidence of chronic viral infection.

2 *What is the likelihood that Maria has developed chronic infection with either hepatitis B or C? (Compare the risks with hepatitis A.)*

Maria has $>10^3$ copies of replicating hepatitis B DNA and hepatitis C RNA in her blood and is therefore chronically infected and infectious to others. When she learns the diagnosis, Maria becomes concerned that she may transmit the virus to her baby.

3 *Can hepatitis B or C be passed on by vertical transmission? What does this term mean? Can clinical intervention prevent transmission?*

Maria's consultant warns her that she must have a liver biopsy to establish the stage of her disease. There is no way of knowing how long she has had chronic viral hepatitis and she is at risk of cirrhosis.

4 *Which three histological features are essential for the diagnosis of cirrhosis?*

Unfortunately Maria's liver biopsy reveals that she is cirrhotic. Her consultant warns her that she is at risk of developing portal hypertension, meaning that the circulation by-passes the liver.

5 *Name at least three sites at which portal–systemic anastomoses develop in cirrhotic patients with portal hypertension and the most severe complications likely to occur due to this process.*

The bad news does not end there. She must be screened in case she develops hepatocellular carcinoma.

6 *Name two features that would raise suspicion of a developing hepatocellular carcinoma in a cirrhotic patient.*

Answers

Case 1

1 The likely diagnosis is myocardial infarction. The risk factors are:
- Smoking.
- Hypertension.
- Diabetes mellitus.
- Family history.
- Hypercholesterolaemia.
- Previous ischaemic heart disease.
- (Also male gender.)

2 The ECG shows sinus rhythm with a rate of approximately 100 beats per minute. The axis is normal. There is ST elevation in leads V2–V6 and leads I and aVL. T wave inversion is also seen in these leads. The ECG shows the changes of an acute myocardial infarction that extensively involves the anterior, septal and lateral regions of the left ventricle.

3 Acute rupture of the interventricular septum or mitral regurgitation secondary to rupture of a papillary muscle are likely to have happened. Distinction between these two entities on clinical features alone can be difficult. Ventricular rupture does not fit well as this would rapidly produce cardiac tamponade and a cardiac arrest.

4 Both the papillary muscles and the interventricular septum are supplied by the left anterior descending coronary artery. Infarction in this territory can include infarction of either of these structures. The ensuing necrosis weakens the tissue, rendering them susceptible to rupture, particularly in the context of a heart that may be beating abnormally due to other effects of the myocardial infarction. There is usually an interval of a few days between the infarct and the rupture as the process of necrosis requires time to become established.

5 Beta-blockers can decrease the incidence of ventricular rupture, possibly by a negative inotropic effect. Early administration of thrombolysis at the time of the infarct is also helpful as it can reduce the volume of myocardium that is infarcted.

6 Atherosclerosis of the coronary arteries.

7 Other organs that might be affected are:
- Brain: cerebrovascular accident and transient ischaemic attacks.
- Lower limbs: peripheral vascular disease.
- Kidneys: renal artery stenosis.
- Gastrointestinal tract: mesenteric ischaemia.

8 Other complications include:
- Death.
- Arrhythmias (bradycardias or tachycardias).
- Cardiac failure.
- Rupture of the free ventricular wall.
- Rupture of the interventricular septum.
- Rupture of a papillary muscle.
- Papillary muscle dysfunction.
- Mural thrombus and embolic events.
- Ventricular aneurysm.
- Pericarditis.
- Dressler's syndrome.

See Chapters 35 and 36.

Case 2

1 The patient is hyponatraemic and hyperkalaemic with a high–normal urea. The fasting glucose is low. There is mild hypercalcaemia.

2 The combination of hyponatraemia, mild hyperkalaemia, borderline raised urea, mild hypercalcaemia and fasting hypoglycaemia are all features of adrenal cortical insufficiency. Postural hypotension and general lethargy are also encountered in this condition. The sodium and electrolyte disturbances are due primarily to a loss of aldosterone. The hypercalcaemia and hypoglycaemia reflect cortisol deficiency, as does the mild impairment in renal function.

3 Thyroid-stimulating hormone (TSH), thyroxine (T4), follicle-stimulating hormone (FSH), luteinising hormone (LH) and testosterone levels are all low. The patient's blood results imply hypothyroidism and hypogonadism. However, in both these cases, as well as the hormones produced by the target organ, the stimulatory hormones (TSH and FSH/LH) are also low. In primary failure of the thyroid and testes, these stimulatory hormones would be expected to be elevated in an attempt to restore normal thyroxine and testosterone levels. Therefore, this indicates that the endocrine organs are failing due to a deficiency of the hormones that normally stimulate and regulate them.

4 The patient has hypopituitarism (typically this term refers to the anterior pituitary). The causes are as follows:
- Trauma.
- Surgery.
- Meningitis.
- Encephalitis.
- Syphilis.
- Intracranial tumour including craniopharyngioma.
- Metastases.
- Infarction.
- Sarcoidosis.
- Langerhan's cell histiocytosis.
- Haemochromatosis.
- Radiation.
- Chemotherapy.
- Anorexia nervosa.
- Hypothalamic dysfunction, which can produce secondary hypopituitarism.

5 The anterior pituitary secretes growth hormone (GH), TSH, adreno-corticotrophic hormone (ACTH), FSH, LH and prolactin.
- TSH, FSH, LH and prolactin can be assessed by blood levels. Care must be taken in females to correlate the levels of FSH and LH with the normal range for the phase of the patient's menstrual cycle.
- GH function can be evaluated using the insulin stress test. This involves inducing hypoglycaemia with insulin. A normal patient should mount an effective response to restore glucose levels and this will include release of GH. This test needs to be carried out carefully, with full resuscitation facilities available due to the dangers of hypoglycaemia.
- ACTH and the adrenal cortex can be evaluated with a synacthen test in patients in whom cortisol deficiency is suspected. Random levels are often unhelpful due to the natural variation in cortisol levels throughout the day, although an 8 a.m. cortisol can be a useful initial, simpler investigation. In the synacthen test, synthetic ACTH is given. In a patient in whom the cortisol deficiency is due to primary adrenal failure, there will be no response and the cortisol levels will not rise. In a patient in whom the cortisol deficiency is secondary to a lack of ACTH, the adrenal glands remain capable of responding to ACTH and cortisol levels increase. However, if the ACTH deficiency is chronic,

there will be secondary atrophy of the adrenal glands, so the response may be delayed and this must be borne in mind when determining the duration of the test.
• The insulin stress test can be employed to evaluate the pituitary adrenal axis as well as GH secretion, but the synacthen test is less hazardous and is preferred in situations in which only the pituitary adrenal axis is of concern (such as Addison's disease).
  See Chapters 88, 89 and 92.

Case 3

1 A fibroadenoma is a benign tumour of the breast that is composed of ducts and stroma. *See Chapter 105 for further details.*
2 Fibrocystic disease is a benign disorder of the breast in which there is cystic dilatation of the terminal duct lobular units of the breast in association with fibrosis and sometimes apocrine metaplasia. *See Chapter 105 for further details.*
3 A carcinoma is a malignant tumour of epithelium. *See Chapter 24 for further details.*
4 Most breast carcinomas are either ductal or lobular. The receptor status is important as it suggests that hormonal therapy with anti-oestrogens may be beneficial. *See Chapter 106 for further details.*
5 The following features are of interest:
• Confirmation of the type of the carcinoma and its grade.
• The pathological stage.
• The presence or absence of lymphovascular invasion.
• The status of the surgical margins.
• The status of the lymph nodes.
These parameters are common to many malignant tumours. *See Chapters 24, 28 and 106 for further details.*
  If receptor status has already been established on a biopsy, it may not need to be repeated on excision specimens.
6 Bilateral pleural effusions.
7 Prostate, kidney, thyroid and lung. *See Chapter 101 for further details.*

Case 4

1 The patient has a right-sided upper motor neurone lesion pattern of signs. *See Chapter 85 for further details.*
2 Epilepsy in the form of focal, partial seizures. Epilepsy is a tendency to recurrent seizures. Not all seizures are of the classic grand mal type.
3 The patient has had a generalised seizure. In view of the patient's established tendency to repeated seizures, a diagnosis of epilepsy is reasonable. However, a new onset of epilepsy in a patient of this age is unusual in the absence of an underlying cause. Various metabolic and other disturbances can induce seizures, but in this patient's case he also has focal, localising neurological signs to the upper motor neurone system for his left arm. This combination of focal neurology and seizures suggests an underlying mass lesion. In addition, the evolution of the patient's seizure type from focal to generalised may reflect an increase in the size of the tumour.
4 The basic classification of tumours is into the divisions of benign and malignant. Malignant tumours may be either primary or secondary. *See Chapter 24 for further details.*
5 The following complications can be caused by a brain tumour:
• Headaches.
• Seizures.
• Focal neurological deficits.
• Hydrocephalus.
• Raised intracranial pressure.
• Confusion.

See Chapter 83 for further details.
6 The following non-neoplastic lesions can behave as space-occupying lesions:
• Haemorrhage (either intracerebral or outside the brain).
• Oedema (as can occur with a thromboembolic infarct).
• Abscess.

Case 5

1 The following information should be sought:
• Degree of exercise intolerance, usually gauged as the distance that can be walked on the flat and the number of flights of stairs that can be climbed.
• All employment, current and previous.
• Hobbies (e.g. keeping pigeons).
• Presence of any pets.
• History of any respiratory diseases, allergies or eczema.
• Family history of respiratory diseases, allergies or eczema.
• Exposure to asbestos.
• Exposure to chemicals and dusts.
This information is part of the history for anybody who presents with a respiratory problem.
2 Chronic obstructive pulmonary disease should be considered. The peak expiratory flow rate should be measured.
3 An obstructive defect. Note that the patient's flow rates are much lower than normal and that the total volume of air that is moved in and out of the lungs during one respiratory cycle is also much less than normal.
4 Features that suggest severe dyspnoea include the following:
• Inability to talk in complete sentences.
• Use of accessory respiratory muscles.
• Tachypnoea.
• Cyanosis.
• A peak expiratory flow rate of under 50% of the predicted one.
The diagnosis is an infective exacerbation of COPD.
5 The blood gases show a decreased Po_2, elevated Pco_2 and decreased pH, indicative of a respiratory acidosis and type 2 respiratory failure. This is serious as it indicates exhaustion has occurred. The greater diffusing capacity of carbon dioxide means that hypercapnia tends to develop later than hypoxia in pulmonary disease. In the setting of an exacerbation asthma or COPD, this indicates exhaustion in maintaining the increased respiratory effort. It can also denote severe, end stage lung disease.
6 The main types of COPD are emphysema and chronic bronchitis, which often overlap. *See Chapter 45.*
7 Many infective exacerbations of COPD are caused by *Haemophilus influenzae*, but other organisms that produce pneumonia may also be responsible. The body's response is that of acute inflammation. *See Chapters 13, 16 and 42 for further details.*
8 Bronchial carcinoma. Both COPD and bronchial carcinoma are caused by smoking.
9 Small cell carcinoma and non-small cell carcinoma (squamous cell carcinoma, adenocarcinoma, large cell carcinoma).
See Chapter 47 for further details.

Case 6

1 The patient has arthralgia, a photosensitive rash in the so-called butterfly or malar distribution, proteinuria and is a young adult female. This combination is very suggestive of systemic lupus erythematosus.
2 An autoantibody screen, in particularly looking for antibodies

against double-stranded DNA. Positive anti-ds-DNA antibodies are common in SLE.

3 Renal disease is common in SLE (around 50% of patients have some form of renal abnormality). While many definitions of the nephrotic syndrome stipulate specific levels of proteinuria in 24 hours, a useful alternative concept is that the degree of proteinuria required to define nephrotic syndrome is that necessary to cause oedema. This patient has proteinuria and oedema, so nephrotic syndrome should be suspected. A formal 24-hour urinary protein evaluation should be performed.

4 Renal disease in SLE is classified into five categories:
• Type I: minimal change.
• Type II: mesangial glomerulonephritis.
• Type III: focal proliferative glomerulonephritis.
• Type IV: diffuse proliferative glomerulonephritis.
• Type V: membranous nephropathy.
See Chapter 66 for further details.

5 The following complications can occur:
• Hypoalbuminaemia.
• Peripheral oedema.
• Ascites, pleural and pericardial effusions.
• Hypercholesterolaemia.
• Hypercoagulability.
• Increased risk of infection.
See Chapter 66 for further details.

6 The decreased reflexes and the absence of hypertonia suggest a lower motor neurone lesion. Furthermore, the distribution of the weakness is not typical of a CNS/upper motor neurone lesion. *See Chapter 85 for further details.*

7 (C5)C6, C7 and C8.

8 The radial nerve.

9 The patient has a lesion of the radial nerve. This case illustrates one of the basic concepts in neurology, that of localising a lesion. Knowing where a lesion is can help to determine the diseases that may cause it (and vice versa). To do this, knowledge of the neuroanatomy of the motor and sensory pathways is vital. This must include understanding of the upper and lower motor neurone systems, familiarity with the motor and sensory distributions of each of the spinal nerve roots and knowing the motor and sensory distributions of each of the main peripheral nerves, together with the spinal nerve roots that contribute fibres to the nerve. This can be supplemented by also knowing the typical features of common lesions (e.g. palsies of the radial, median and ulnar nerves).

Peripheral neuropathy can be found in a minority of patients with SLE.

10 Although SLE is a complex disease, current theories indicate that it features a combination of immune complex-mediated processes and vasculitis. *See Chapters 9, 19 and 31 for further details.*

11 SLE is one of a group of diseases that can produce a wide variety of clinical features. Arthralgia and skin rashes are characteristic, especially when combined with renal dysfunction. Alopecia is relatively common. Patients may have a prothrombotic tendency. Recurrent abortions affect around 30% and are due to the lupus anticoagulant, which, despite its name, is also implicated in hypercoagulability. Neurological features occur in 50–60% and include cognitive problems and psychosis. *See Chapters 29 and 99 for further details.*

Case 7

1 The patient can be reassured that he has a benign peptic-type gastric ulcer and that no cancer was seen. In general, the appearance of an ulcer at endoscopy can give a good idea whether it is a peptic ulcer or a malignant tumour, but biopsy confirmation remains vital.

2 *Helicobacter pylori* is implicated as the causative agent in the vast majority of duodenal peptic ulcers but is seldom involved in oesphageal ulcers. Over half of gastric peptic ulcers are *H. pylori*-related. *See Chapter 50 for further details.*

3 The patient should be warned to avoid drinking alcohol while taking metronidazole because the drug interferes with the metabolism of ethanol with the result that high levels of ethanal accumulate. Ethanal (acetaldehyde) can produce an unpleasant reaction that includes hypotension and flushing. *See Chapter 58.*

4 The follow-up endoscopy is required to ensure that the ulcer has healed. A non-healing ulcer would raise the possibility of an additional cause, such as a malignancy that was not sampled in the biospy.

5 Gastro-oesophageal reflux disease. There is likely to be a hiatus hernia. *See Chapter 51 for further details.*

6 The mucosa is glandular mucosa. The normal oesophagus is lined by stratified squamous epithelium. The diagnosis is Barrett's oesophagus. (The biopsy is unusual in that it includes a native oesophageal duct and gland, which is in the submucosa unlike gastric glands. The presence of this structure confirms that the biopsy is genuinely of oesophageal origin. The ducts open through the normal squamous epithelium.) *See Chapter 51 for further details.*

7 Metaplasia. *See Chapter 23 for further details.*

8 The causes of an obstruction to a tubular organ such as the oesophagus can be considered in four categories: lesions in the lumen, lesions in the wall, lesions extrinsic to the tube and the neuromuscular function of the organ. The last of these is particularly important in the oesophagus as swallowing is a complex action. Causes include the following:

• Intraluminal	Benign oesophageal stricture
• Mucosal	Hiatus hernia
	Oesophageal malignancy
	Benign neoplasm
	Plummer–Vinson syndrome
	Schatzki ring
	Oesophagitis
• Wall	Pharyngeal pouch
	Oesophageal malignancy
• Extrinsic	Goitre
	Bronchial carcinoma
	Mediastinal tumour
	Enlarged left atrium
	Aortic arch aneurysm
	Aberrant mediastinal vascular anatomy
	Peritonsillar abscess
	Pharyngeal pouch
• Motility	Achalasia
	Chagas' disease
	Scleroderma
	Cerebrovascular accident
	Multiple sclerosis
	Motor neurone disease
	Myasthenia gravis
	Parkinson's disease
	Myopathy
	Diffuse oesophageal spasm

Some of the causes, such as a malignant tumour, can be allocated to more than one category as they may act by more than one mechanism.

Motility disorders tend to yield dysphagia for solids and liquids. The other categories, which are all variants of physical obstruction, show a greater degree of dysphagia for solids over liquids because peristalsis remains functional and liquids can more easily negotiate an obstruction than solids. However, in advanced mechanical obstruction, dysphagia for liquids will occur and the division is in any case not absolute.

9 Oesophageal adenocarcinoma. The patient has Barrett's oesophagus and this can be complicated by adenocarcinoma. *See Chapter 51 for further details*. His previous history of *H. pylori* is unlikely to be relevant to his oesophageal disease.

Case 8

1 The cardinal features of inflammation are calor, rubor, tumor and dolor:
• Calor: heat due to increased blood flow, due to vasodilatation mediated by prostaglandins and LTB4.
• Rubor: redness due to vasodilatation, mediated by prostaglandins and LTs (SRS-A).
• Tumor: swelling due to fluid exudation through newly permeable blood vessels, mediated by histamine, bradykinin and prostaglandins. They cause endothelial cell contraction which enlarges the gaps between each cell.
• Dolor: pain due to prostaglandins and kinins.
See Chapter 8 for further details.

2 This is pus, an exudate containing polymorphonuclear neutrophils (PMNs) and plasma proteins, such as fibrin. Exudates contain protein, transudates do not. The exudate forms because the contraction of endothelial cells allows plasma proteins to escape from the circulation; the hydrostatic pressure in the vessel is increased as vasodilatation supplies more blood to the area.

The blood cells are too large to escape by such passive mechanisms and must be attracted from the circulation by upregulation of adhesion molecules such as selectins, intercellular adhesion molecules (ICAMs) and integrins. They are activated by adhesion and exit through the enlarged gaps using pseudopodia.

The PMNs follow a concentration gradient of chemokines, such as complement C3b and C5b, plus any bacterial fragments that may have entered the wound site. The PMNs phagocytose opsonised material and die within hours, releasing toxic chemicals into the tissues, causing further tissue damage, which is added to the fibrinopurulent exudate. *See Chapters 2 and 13 for further details*.

3 The body's temperature is regulated by the hypothalamus and is normally 37°C. A rise in temperature in response to injury, inflammation or infection (or all three) is due to the actions of interleukin-1, interleukin-6 and prostaglandins on the hypothalamus, which reset the temperature regulation centre.

Aspirin is derived from willow bark and is an antipyretic, anti-inflammatory drug that blocks cyclo-oxygenase. Prostaglandins are derived from arachidonic acid in the membranes of inflammatory cells and platelets and the breakdown pathway includes two main arms: (i) cyclo-oxygenase, producing thromboxane and prostaglandins, and (ii) lipoxygenase, producing leucotrienes. Interestingly, aspirin and other antipyretics will only reduce an abnormally high temperature, and do not lower a normal temperature. (Paracetamol acts directly on the temperature-regulating centre and does not block cyclo-oxygenase.)
See Chapters 8 and 13 for further details.

4 This is granulation tissue, the tissue of healing and repair. The scab is formed of a protective layer of hardened plasma proteins and coagulum from the clotting cascade and beneath it a new layer of epidermis grows. In the wound bed, fibroblasts lay down collagen and angiogenic factors

attract new vessels to grow in from nearby capillaries – it is these delicate loops of new vessel that cause the punctuate appearance. *See Chapter 15 for further details*.

5 Scars are the end stage of repair and occur when tissue has been irreplaceably lost. Collagen contracts, pulling the wound edges together and reducing the extent of the scar. The epidermis regenerates, but adnexal structures such as sweat glands and hair follicles are not formed. The skin is thinner than usual and the site is indented. If scar contracture occurs across a joint (for instance after burn healing), restricted movement may occur due to joint deformity. *See Chapter 15 for further details*.

Case study 9

1 Cystic fibrosis. A sweat test can be undertaken.

2 Cystic fibrosis is an autosomal recessive condition, the gene for which is located on chromosome 7.

3 Autosomal recessive diseases are usually enzyme based. Most enzymes work at sufficient efficiency and capacity that half normal levels still provide adequate function.

4 Inherited conditions that affect structural proteins are usually autosomal dominant. The same degree of spare capacity and independent function as with enzymes is not present and so even 50% of the protein being abnormal produces disease.

5 Brochiectasis with recurrent infections. *Pseudomonas aeruginosa* is commonly responsible for infective exacerbations in cystic fibrosis.

6 The pattern of motor features in the left upper limb is that of an upper motor neurone lesion, which localises the lesion to the spinal cord or right primary motor cortex. The spread from the hand to the forearm indicates that the process is extending. The associated twitches are not fasciculations, but are partial epilepsy. In the context of bronchiectasis, a brain abscess is probable as a space-occupying lesion in the right primary motor cortex, in the hand and arm region that produces both the motor features and acts as the seizure focus.

7 In addition to bronchiectasis, brain abscesses are more likely in cases of skull fracture, sinonasal and middle ear/mastoid complex infection, congenital cyanotic heart disease and infective endocarditis.

8 There is a catch to this question. The patient is homozygous for cystic fibrosis and, as it is an autosomal condition, he would transmit a defective allele to any children. However, cystic fibrosis is frequently associated with defects in the vas deferens such that affected males are infertile. Thus, it is very unlikely that the patient will father any children. If he did, all would receive an abnormal allele.
See Chapters 22, 43 and 84 for further details.

Case study 10

1 The following are the main routes by which adults catch different types of hepatitis:
• Hepatitis A: faecal–oral transmission, e.g. from mussels or oysters in shallow sea beds contaminated by the discharge of faecal effluent.
• Hepatitis B: mainly via the blood, as in intravenous drug users, needlestick injury in health care workers and blood transfusion (prior to screening). Also via other body fluids: semen, saliva and tears to some extent.
• Hepatitis C: almost always via the blood, typically in intravenous drug users or blood transfusion (prior to screening).
• Hepatitis D: the delta virus is incomplete and only causes disease if the patient is also infected with hepatitis B. Routes of infection are the same as for hepatitis B.
See Chapter 60 for further details.

2

• Hepatitis A: no risk, as it is a fulminant disease with no chronic effects ('kill or cure').
• Hepatitis B: 10% risk in adults of developing chronic infection (contrasts with childhood infection).
• Hepatitis C: 70–80% risk of chronic disease.
See Chapter 60 for further details.
3 Caesarian section is effective in preventing vertical transmission, which occurs due to trauma at the time of birth or in the perinatal period. Infection in early childhood may be from play with infected children. Viral hepatitis is not thought to cross the placenta.

HAV is not passed on in this way. HBV is more likely than HCV to be transmitted by vertical transmission: the risks are highest when there are high circulating levels of replicating virus in the bloodstream. HBV is passed on in around 50% or more of chronically infected mothers; the risk is around 5% in HCV. Many of the cases of HCV that are transmitted vertically are in patients with HIV/AIDS.

The risk of the child developing chronic disease is 90% in those infected with HBV at birth and 50% with childhood infection. Vaccination against HBV is effective, but no vaccine is yet available for HCV. *See Chapter 60 for further details.*
4 The three histological features are:
• Fibrous septa: fibrous septa are formed and disrupt the normal lobular/acinar liver architecture and prevent normal blood flow from the portal tracts towards the central vein.

• Regenerative nodules: these are formed as the liver attempts to repair itself and replace the cells damaged by the inflammatory reaction to the initiating stimulus. The fibrous septa impede the process and prevent resolution (restitution to normality), which is possible if a liver receives one acute, massive insult such as fulminant hepatitis A infection. (The liver is an example of a 'permanent' tissue, capable of repair but not constantly undergoing cell turnover.)
• Diffuse involvement of the **entire** liver by the cirrhotic process: there are several conditions in which cirrhosis-like changes can occur in a limited area, the best known of which is focal nodular hyperplasia.
See Chapters 3, 56 and 60 for further details.
5 The sites of portal–systemic anastomosis are:
• Left gastric vein (portal) and lower oesophageal veins (systemic).
• Superior (portal) and inferior (systemic) rectal veins.
• Retroperitoneum (mesenteric veins meet systemic veins in the abdominal wall).
• Periumbilical region – the old ligamentum teres carries the umbilical vein (portal), which anastomoses with the anterior abdominal wall veins (systemic).

Oesophageal varices are the most likely to cause problems due to rupture and torrential haemorrhage, with a 40% mortality risk. *See Chapter 61 for further details.*
6 An enlarging nodule on ultrasound scanning and a rising serum α-fetoprotein level. *See Chapter 63 for further details.*

Glossary

Acute: an adjective that indicates a rapid onset and implies a limited duration (cf. chronic).

Adenocarcinoma: a malignant tumour of glandular epithelium.

Adenoma: a benign tumour of glandular epithelium.

Allele: one copy of a gene (either paternal or maternal). With the exception of the genes that are found on the sex chromosomes in males, all nucleated cells in the body possess two alleles for each gene. A few genes, such as those for the α-chain of globin, are duplicated on a chromosome.

Aneuploid: an adjective assigned to a cell which has a chromosome number that is not an integer multiple of 23 (in humans).

Angiosarcoma: a malignant tumour derived from endothelial cells.

Apoptosis: a form of cell death in which the cell activates mechanisms to kill itself. It is also known as programmed self death. Apoptosis is often not associated with an inflammatory response to the death of the cell (cf. necrosis). However, inflammatory cells, particularly T cells, can induce apoptosis.

Atrophy: a reduction in the size of a tissue or organ. Atrophy is often due to the removal of a stimulus that maintains the size of the tissue or organ (e.g. use maintains muscle bulk and disuse leads to atrophy; removal of adrenocorticotrophic hormone results in atrophy of the adrenal cortices).

Autosome: any of the 22 non-sex chromosomes.

Carcinoma: a malignant tumour of epithelium.

Caseation: a particular kind of necrosis that is highly suggestive of tuberculosis. The term relates to the macroscopic resemblance of the necrosis to soft cheese.

Chondroma: a benign tumour of cartilage-producing cells.

Chondrosarcoma: a malignant tumour of cartilage-producing cells.

Chronic: an adjective that indicates a relatively slow onset and implies longstanding, persistent disease (cf. acute).

Coagulative: an adjective related to necrosis. Coagulative necrosis is the process that occurs in most solid organs and is characterised by the presence of 'ghost cells', which consist of cytoplasmic outlines that have lost their nuclei. Fibrosis usually follows.

Cyst: a cavity that is lined by epithelium. Adjective: cystic, a tumour that has the configuration of a cyst.

Cystadenocarcinoma: a cystic malignant tumour of glandular epithelium.

Cystadenoma: a cystic benign tumour of glandular epithelium.

Diploid: an adjective that specifies that a cell possess 23 pairs of chromosomes (46 chromosomes in total). Most normal human cells in the body, other than gametes, are diploid.

Diverticulum: an invagination of the mucosa of a hollow muscular organ into the wall of that organ with protrusion through the smooth muscle. Plural: diverticula.

Dysplasia: (1) Abnormal growth and maturation of an epithelial tissue, where the abnormal cells are confined to the epithelium and do not invade beyond it. Dysplasia in this context implies the first stages of the development of a neoplasm and is a neoplastic process. (2) Historically, dysplasia could refer to more general disorders of growth, without necessarily having neoplastic implications and is still occasionally encountered in this context (e.g. malformed, dysplastic kidneys).

Erythropoiesis: the synthesis of erythrocytes by the bone marrow.

Exon: a segment of DNA that is encoded (**ex**pressed) into mRNA.

Fistula: an abnormal communication between two epithelial surfaces.

Gene: a segment of DNA that encodes a protein.

Gene expression: transcription of an exon segment of DNA into mRNA, to be translated into a protein by ribosomes within the cytoplasm.

Genotype: the complete genetic composition of an individual, including both sets of chromosomes.

Granulation tissue: granulation tissue is an early reparative response and is composed of new capillary blood vessels with fibroblasts and fibrous tissue.

Granuloma: a collection of activated macrophages. Granulomas are a characteristic finding in a variety of diseases.

Haemangioma: a benign tumour of blood vessels.

Haematopoiesis: the process by which bone marrow generates the cells of the peripheral blood. Adjective: haematopoietic.

Haploid: an adjective that indicates that a cell possesses 23 single chromosomes. The term is most commonly used with regard to human gametes.

Hyperplasia: an increase in the number of endogenous cells within a tissue or organ.

Hypertrophy: an increase in the size of individual endogenous cells within a tissue or organ, often leading to a macroscopic increase in the size of the organ. For example, skeletal muscle can hypertrophy after repeated exercise. The number of cells is unchanged.

Intron: an **int**ervening segment of DNA that is not transcribed into mRNA. Much of the DNA sequence is composed of introns.

Karyotype: the chromosomal make-up of an individual.

Leiomyoma: a benign tumour of smooth muscle.

Leiomyosarcoma: a malignant tumour of smooth muscle.

Leukaemia: a malignant tumour derived either from lymphoid or haematopoietic precursors in which the malignant cells are present in the bone marrow and the peripheral blood.

Liquefactive: an adjective used to describe necrosis in the brain.

Locus: the position of a gene on a chromosome.

Lymphoma: a malignant tumour of lymphocytes.

Malignant: an adjective that relates to tumours and indicates that they can invade and metastasise. Noun: malignancy.

Megakaryopoiesis: the synthesis of platelets, via the production of megakaryocytes, by the bone marrow.

Melanoma: a malignant tumour of melanocytes.

Metaplasia: the transformation of one cell type to another.

Metastasis: a deposit of a malignant tumour that is distant from the site of the original tumour and is not in anatomical continuity with it. Also used to indicate the concept of distant tumour spread. Plural: metastases. Verb: metastasise.

Mutation: an alteration in the genetic sequence which may occur at either the level of a chromosome or at the DNA level. Mutations at the DNA level may involve several genes, a segment of a gene or just a single base. Most mutations are deleterious, but, rarely, mutations can be beneficial.

Myeloid: (1) A collective term for the bone marrow cells that give rise to erythrocytes, platelets and peripheral blood leucocytes. (2) An adjective used as a synonym for myelopoietic.

Myeloma: a systemic malignant tumour of plasma cells in which the plasma cells are present in the bone marrow.

Myelopoiesis: the synthesis of the leucocytes of the peripheral blood (neutrophils, eosinophils, basophils and monocytes/macrophages) by the bone marrow.

Necrosis: the death of cells due to destruction of the cell by an external cause. Necrosis is typically associated with inflammation (cf. apoptosis).

Neoplasm: an alternative name for a tumour.

Osteosarcoma: a malignant tumour of bone-forming cells (specifically osteoid-synthesising cells).

Papilloma: a descriptive noun for types of tumours. A papilloma has a smooth contour and protrudes from the surface of the tissue of origin. This can include a projection within the lumen of a hollow organ. Adjective: papillomatous.

Phenotype: the appearances and functions resulting from expression of the genome. The term is closely related to genotype. For example, a person may have a genotype in which they have one allele for blue eyes and one for brown eyes. Their phenotype will be brown eyes.

Plasmacytoma: a discrete tumour formed by plasma cells.

Polyp: a descriptive noun for a protuberance above an epithelial surface. Adjective: polypoid.

Polyploid: an adjective that describes a cell that has a chromosome number that is an integer multiple of 23 (in humans).

Primary: a noun used to describe the initial tumour mass of a malignant tumour at its site of origin (cf. secondary).

Sarcoma: a malignant tumour of mesenchymal soft tissue.

Secondary: a noun used to describe a metastatic deposit of a malignant tumour (cf. primary).

Sex chromosome: the X or Y chromosome.

Sinus: a blind-ended, often dilated, invagination from an epithelial surface.

Small cell carcinoma: a malignant tumour derived from epithelial neuroendocrine cells.

Squamous cell carcinoma: a malignant tumour of stratified squamous epithelium.

Telomere: a repeated sequence of DNA that is found at the ends of the chromosomal arms and is important for cell replication and senescence by providing a binding site for DNA replicating enzymes to initiate duplication of the chromosome.

Teratoma: a tumour that contains elements that are derived from all three embryological layers.

Transcription: the process by which DNA is converted into mRNA.

Translation: the mechanism by which the base sequence of mRNA is converted into an amino sequence by ribosomes.

Tumour: a mass that is formed by an abnormal proliferation of cells. An alternative name for a neoplasm.

Reference ranges

Please note that reference ranges (also known as normal values) vary from hospital to hospital. The reference range can also be different between males and females, adults and children, or between different ethnic groups. The following are given as a general guide only and for use with the case histories.

Biochemistry

Na^+:	135–145 mmol/L
K^+:	3.5–5 mmol/L
Urea:	2.5–6.7 mmol/L
Creatinine:	70–170 µmol/L
Glucose:	3.5–5 mmol/L (fasting)
Ca^{2+} (corrected):	2.1–2.65 mmol/L
Bilirubin:	0–17 µg/L
GGT:	0–50 IU/L
(gamma glutamyl transferase)	
ALT:	0–52 IU/L
(alanine aminotransferase)	
Alkaline phosphate:	30–100 IU/L
Albumin:	35–48 g/L

Blood gases (room air)

pH:	7.35–7.45
Po_2:	11.0–12.6 kPa
Pco_2:	4.7–6.0 kPa
HCO_3^-:	19–24 mmol/L

Haematology

Hb (female):	11.5–15.5 g/dL
Hb (male):	13–18 g/dL
WCC:	$4–11 \times 10^9$/L
(white cell count)	
Platelets:	$150–450 \times 10^9$/L
MCV:	75–95 fL
(mean corpuscular volume)	
MHC:	28–33 pg
(mean haemoglobin concentration)	
MCHC:	32–36 g/dL
(mean corpuscular haemoglobin concentration)	

Hormones

TSH:	0.5–5 mU/L
(thyroid-stimulating hormone)	
T4:	70–140 mmol/L
(thyroxine)	
FSH:	5–20 IU/L
(follicle-stimulating hormone)	
LH:	5–20 IU/L
(luteinising hormone)	
Testosterone:	3–10 ng/L

Index

subdural haemorrhage 180, *180, 190*
subendocardial myocardium 86
substantia nigra 187
sudden death 96–7
sun exposure 225
suppurative chronic inflammation *38, 39*
survival, neoplasia *66*, 67
sweat glands *102*
sympathetic nervous system 81
synapses, neuromuscular *212, 213*
syncytiotrophoblast *160, 161*
syndrome of inappropriate ADH secretion (SIADH) 192–3, *192*
synovial joints *214*, 215
syphilis *70*, 71
systemic hypertension *80*, 81
systemic immune responses *50*, 51
systemic lupus erythematosus (SLE) *48, 49*
   fibrosing alveolitis 109
   secondary glomerulonephritis 151
systemic vasculitis *74*, 75, 151
systemic venous thrombosis 90, *91*, 93

Takayasu's arteritis *74*, 75
tamponade 97
Tc (cytotoxic T) cells *30*, 31, *114*, 115
T cell lymphomas *206*, 207
T cell receptor (TCR) *30*, 31, *32*, *46*, 47
T cells *30*, 31
   chronic inflammation *38, 39*
   immunity overview *50*, 51
   immunodeficiency disorders *42*, 43
   leukaemia 210
   reticuloendothelial system *34*, 35
   tolerance *46*, 47
teeth *204*
telomerases 63
telophase *52*
temperature extremes *20*, 21, 37
teratoma *160, 161, 164*, 165
terminal duct lobular unit (TDLU) *226*, 229
terminology 240 1
   cell division 53
   neoplasia *58, 59*
   skin disorders 220
tertiary hyperparathyroidism 199
tertiary syphilis *70*, 71
testicular cancer *160, 161*
tetanus 185
tetralogy of Fallot *78, 79*
thalassaemia *210*, 211
T helper (Th) cells 39
thrombin 88
thrombocytopaenia 211
thromboembolus *146*
thrombolysis 87, 90
thrombosis 88–9, *89*–90
   atherosclerosis *83*, 84
   bowel 123
   cerebrovascular accidents *176*, 177
   embolism *91*, 92–3
thymus *46*, 47, 213
thyroid *194*, 195, 196–7, *196, 204*
thyroid-stimulating hormone (TSH) *192*, 193

tissue damage
   acute inflammation *36*, 37
   alcohol 23
   clinical signs *26*
   drugs *22*, 23
   environmental toxins *20*, 21
   nutritional disorders *24*, 25
   tobacco *22*, 23
   types/effects *16*, 17
   see also necrosis
tissue factor (TF) *88*, 90, *92*
tissue types 17
TNFR1 receptor *18, 19*
TNM (tumour, nodes, metastases) system 67
   breast carcinoma 229
   cervical cancer 171
   lung cancer 111
   prostate cancer 163
   renal carcinoma 157
   uterine cancer 169
tobacco *22*, 23
tolerance *46*, 47
tongue *204*
tonsil *204*
tophi *214*, 215
toxic chemicals 21, *22*, 23, 155
toxic megacolon 125
transferrin *72*, 73
transitional epithelium 17, 157, *158*, 159
transplantation 33
transport, normal cell *12*, 13
transposition of the great vessels *78*, 79
transudates *14*, 15
trauma see injury
T regulatory (CD8+) cells *30*, 31
Treponema pallidum 71
tricuspid valve *94*, 95
trophoblast *172*, 173
trypsin *142*, 143
tuberculosis (TB) *104*, 105
   granuloma *38, 39*
   hypersensitivity *48, 49*
   tuberculous meningitis 184
   tubulointerstitial disease 155
tubular adenoma *126, 127*
tubules, kidney *146*, 147
tubulointerstitial diseases *154*, 155
tubulovillous adenoma *126, 127*
tumour necrosis factor (TNF) *18*, 19
   acute inflammation *36, 37*
   cachexia *24*, 25
   immunity overview *50*, 51
   natural immunity *26*, 27
tumours
   classification *58, 59*
   formation *60*, 61
   see also benign tumours; malignant disease; metastasis; neoplasia; TNM
tumour suppressor genes *62*, 63, *126*, 127
tunica intima *83*, 84
Types I/II/III/IV hypersensitivity *48*, 49

ulceration, peptic *116*, 117
ulcerative colitis *124*, 125
unfixed antigens *48, 49*

unstable angina 86
upper motor neurone lesions 187, *187*
urachal remnants *146*, 147, 159
uric acid *214*, 215
urinary tract abnormalities *146*, 147
urothelial transitional cell carcinoma *158*, 159
usual interstitial pneumonia (UIP) 109
uterus 166–7, *166, 168*, 169

vaccination 67, 105
valvular disease, cardiac *94*, 95
varices, oesophageal 141
varicocele, left-sided 157
vascular compression, intracranial 179
vascular disorders 221
   cerebrovascular accidents *176*, 177, *178*
   dementia *190*, 191
   diabetes mellitus *202*
   kidney diseases *146*, 147
   pulmonary 98–9, *98*
   vasculitis *74*, 75, 123, 151
Vater, ampulla of *142*
veins
   normal *76*, 77
   thrombosis 90
      bowel 123
      embolism *91*, 92–3
ventricular septal defect (VSD) *78*, 79
ventricular vibrillation 21
vertebrobasillar arteries *178*
villous adenoma *126*, 127
viral infection
   chronic inflammation 39
   defences against *42*, 43
   DeQuervain's thyroiditis 195
   encephalitis 184–5
   hepatitis *136*, 137 8
   Hodgkin lymphoma 207
   major histocompatibility complex *32*, 33
   meningitis 184, 185
   tubulointerstitial disease 155
Virchow's triad 89, *89*
visual field defects 193
vitamin D deficiency 217
volvulus *122*, 123
von Willebrand factor (vWF) *76*, 77, *88*, 90

Warthin's tumour 205
water, drowning 21
watershed zone infarction *16*
Wegener's granulomatosis *74*, 75
Werner's syndrome 199
Wernicke's encephalopathy *186*
white pulp (spleen) *34*, 35
Willis, circle of 181
Wilm's tumour *174*, 175
Wilson's disease *72*, 73, *186*, 187
wound healing *40*, 41, *202, 203*

X-linked disorders *54*, 55, 213
Xp21 gene 213

yolk sac tumour *160*, 161

Ziehl–Neelsen stain *104*